D0643582

Communities of Care

Recent and Related Titles in Gerontology

Stuart H. Altman and David I. Shactman, eds.
Policies for an Aging Society

Robert H. Binstock, Leighton E. Cluff, and Otto von Mering, eds.
The Future of Long-Term Care: Social and Policy Issues

Leighton E. Cluff and Robert H. Binstock, eds.
*The Lost Art of Caring: A Challenge to Health Professionals,
   Families, Communities, and Society*

Tom Hickey, Marjorie A. Speers, and Thomas R. Prohaska, eds.
Public Health and Aging

Robert B. Hudson, ed. *The New Politics of Old Age Policy*

John P. Marsden. *Humanistic Design of Assisted Living*

Nancy Morrow-Howell, James Hinterlong, and Michael Sherraden, eds.
Productive Aging: Concepts and Challenges

Karl Pillemer, Phyllis Moen, Elaine Wethington, and Nina Glasgow, eds.
Social Integration in the Second Half of Life

Benyamin Schwarz and Ruth Brent, eds.
Aging, Autonomy, and Architecture: Advances in Assisted Living

Joseph White. *False Alarm: Why the Greatest Threat to Social Security and
Medicare Is the Campaign to "Save" Them*

Sheryl S. Zimmerman, Philip D. Sloane, and J. Kevin Eckert, eds.
Assisted Living: Needs, Practices, and Policies in Residential Care for the Elderly

Robert H. Binstock, Consulting Editor in Gerontology

Communities of Care

Assisted Living for African American Elders

Mary M. Ball
Molly M. Perkins
Frank J. Whittington
Carole Hollingsworth
Sharon V. King
Bess L. Combs

Gerontology Institute, Georgia State University
Atlanta, Georgia

Foreword by May L. Wykle

The Johns Hopkins University Press
Baltimore

© 2005 The Johns Hopkins University Press
All rights reserved. Published 2005
Printed in the United States of America on acid-free paper
9 8 7 6 5 4 3 2 1

The Johns Hopkins University Press
2715 North Charles Street
Baltimore, Maryland 21218-4363
www.press.jhu.edu

Library of Congress Cataloging-in-Publication Data

Communities of care : assisted living for African American elders
/ Mary M. Ball . . . [et al.].
        p.   cm.
   Includes bibliographical references and index.
   ISBN 0-8018-8194-3 (hardcover : alk. paper)
      1. Older African Americans—Long-term care—Case studies.
2. Congregate housing—United States—Case studies.
      [DNLM: 1. Assisted Living Facilities—Aged—United States.
2. African Americans—psychology—Aged—United States. 3. Per-
sonal Autonomy—Aged—United States. WT 27 AA1 C734 2005]
I. Ball, Mary M.
      HV1461.C646 2005
      362.61'089'96073—dc22   2004030326

A catalog record for this book is available from the British Library.

*To the providers, residents, and families whose work,
commitment, and love made these six personal
care homes authentic communities of care*

Contents

Foreword

Aging African Americans are often haunted by the thoughts of spending their last days in an uncaring institutional setting. My grandmother, a proudly independent woman, would threaten to "go live in the poor house" as a ploy to keep her family in line. In a fierce drive to preserve her independence, she absolutely rejected any thoughts of living in a nursing home because for decades she had cared for many of us in her own home. Most elder African Americans (93%) are cared for at home by their children or relatives and perceive placement in institutions as an insult to the "hands that raised, comforted, and fed them." This prevailing thought of ingratitude was held by the community, particularly the church. Although seldom expressed, the notion of obligation was reinforced in subtle ways. Without a sanctioned alternative, family caregivers faced a serious dilemma, especially when caregiving became an overwhelming burden.

The plight of black elders and the struggle to care for them have roots in slavery. Anxiety regarding the abandonment of those elders who no longer had a meaningful work role prompted families to find ways to protect them in their last days. Thus, black families have a long history of taking care of their elders. This caring practice undoubtedly came from original African society, which demonstrated respect and reverence for older persons. Caring for elders, blood related or not, became a norm in the culture of blacks in the United States. Older black Americans were the source of family history and set ethical, religious, and moral standards for the group. Elders, who provided love and strength for younger members, were instrumental in sustaining a relationship that incorporated the past, present, and future. They were proud of their stamina considering that they had survived slavery with a sense of family still intact.

After slavery, black Americans established small homes for the aged for families who could no longer provide care. A good example of such a home comes from the history of the Eliza Bryant Center, in Cleveland, Ohio, which was established originally in 1896 as the Cleveland Home for Aged Colored People. Eliza Bryant, whose mother was freed from slavery in 1857, campaigned for a place to care for sick and disabled black elders because, at that time, white homes would not admit blacks. Today, the Eliza Bryant Center is a 100-bed facility providing for predominantly African American elders.

It is no wonder that these small, community board-and-care homes were acceptable to older African Americans and their friends and families. During the time when racial bias was legal, these centers represented an ideal place of care for families unable to look after loved ones who could no longer live independently. Some families opened their own homes and took in elders as boarders. Consequently, most of the residents were able to adjust to the domestic atmosphere, creating a new family of individuals in similar circumstances. Although they were not always perfect, these facilities were referred to as "mom and pop" homes and were widely accepted in the black community. Both black and white organizations provided these homes with financial support to care for African American elders, and today the homes are part of a wider system of regulated care for elders.

Black elders are poorer, are sicker, and suffer more from health disparities than do their white counterparts. Therefore, they experience a different set of problems when it comes to finding appropriate and affordable environments of care. Rapid changes in long-term care, coupled with an increase in longevity, have occurred over the past 30 years, particularly among minorities. Subsequently, there is a growing demand by the public for quality standards of institutional care. Older adults are sometimes torn between the condition of becoming a "burden" to loved ones and the prohibitive cost of living in a nursing facility. Further complicating placement decisions is a lack of affordable, accessible, and culturally supportive care environments. Adequate community services can help provide the type and quality of care that black elders need and also make available care settings that families can trust. With the ever-accelerating cost of living, it remains difficult to find appropriate care systems for older minorities. Despite our best efforts, we know that the number of small homes in the community is insufficient for fulfilling the needs of black elders. Research has shown that community homes can provide the right type of environmental fit for residents. Older persons live longer, which creates a crisis in caregiving, while the ardent task of providing culturally competent services remains. Finding alternative living environments for elderly persons is one of our greatest challenges in health care. Qualitative studies of the adjustment of black elders in long-term care institutions will fill an essential need.

May L. Wykle, R.N., Ph.D., FAAN, FGSA
Dean and Florence Cellar Professor of Gerontological Nursing
Frances Payne Bolton School of Nursing
Case Western Reserve University
Cleveland, Ohio

Preface

> At this Home Place, I never measured my love or my service by who you were. Every woman becomes a queen and every man becomes a king. What I do for one, unless the needs are more or less, I do for all.
> —ESTHER ADAMS, OWNER OF PEACH BLOSSOM

This book is about African American communities of care. Here, the "communities" are the six assisted living facilities that are home to the African American elders whose stories we tell. Each facility is unique—in size, appearance, and neighborhood, in the types of residents who live there, and in the care provided. All, however, are places where individuals have found what they needed: a community of care. These care communities are an important, and often necessary, long-term care option for African American elders.

We examine the daily lives of the people who live, work, and visit in these care communities, drawing from two in-depth, qualitative studies of assisted living carried out between the spring of 1999 and the fall of 2001. The goal of the studies was to find out how to maximize the independence and autonomy of assisted living residents; each entailed yearlong data gathering in diverse assisted living settings by a team of researchers. The first study, funded by the AARP Andrus Foundation, was set in five small homes located in metropolitan Atlanta. All of the homes were owned and operated by African Americans, and more than half of the residents and their caregivers were poor. Each of these five homes is represented in this book. The second study was supported by the National Institute on Aging and included homes that differed in size, location, resources, and race of residents and providers. Only one home from the second study is included in this book—a large, corporately owned home that served the more affluent African American community. Each of this book's six authors participated in the data gathering and analysis for both studies and in the writing of these chapters. We endeavor to render an understanding of life in these African American communities of care and of the meaning they have for their members.

The book has 12 chapters and is divided into four parts. Part I, the introduction, begins in chapter 1 with a review of the background of our studies,
including our own earlier investigations of long-term care for both minority
and nonminority older people as well as the published studies of other researchers on the use of long-term care facilities by African Americans. We describe our research goals and the qualitative methods used to collect and analyze our data. We pay special attention to the composition of the research
team and how it worked, both individually and as a unit, to fit into the life of
the homes that served as our research sites and how we were able to obtain
valid observations and information. In chapter 2 we provide a detailed profile
of each of the six African American communities we studied, including their
owners, staff, and residents. We focus on both institutional and personal
characteristics, comparing the homes with other facilities in Atlanta, the state
of Georgia, and the nation.

Part II recounts the journey of becoming a resident. It begins in chapter 3
with case histories that typify a range of life experiences. We describe residents'
opportunities for education, health care, and employment and discuss the effects of race and poverty on their past and present lives and future needs for
care. Chapter 4 moves to an examination of the circumstances surrounding
decisions to seek formal long-term care and the choice of the assisted living
setting. We describe typical moving situations, and we discuss the roles of residents, family members, and providers in decision making and the influence
of race and culture. The chapter concludes with an exploration of residents'
early experiences in the home and the adaptation process. Throughout this
section of the book, we discuss the many influences that determine residents'
common and divergent paths.

In part III we examine the components of care provided in these communities, beginning in chapter 5 with a discussion of the facility care providers.
Many paths have led these individuals to own or work in assisted living facilities, and we describe the business of caring in relation to the unique cultures
and modes of operation in each home. The particular challenges of the African
American owners and operators of the small homes who serve largely low-
income African American elders are brought into focus. Part III also depicts the
as yet uncharted experiences of providers in large, corporately owned African
American assisted living facilities. Residents here have a different vantage
point, and chapter 6 explores how these African American elders experience
the role of care receiver. The chapter describes residents' attitudes toward being

helped and toward the care they receive, and it explores the strategies they have developed for self-care and protection of their sense of independence.

In chapter 7 we focus on the role of "kin-work" in residents' day-to-day lives and in the creation of a community of care. We examine residents' relationships with their families and the effect of family involvement on the care of residents. We discuss the influence of race and culture on family roles, as well the effect on family support of other factors, including residents' disabilities and attitudes; family members' own lifestyles, attitudes, and health problems; relationships between residents and families; providers' expectations; and the overall environment of the home. Part III continues with chapter 8, a discussion of how the wider community contributes to the residents' care world. Residents connect to the community through a variety of "bridges," including senior centers, mental health programs, churches, and facility-sponsored activities. We examine these community activities, the effect they have on residents' overall quality of care and life, and the influence of race, culture, and facility size and resources on the overall resident experience.

Chapter 9 focuses on the concept of autonomy as it applies to the assisted living environment. We describe different types of autonomy that are possible for residents, discuss the choices most important to residents' quality of life, and identify the barriers and supports for autonomy in each care setting. In chapter 10 we discuss the challenges residents face in continuing to live in these assisted living communities as they increase in age and frailty. We describe their trajectories of physical and mental decline, and we identify factors that determine the capacity of both residents and providers to manage decline. Part III presents a comprehensive look at assisted living facilities as communities of care and lays the foundation for the concluding chapters in part IV.

In chapter 11 we examine how residents define and find meaning in assisted living. Achieving a meaningful existence in this care environment involves an interplay between continuity and change; being open to change is as important as staying connected to the past. We discuss the tradition of mutual support and collective unity that remains active after the move into assisted living and is an important source of strength and meaning in residents' lives as they continue their transition. In the book's final chapter, we discuss the public policy implications of our findings for residents, for providers, and for family members. The chapter concludes with a set of specific recommendations based on our findings.

Acknowledgments

The material presented in this book derives from two projects. The first was funded by the AARP Andrus Foundation and the second by the National Institute on Aging (R01AG16787-01). We are grateful to both organizations for their support.

We have been helped by many people in carrying out our research and writing this book. First, we are indebted to the owners of these six communities, who allowed entrée to their homes, and to the residents, providers, and family members who shared their thoughts and lives with us. We appreciate their effort and their candor in answering our questions, and we hope that this book will in some way contribute to improving the lives of those who live and work in assisted living.

We are indebted to Dr. Margaret Counts-Spriggs, at the Whitney M. Young School of Social Work, Clark Atlanta University, and Dr. Makunga Akinyela, of the Department of African American Studies, Georgia State University, who served as consultants on issues of race and culture for this project. We appreciate the time they spent visiting these communities and their special contributions to our data analysis. We also want to thank Dr. Bettye Rose Connell, at the Rehabilitation Research and Development Center, Atlanta VA Medical Center, who conducted the environmental assessment at Oak Manor, and Regina Davis and Nelta Clements, who assisted with fieldwork at Oak Manor.

Our friends in the Atlanta Long-Term Care Ombudsman Program were invaluable in helping us select study facilities and gain the cooperation of their owners. We are grateful for their assistance. We acknowledge the support and insight of our research advisory committee, who helped guide our research objectives and project design. They include representatives of the Georgia Long-Term Care Ombudsman Program, the Georgia Office of Regulatory Services, the Georgia Community Care Services Program, the Georgia Chapter of the Assisted Living Federation of America, the Assisted Living Association of Georgia, and administrators of local assisted living facilities.

We thank the directors of the senior centers, adult day health programs, and mental health programs attended by some of the residents of these six homes for the opportunity to visit their centers and learn about their programs.

Finally, we owe a debt to our families, friends, and pets. We are grateful for their understanding and patience during the writing of this book.

Communities of Care

Part I / Introduction

CHAPTER 1

The Genesis of the Book

This book is about long-term care. It is also about older, frail African Americans and their families and paid caregivers. Most of all, it is about the communities that grow up around these elders, enveloping and supporting them in their declining years—what we have termed "communities of care." The story begins with a brief discussion of the political and economic context of the investigation, describing a societal aging policy that is struggling gamely, but weakly, to catch up with the requirements of the lengthening lives of its citizens and a burgeoning, modern long-term care industry.

The Long-Term Care Context

As the population of all modern societies continues to age and the number of elders rises, the social burden of caring for an increasingly older and often disabled population also grows. The American delivery of long-term care is hardly systematic, but its vast collection of highly differentiated care arrangements does provide an array of essential services when families, who still provide most needed care to elders (Jenkins, 2001; Shanas, 1979; Stone, Cafferata, & Sangl, 1987), are absent or overwhelmed by their responsibilities. To the long-standing institutions and arrangements we inherited from the nineteenth and the first half of the twentieth centuries, we have grafted several new "care inventions" that arose from either the creative genius of professional caregivers or the entrepreneurial spirit of business people.

In the 1950s and 1960s, the almshouses, poor farms, and nursing homes that had long served society's poor, weak, and old through public welfare efforts and private charity began to be transformed into modern, bureaucratic service businesses aimed at the growing market of the sick and old, who would no longer die of pneumonia or some other quick-acting infection. The days when Sir William Osler, the influential Canadian physician, reportedly described pneumonia as the old man's friend were long gone. A care market to serve the growing number of surviving frail elders was identified and created by an informal, almost invisible collaboration between the federal government and the private sector. Government experimentation and allocations for public housing, social services, and loans and grants aimed at private congregate housing for vulnerable populations were supplemented in the private market by a ready supply of capital. Innovations such as senior centers, meals-on-wheels, adult day care, and hospice and a burgeoning demand for home care led during the 1970s and 1980s to a proliferation of long-term care options that presented a confusing array of services and payment plans. Few seniors were wealthy enough to afford the best care money could buy, while the masses were finding the supply of government-sponsored services to be inadequate to their needs. Gradually, through the 1990s, the elders of the "greatest generation" and their children who had enjoyed the benefits of postwar prosperity found the private senior housing and care markets to be increasingly attractive and financially accessible. At the same time, the burden of care on poor and working-class families was overtaking government's ability to help and the public's willingness to pay. These countertrends created what Carroll Estes has called the "no-care zone" (Estes et al., 1993) and contributed to a further fragmentation of long-term care services.

Today, we find ourselves with an expensive and increasingly inadequate supply of supportive housing, home-delivered services, and institutional care. Although most nursing homes now are closely regulated, standardized, and certainly more professional than those of 30 to 40 years ago, they remain for most of us the wicked witch of the long-term care market. The nursing home is where no one wishes to "end up," though nearly half of us will, at least briefly, at some time in life (Kemper & Murtaugh, 1991). When late-life needs become chronic and the nursing home specter is on the horizon, some of us can delay or prevent nursing home placement altogether by entering an assisted living facility—the setting for this book. If we are well-off, we can choose from a surfeit of attractive and pricey places, with all the "move-in" incentives found in the mass apartment market. This is the visible market with which most readers of this book are familiar. The facilities resemble luxury apartments and are usually located in or near well-heeled neighborhoods.

Other facilities represent a different world entirely. Their neighborhoods tend to be modest, sometimes even run-down, their clients poorer, their owners stretched physically and financially to near the breaking point, and their profits often vanishingly small. Their role in the long-term care system, however, is no less important than the up-market facilities, because their communities depend on them for services many families can no longer provide. They often are called board-and-care homes, group homes, or, as in Georgia, personal care homes. The homes we report on in this book embody both these assisted living worlds.

The World of Assisted Living

Assisted living facilities (ALFs) are a type of supportive housing that falls somewhere between private homes and nursing homes (Hawes, Rose, & Phillips, 1999). In this middle ground can be found a wide range of facilities. They vary from state to state in what they are called and how they are licensed and defined, but for the most part, ALFs are nonmedical, community-based living environments that provide shelter, meals, and 24-hour protective oversight and personal care services to residents (Hawes, Rose, & Phillips, 1999). Some have tried to clarify the assisted living muddle by cataloging homes as either assisted living or board and care (Mollica et al., 1995), *assisted living* referring to facilities that have private rooms with cooking capacity, service plans geared to individuals, and philosophies that promote independence, control, and choice and *board and care* generally meaning homes that allow multiple occupancy bedrooms and shared bathrooms. The reality is that these care facilities defy classification; while we have been writing this book, both the industry and policy makers have been struggling with how best to define, regulate, and pay for this care species so that assisted living does not follow the path of its nursing home cousin.

In 2002 these care homes numbered 36,399, with 910,486 units or beds—an increase of 14.5% over the year 2000 (Mollica, 2002). Assisted living facilities range in size from 2 to more than 1,400 beds; most of the residences are small (2–10 beds), but most residents live in medium-sized (11–50 beds) or large (51 or more beds) homes (Hawes et al., 1995). Payment for assisted living comes from four different sources: personal funds of residents and their families; the federal Supplemental Security Income (SSI) program; the State Supplemental Payments program; and Medicaid waiver community care programs.* Unlike nursing homes, ALFs receive most of their payments not from Medicaid but

*Section 1915(c) of the Social Security Act authorizes the waiver of certain Medicaid statutory requirements. These waivers enable states to cover a broad array of home and community-based services (HCBS) for targeted populations as an alternative to institutionalization. Centers for Medicare and Medicaid Services, www.cms.hhs.gov/medicaid/1915c/history.asp (September 16, 2004).

from the pockets of those who inhabit them. Most public payments for ALFs are low, and, although in 2002 forty-one states provided some type of Medicaid-reimbursed services in ALFs, a relatively small number of beneficiaries is served in this setting—about 102,000 (Mollica, 2002). Almost all assisted living model homes are completely privately funded, albeit with widely varying fees, and they tend to cater to a higher social class and more affluent lifestyle than homes following the board-and-care model. The National Center for Assisted Living (2001) reports an average monthly fee of $1,873, with two-thirds of facilities charging between $1,000 and $2,500, 15% charging more than $2,500, and 5%, more than $3,500. One study conducted in the early 1990s of small board-and-care homes found median monthly fees ranging from $423 to $923 (Morgan, Eckert, & Lyon, 1995).

Over the past couple of decades, ALF residents have become increasingly older and sicker, on average, and more like those found in nursing homes (Hawes et al., 1995, 2003; Yee, Capitman, & Sciegaj, 1996). A recent national study estimates that approximately one-fourth of residents need help with three or more activities of daily living (ADLs) and have moderate to severe cognitive impairment (Hawes, Rose, & Phillips, 1999).

Although we do not know a lot about African Americans living in ALFs, we do know that most live in homes with fewer than 25 beds (Hawes et al., 1995; Morgan, Eckert, & Lyon, 1995; Mutran et al., 2001). The limited information we have about ALFs with majority African American populations suggests that these homes have lower monthly charges and a higher proportion of male residents and that compared with their white counterparts, African American residents have fewer close relatives listed as next of kin, are more likely to have public financial support, and tend to be more satisfied with the quality of care, particularly in the family-type homes (Morgan, Eckert, & Lyon, 1995; Mutran et al., 2001).

Assisted Living in Georgia

In Georgia, the setting for our book, assisted living facilities are called "personal care homes" and include the whole spectrum of assisted living (AL) in this licensing category, with no limitations on size of home or age of resident (except they must be over the age of 18). Georgia has 1,720 licensed facilities with 25,906 beds (Office of the State Long-Term Care Ombudsman, 2004), and homes are designated as family (2–6 beds), group (7–15 beds), or congregate (16 or more beds). As is true of ALFs across the nation, the majority are small, but most residents live in larger homes. Sixty-five percent of the homes in the metropolitan Atlanta area have 2 to 6 beds, and 41% of residents statewide live in homes with fewer than 25 beds (Victoria Flynn, director, Georgia Personal Care Home Program, pers. comm.). Residents of Georgia's ALFs are similar in age and disability to those in the national profile (Ball et al., 2000; State Health Planning Agency, 1993).

African Americans and Long-Term Care

Older African Americans do not inhabit the world of either nursing homes or assisted living to the same extent as white elders. Numerous reasons have been posited for this differential use. Need is not one of them. The number of older African Americans (8% of the population aged 65 and over in 2000) is expected to increase by 131% over the next 30 years, compared with a growth rate of 81% for older whites (Administration on Aging, 2002). Functional status, the accepted benchmark for predicting the need for long-term care (Harel & Noelker, 1995; Wolinsky et al., 1993), also is worse among African American elders. Older African Americans tend to have poorer health (Belgrave & Bradsher, 1994; Binstock, 1999) and higher rates of chronic disease and disability (Wallace et al., 1998) than white elders. In 2000 older African Americans were more likely than older whites to rate their health as fair or poor (42% compared with 26%), a strong predictor of disability (Administration on Aging, 2002). Although data from the 1999 National Long-Term Care Survey shows a decline in disability from 1994 to 1999 for blacks aged 65 and over, including a greater decline for elderly blacks than whites, the prevalence of disability was still higher among blacks than whites (24% versus 19%) (Manton & Gu, 2001).

Socioeconomic status contributes to the vulnerability of older African Americans. Disability rates are higher among less educated African American older persons (Manton & Gu, 2001), and disease and impairment are more common among elders with low incomes (Jackson & Perry, 1989; Markides, 1989). Poverty rates are higher among elderly African Americans (22%) than white elders (9%). The predominance of poverty and women among elderly African Americans and the greater likelihood that older African American women are unmarried and poor all contribute to the differences in health status of blacks and whites (Administration on Aging, 2002; Jackson & Perry, 1989). This variation by race in the impact of aging—often referred to as the "double jeopardy" of being old and black—is primarily the result of the experience of racism throughout the life course (Jackson, 1985; Markides, 1983). Throughout this book, there is evidence of this double jeopardy in the lives of our informants.

Still, even in the face of greater apparent need, older African Americans are more likely than elderly whites to resist moving to formal long-term care settings. Their rate of nursing home use is between one-half and three-quarters that of elderly whites (Gaugler et al., 2003; Murtaugh et al., 1997; Wallace et al., 1998), and what we know about the race of assisted living residents tells us that only a small minority are black (Brooks, 1996; Hawes et al., 1995; Mui & Burnette, 1994).

Various explanations for this differential use have been proposed. A common argument for lower nursing home use among African Americans is that they have stronger family ties and traditionally care for their elders at home (Belgrave, Wykle, & Choi, 1993). Supports for this culturally based argument usually rest on the fact that African American elders are less likely than elderly whites to live with a spouse, to live alone, or be heads of households and are more likely to live with other relatives (Federal Interagency Forum on Aging-Related Statistics, 2000). Some consider such culturally based inferences to be purely speculative, given the lack of information about cultural preferences and evidence that other factors, such as income, are more important than health in determining living arrangements (Belgrave & Bradsher, 1994). Moreover, elderly African American women are more likely than whites to be heads of households, which may mean that they are giving rather than receiving care and could be a factor in decisions about their own their long-term care (Belgrave, Wykle, & Choi, 1993).

In both African American and white families, support of elders delays a move to a nursing home, though the relative importance of informal support for each is uncertain. Some studies have found that African American elders rely more on informal support than do whites (Jenkins, 2001; Mitchell & Register, 1984; Mutran, 1985), and family care enables them to postpone nursing home use to later ages (Cagney & Agree, 1999), while other findings indicate that white elders rely more on their families for care at home (Belgrave & Bradsher, 1994; Mutran et al., 2001). Groger (1994) suggests this lack of accord in findings stems from the different types of data used and variations in how support is defined.

Other research challenges cultural explanations and instead offers structural factors to account for differential nursing home use. Most studies find no significant relationship between household or family income and the risk of entering a nursing home, but Medicaid coverage may confound the relationship between social class and nursing home use (Cagney & Agree, 1999). Both people who are well-off and those who are very poor and have Medicaid coverage tend to have higher rates of institutionalization (Headon, 1993). At the same time, the greater reliance of older African Americans on Medicaid puts them at higher risk than whites of being denied admission to nursing homes that give preference to more lucrative private-pay residents, suggesting a partial explanation for the racial disparity (Belgrave, Wykle, & Choi, 1993). Another possible reason is that physicians and social service personnel refer fewer African Americans to nursing homes because of their perception that nursing homes are less culturally acceptable to blacks (Cagney & Agree, 1999; Morrison, 1995). In addition, the lower opportunity cost of the African American informal caregiver's time relative to that of white caregivers has been suggested as a contributing cause of African Americans' lower nursing home use (Headon, 1992). However, one study examining the attitudes of older African American women toward future nursing home use indicates that elders' concerns about overburdening their families lead to more positive attitudes toward this possibility (Schoenberg & Coward, 1997).

A final factor may be the nature of the long-term care market. Because most nursing homes are predominantly white, older African Americans may, in fact, feel unwelcome there. Residential segregation also may limit the availability of nursing homes (Wallace et al., 1998). A four-state study finds African Americans tended to be concentrated in predominantly African American facilities located in African American communities (Howard et al., 2002). In addition, evidence shows that quality of care is lower in nursing homes serving the African American community (Wallace, 1990) and that minorities are much more likely to be residents of public facilities, possibly because hospital discharge planners typically refer poor elders to such facilities (Morrison, 1995).

The limited information we have about African Americans in ALFs suggests similar structural explanations for their lower use of this care setting, such as the higher poverty rates among African Americans (Brooks, 1996; Hall, 1993; Morrison, 1995). However, one study of small board-and-care homes in Baltimore and Cleveland finds proportionately more older African Americans living in these homes than in nursing homes (Morgan, Eckert, & Lyon, 1995), suggesting that smaller ALFs that have lower fees and are minority owned are more financially and culturally attractive to African American elders. Available information also tells us that ALFs are segregated by race even more than nursing homes (Ball et al., 2000; Howard et al., 2002; Mutran et al., 2001), a fact that may derive from Medicaid and Medicare nondiscrimination policies operative in most nursing homes but in few ALFs because of the limited federal funding in the latter setting (Mutran et al., 2001). The Cleveland-Baltimore study of small homes also finds that homes were segregated by race of the operator (Morgan, Eckert, & Lyon, 1995).

Many questions about long-term care use by African American elders are left unanswered, but this group's need for long-term care services of some kind is undeniable. Assisted living facilities are thought to be more attractive than nursing homes to all disabled elders, regardless of race or ethnicity, because of their less institutional nature.

Background of the Study

This book has evolved from a long history of collaborative research by its authors focusing on the quality of life in long-term care. In the initial study (1989–91), Ball and Whittington focused on the home care experiences of poor elderly African Americans receiving services from Georgia's home and community-based Medicaid waiver program. This ethnographic study emphasized the importance to these poor elders of holding on to their remaining independence and staying in their homes and in control of their lives. It also pointed out the significance of the entire care "community," made up of families and friends, agency workers, and the elders themselves, in the struggle to keep frail older persons in their own homes and communities (Ball & Whittington, 1995).

We next turned our attention to the experiences of elders living in assisted living communities. Our first study of ALFs (1996–97) investigated risk factors for mental health and substance abuse problems among residents (almost all of them white and over the age of 65) in three suburban Atlanta counties. This study identified 11 components of quality of life, as defined by the residents, and confirmed that holding on to independence and autonomy and retaining connections with the wider community remain vital to elders' quality of life even after moving to assisted living (Ball et al., 2000, Ball et al., 2004b). This study further demonstrated the importance of achieving goodness of fit between the resident and the facility's social and physical environment— where the care a resident needs and desires dovetails with a provider's own resources and priorities. A subsequent study (1997–98) examined the quality of life of disabled veterans living in ALFs (Whittington et al., 1998). Compared with the previous study, the resident sample was younger (37% under the age of 65), more racially diverse (56% African American), and poorer (20% received SSI). Findings from this study suggest that economic status has greater influence than race on residents' quality of life.

These preliminary studies laid the groundwork for the two investigations that are the basis of this book. Together with findings from other long-term care research, they demonstrated the need for in-depth exploration of the lived experience of African Americans in assisted living, of the forces that lead them to chose this long-term care option and their particular facilities, and of the outcomes of these choices for them and their families.

Study Methods

Two in-depth, qualitative studies of assisted living carried out between the spring of 1999 and the fall of 2001 are the basis of this book. For both the studies, we used an ethnographic approach (Muller, 1995) to understand life in these assisted living communities. Our goal was to identify and describe the intensity and range of daily experiences, activities, perceptions, interactions, and decision making—formal and informal—as they occurred within these homes.

Choosing the Communities and Gaining Access

We used "purposive" sampling (Patton, 1990) to choose facilities where we could learn the most about the issues of central importance to both studies—how to maximize independence and autonomy in assisted living. The homes in the first study (Study I) were all owned and operated by African Americans, and all or most of their residents were African American. These homes varied in resources, socioeconomic status of residents, and size—all factors thought to influence residents' independence and autonomy. We selected three small family model homes (2–6 beds), based on the high proportion (74%) of this type of home among ALFs in the nine-county metropolitan Atlanta area, and two larger facilities (7–15 beds). All five of these homes served residents with low to moderate income. At the time of Study I, none of the homes in the metropolitan Atlanta area serving primarily African American residents was large (more than 25 residents) or had higher-income residents. Although Study II homes varied in race of residents, owners, and staff, geographic location, and ownership, the data for this book are derived only from the one home in the study in which all residents were African American. This home, which opened in fall

1999, was conceived and built to provide affluent African Americans a long-term care option similar to that of whites—a high-amenity facility located in their own community. The Study II home was relatively large (75 beds), corporately owned, and located in a middle-class African American neighborhood.

Although for both studies it was relatively easy to identify ALFs in the Atlanta area that were owned and operated by African Americans and met our inclusion criteria, finding owners willing to be subjected to our scrutiny for a year was more challenging. Our strategy for Study I, which proved successful, was to call upon our colleagues in the Atlanta Long-Term Care Ombudsman Program (an advocacy program for residents of long-term care facilities) to provide information about potential study homes, suggest owners who might be willing to participate, make preliminary contacts, and accompany members of the research team on initial visits. These visits provided an opportunity for us to experience the homes firsthand and explain to the owners who we were and what our study was about. As it turned out, three owners readily agreed, and a fourth, who had heard about the project, lobbied to participate. Only the owner of one of the larger homes (13 beds) initially resisted, agreeing to participate only after speaking with two owners who had already experienced several weeks of research visits. To gain access to the Study II home, we met with the executive director and representatives of the corporation, all of whom were eager to be a part of the study. Detailed descriptions of these settings are found in chapter 2. We refer to the homes by fictitious names: Rosie's Loving Care, Peach Blossom, Blue Skies, Greene's Personal Care Home, and Sunshine House (Study I) and Oak Manor (Study II).

Team Strategy

We used a team strategy in both studies. One or more team members collected data in each home, and we conducted analysis as a group. Eight investigators—the six authors of this book and two graduate students—participated in the study of these six communities. One investigator was assigned to each of the small family model homes, two to each of the larger family model homes, and three to the large home in Study II. Mary Ball was the lead investigator for two of the family model homes in Study I and the large Study II home.

Protecting Participants

Before entering the homes as researchers, we obtained informed consent from owners for general access to their homes to observe activities and interact informally with them, the residents, and their staff. We then elicited separate consent from residents whose personal records we reviewed and from residents, providers, and family members or friends of residents whom we interviewed. In cases of guardianship, family members or social workers gave consent.

We use fictitious names for all individuals and homes throughout the book to protect the identities of participants. In selecting names, we tried to remain true to the character of homes and participants by referring to people as they were referred to in real life (that is, by first name, last name, or nickname) and by choosing names for homes that are typical of the size and type of home. In some cases we altered information (for example, place of birth) to further camouflage participants, but we took care not to change characteristics that would materially affect interpretation of data or conclusions.

Establishing Rapport and Reciprocity

In qualitative research, success in obtaining comprehensive and accurate data depends on the researcher's ability to develop trusting relationships with informants. In each of the homes, relationships developed gradually. For example, during the first two months of the study, the owner of Greene's Personal Care Home required researchers to notify her before visiting, staff were watchful of what they said and did in the researchers' presence, and residents were reserved in their interactions. After this initial period, the two investigators were permitted to visit the home freely; by the end of the study, their presence was barely noticed by staff, and residents looked forward to and enjoyed their visits. In contrast, the owner of Sunshine House, who worked full-time at another job, maintained certain restrictions throughout the study, which limited both the quality and quantity of data. The most challenging were the limitation of field visits in the early months to times when his manager was on duty, typically the night shift; the requirement of a monthly calendar of scheduled visits; an unwillingness to help researchers contact family members for interviews; and the refusal to allow us access to resident records.

A key factor in the development and maintenance of rapport was our informants' perceptions of our sincere interest in them as individuals. The owner of Rosie's Loving Care told us, "I think [the research experience] was fantastic. It was such an interest that you showed and the love and devotion that you showed to the people. It seemed genuine to me." What researchers gave to each home also influenced relationships. Throughout the course of the study period, we all provided a variety of goods and services: we brought fruit, candy, and home-baked pies, cooked entire meals, bought Christmas presents for residents, put up a Christmas tree and decorations, helped residents find a source for free eyeglasses and access to a senior center, furnished art supplies, and even made curtains. Relationships continue. Three years after our official departure, we "adopted" Greene's at Christmas, and the lead investigator for Oak Manor is a regular volunteer there at biweekly Bingo nights.

Although five of the eight researchers who visited the homes were white and most residents and all providers were African American, we believe that race was not a significant barrier in learning the truth about these communities. We recognize that it may not be possible for a white person to understand fully the African American experience, but we believe the extended research period and the rapport that developed between white researchers and African American residents and providers minimized this gulf. As the provider in Peach Blossom told the investigator, "I don't think your being white had anything to do with it. You know about cultural differences. Because of your knowledge it went very well. I have had people come in and start asking a bunch of questions. You did everything very diplomatically and [the residents] were very comfortable. I have been a black woman for 71 years, and there are some things another race may not know as well as I, but I shared the truth."

Notably, we faced the most significant problems with data collection in the two homes in which the three African American investigators were based. As noted, the owner of Sunshine House restricted access to the home and residents, and all three researchers working at Oak Manor (one white and two African American) encountered resistance from some residents. This resistance had several origins. First, residents at Oak Manor, compared with those at the smaller homes, were, in general, more educated and knew about the historical experiences of African Americans in research—for example, the Tuskegee experiment. They also were more willing to assert themselves with the facility management and the researchers. The other barrier, and most likely the primary one, was one extremely vocal resident who had considerable influence over facility management and some residents. At the resident council meeting where the lead investigator (who was white) introduced the project to the residents, he reviewed the history of adverse treatment of African Americans by whites and chastised our university for what he considered its insensitivity to a neighboring African American community (not the one where the facility was located), although he assured the researcher he had nothing against her personally. This resident had particular concerns about researchers' having access to residents' health records, and only after we agreed not to look at residents' records were we able to move forward with the project. Despite this rocky start, we encountered no further hurdles in this home, and the resident opposition leader was the first interview participant.

Collecting Data

To learn about these communities, we used four data-collection methods: participant observation, informal interviewing, in-depth interviewing, and review of resident records and facility documents. The formal data collection period extended for 17 months in Greene's, 13 months in Rosie's, Peach Blossom, Blue Skies, and Oak Manor, and 12 months in Sunshine House. This prolonged period allowed us to observe the range of life experiences and routines in all the homes through at least a full calendar year, including, for example, observances of religious and secular holidays and other personally significant events. In addition, we were able to observe the introduction of new residents and their adjustment to their new communities, as well as how decisions were made about residents' leaving. We visited homes approximately weekly at different times throughout the week. Visits ranged in length from 1 to 8 hours (but typically were 2 to 3 hours). In all we made a total of 393 visits and observed for 1,077 hours. Table 1.1 shows the number of visits made and hours spent observing in each home. In addition, four researchers made a total of 53 visits to senior centers and a mental health day program attended by residents.

We recorded observations through field notes, following a detailed guide (developed by the key investigators) that addressed the range of activities (planned and unplanned) and included where and when activities took place,

Table 1.1. *Number of Visits and Hours Spent in Research Homes*

Home	Capacity	No. of investigators	No. of visits	No. of hours
Rosie's	6	1	51	105
Peach Blossom	6	1	53	132
Blue Skies	6	1	60	175
Greene's	13	2	80	186
Sunshine House	13	2	28	53
Oak Manor	75	3	121	426
Total	119	10	393	1,077

who was involved, how they were carried out, what people said (paying attention to the informants' language), and how participants reacted to the world around them. Much of the time was spent just "hanging out" and talking informally with residents, providers, and any visitors in the home. In the small homes, where activities were limited, we spent many hours with residents just sitting or watching TV; we tried to be present when special events occurred, such as a pastor's visit or a birthday party. At Oak Manor, we took part in many of the daily planned activities and joined residents on field trips in the community. Monthly resident council meetings were a rich source of information about life in the home and residents' attitudes. We also accompanied residents to churches, day programs, doctors' offices, grocery stores, and hospitals. As we developed rapport with residents over the course of data collection, we were invited into their rooms and sometimes, with their permission, observed personal care activities.

Informal interviewing was usually unstructured and carried out as part of participant observation. This conversational form of questioning was the only means of interviewing residents who would not agree to more formal interviews or who had cognitive impairment. It also was a convenient way of questioning providers, who often were too busy to sit and talk at length. We recorded all informal interviews through written notes, including verbatim quotes when possible.

We used detailed interview guides to conduct in-depth interviews, and almost all interviews were tape-recorded and transcribed verbatim. Table 1.2 shows the number of residents, providers, and family members and friends we interviewed in each home. We interviewed most residents during the second half of the study period, giving ourselves time first to develop rapport, but were unable to interview as many residents as we planned because of the number with cognitive impairment. In each of the Study I homes, we interviewed the owner or the manager (or both) and at least one other member of the care staff. At Oak Manor, in addition to two executive directors (the first was replaced midyear), we interviewed six other types of managerial staff (for example, activity, food service, and marketing directors), a corporate representative, and three direct care staff. In all homes, we interviewed the person "in charge" early on, to help us get oriented, and then at least one other time during the year. Family and friends of residents provided valuable information, particularly for residents with cognitive impairment. Interviewing family members was quite challenging, since some rarely visited and most led busy lives.

Table 1.2. *Number of Persons Interviewed in Each Home*

Home	Capacity	No. of residents	No. of staff	No. of families and friends
Rosie's	6	3	2	3
Peach Blossom	6	4	2	4
Blue Skies	6	1	2	5
Greene's	13	12	4	3
Sunshine House	13	1	2	0
Oak Manor	75	12	14	9
Total	119	33	26	24

From the resident records, we gathered information about residents' health status, care needs, medications, family contacts, and, in some cases, daily activities. Although certain information is mandated by state regulation, the quality and quantity of these data depended on each home's record-keeping practices. We also reviewed facility documents, including formal admission agreements, written policies and procedures, and marketing materials.

Data Analysis

We used the grounded theory approach (Strauss, 1987; Strauss & Corbin, 1990) to analyze all qualitative data. Because this approach consists of a constant comparative method of inquiry in which data collection, hypothesis generation, and analysis occur simultaneously, we began analysis soon after entering the field and continued long after we had left. An important advantage of grounded theory analysis is its flexibility, allowing researchers to address new findings and modify assumptions made a priori.

The grounded theory method involves two analytical procedures: coding and memoing. Codes are similar to subject areas or topics on which study participants elaborate. In the initial stage of coding, called open coding, we identified emergent themes or concepts based on questions we asked and issues raised by informants and grouped them into categories in terms of their properties and dimensions. As new themes emerged, codes were modified, collapsed, or dropped. In the next stage of coding—axial coding—we related initial categories or subcategories through what Strauss and Corbin (1990) refer to as a paradigm model. This model links categories in a set of relationships denoting causal conditions, context, intervening conditions, action-interaction strategies, and consequences. As part of axial coding, we compared predicted patterns with empirically based patterns (pattern matching). In the final stage of coding—selective coding—we organized major categories around central explanatory concepts or core categories (Strauss & Corbin, 1990). We considered analysis complete when no new or relevant data emerged regarding a category, when category development was dense, and when the relationships between categories were well established and validated.

Using the analytical process of memoing, we recorded methodological and theoretical notes throughout the coding process. Methodological notes helped track problems, changes in research procedures, and issues regarding relationships with participants. Theoretical notes contained insights, observations, interpretations, and questions about the data. In initial analysis, theoretical notes often served as reminders of what information to look for next. At more advanced stages, these analytical memos became more theoretically abstract and complex and included visual representations, such as diagrams and charts.

Data analysis was a team effort. Although individual investigators examined data from the homes they studied, data from all homes were examined by the entire team in weekly meetings. We developed our coding scheme as a group, and at least two people coded the same material, thereby reducing the possibility of coding errors. We also created analytical charts, which all team members used to more thoroughly explore emergent themes and patterns. The final step in our team strategy was a cross-facility comparison of major topics (for example, care provision, environment, social relationships, resident daily routines, and provider roles), which led to identifying core analytical categories. Because of the large volume of data collected by this research, we used a software package (Qualis Research Associates, Ethnograph 5.0) for qualitative data management.

Those variables derived from interviews and record reviews that could be quantified were coded and entered into the Statistical Package for the Social Sciences for analysis. Quantitative analysis was limited to descriptive statistics used to examine characteristics both within and across homes.

Validity, Reliability, and Generalizability in Qualitative Research

In qualitative research, the criteria of validity and reliability are subsumed by Patton (1990) under the concept of credibility, which depends, in part, on rigorous techniques and methods for data collection and analysis. The credibility of our data was achieved through the techniques of negative case analysis, triangulation, memoing, and our team strategy for analysis. Credibility of the data also depends on the credibility of the researcher (Patton, 1990). All the authors of this book are experienced qualitative researchers and have conducted previous research on assisted living.

In qualitative research, the term *transferability* is substituted for generalizability (Lincoln & Guba, 1985). The basis for transferability is the thick description, which presents in close detail the context and meanings of events relevant to those involved (Geertz, 1983). The possibility of transfer to another setting is an empirical question that must be answered by evaluating the situation portrayed by the research as well as the situation being considered for transfer. This study provides the thick description necessary for considerations of transferability to other assisted living settings in Georgia as well as other areas of the United States.

One of the realities of qualitative research is the development of close relationships over time, and ending these bonds can be upsetting, both for researchers and research participants. Although one home closed soon after data collection ended and a number of residents have died or been discharged to nursing homes, at the writing of this book, researchers continue to maintain contact with providers and remaining residents in four of these communities.

CHAPTER 2

The Context of Care

7 a.m. A quiet, average house on a quiet, average residential street. All outward signs suggest that inside is a working-class nuclear family—Mom, Dad, and the kids—groggily preparing for another day at work and school. Yet most passersby would be surprised to learn that inside are mostly old people, in various states of disability and mental alertness; some happy, some sad; some moving carefully through their morning routine in anticipation of the bus that will take them to the senior center, and some hardly moving at all; some looking forward to seeing relatives or friends later in the day, and some bereft of such hopes. For Rosie, who has been up for an hour, this day will be much like all the others during her 10-year career as an assisted living provider: full of effort, concern, anxiety, and satisfaction. Rosie's Care Home, like its residents, is accepted by its neighbors but not really embraced. It occupies a place on the street but is not part of the communal fabric. It serves a function but earns little respect or profit. It is the kind of place that people tend to avoid learning much about but, if it weren't there, would have to be invented.

Visualizing Rosie's, or any of the care homes we studied, as a physical place is not hard; understanding and describing its essence is. At first glance, Rosie's does not appear to be a place of deep emotion; and like most of the homes we studied, it would not be considered very attractive. Some of the homes were even a bit run-down. Outside, though different from one another, they are typical of their neighborhoods and appear to fit in. Their inside look and feel are often not those of "normal" family homes, yet they possess many qualities and routines of family life and their own peculiar sense of normalcy. They certainly are homes, as most of us imagine them, and their owners and staff generally work hard to achieve and maintain that state, or at least its verisimilitude. Although we did not envy the residents, we did feel privileged to visit them and learn from them.

In this chapter we describe the setting of our research, sketching briefly the social context of the study and the collective characteristics of our sample. We also describe each of the six assisted living homes studied, including the neighborhoods within which they are located, showing how these communities influence ownership, residency, and care. In the following chapter, we address in more detail how African American community life shaped the life course of the residents of these six facilities.

The Neighborhoods

Like most large American cities since the Civil War, Atlanta has a sizable African American underclass. Unlike many other cities, however, especially in the South, Atlanta also has had a thriving, vibrant black middle class and even a few black millionaire entrepreneurs. Although not as large as its white counterpart, by mid-twentieth century Atlanta's black educated middle class was widely known and admired among other African American communities, so that Atlanta came to be called "the black mecca." This stable, early middle class was well positioned to take advantage of the civil rights movement of the 1960s and 1970s and its consequent opening of the larger society to black aspiration and achievement. The early black middle class thus spawned a black upper-middle class, populated by physicians, lawyers, professors, engineers, bankers, entertainers, and entrepreneurs. Atlanta's black community is growing more and more economically diverse, following the path already trod by its white counterpart, resulting in significant class differences within the race.

Atlanta also resembles other major American cities in its residential patterns and changes. Until the 1960s, all neighborhoods were rigidly segregated by race, and the cycle of decline and turnover was relatively slow. When federal laws and courts in the 1960s began to demand "open housing," neighborhood transition intensified. "White flight"—the movement of whites farther away from the city center to escape the "encroachment" of newly empowered blacks—became the dominant real estate trend. As whites moved to the suburbs, black families replaced them in both older and newer areas, sometimes able to buy but often only affording to rent. Some newer neighborhoods that had been built after World War II enjoyed an easier transition and remain largely stable and integrated today. Neighborhoods with older housing stock, however, tended to attract absentee landlords who converted the single-family houses to apartment dwellings, boarding houses, and small businesses. These neighborhoods deteriorated and became less and less desirable. In time, many of these older, close-in neighborhoods experienced another transition, as middle-class whites and blacks (some of whom were the children of those who had fled earlier) moved back—or migrated here as Atlanta became an economic magnet in the 1970s and 1980s—in search of more affordable, convenient, racially diverse neighborhoods than those in the suburbs.

An example of such a transitional neighborhood is Ashby Grove, the location of Greene's Personal Care Home. When Greene's was established in 1984, the community was predominantly African American, and homes were modest. Today, young, middle-class families—white and black—are moving into the neighborhood and surrounding residential areas and beginning to refurbish them. Once considered an inner-city slum, the community is quickly gaining a reputation as a "hot," "up-and-coming," "in-town" neighborhood. Property values are rising, and fast-food restaurants, convenience stores, and check-cashing facilities are slowly being replaced by trendy restaurants, art galleries, and shops. Commercial developers are moving into the area and converting old decaying buildings and apartment complexes into luxury lofts, condominiums, and office space. New homes are being built for the first time in a century, and older homes, some dating to the late 1800s, are being restored to their original style. This gentrification may be the enemy of the poor, but it is fervently desired by urban politicians and city officials who covet the increasing tax base.

Sunshine House, however, is situated along Old Canton Road, a busy arterial street that connects Atlanta's downtown with the more affluent black neighborhoods farther from the center of the city. The area, known as Canton Hills, was an all-white neighborhood until the early 1970s, and its housing stock dates from the 1930s and 1940s. Now it sits in a boundary neighborhood linking the older, less desirable, closer-in area with the newer, more stable, obviously middle-class neighborhoods just inside the perimeter highway, a multilane interstate that encircles the city 10 to 15 miles from its center.

Around a bend in Old Canton Road, just past the busy shopping area centered on a large grocery store and several fast-food restaurants, a residential area begins abruptly. The houses are mostly brick, some perched on high banks with wide front lawns, others are set back only slightly from the street, with smaller front yards. The street is heavily traveled, but the houses in this part of Canton Hills are mostly neat and well cared for, and the working- and middle-class community appears stable.

The other facilities in this study are situated in neighborhoods that share some of the history and characteristics of Ashby Grove and Canton Hills. Blue

Skies is located in a formerly all-white suburban area about three miles outside the perimeter that is now predominately, though not entirely, black. Rosie's Loving Care is one block off Old Canton Road in a formerly white middle-class neighborhood, about a mile beyond Sunshine House. Peach Blossom can be found in the Hiram Hill neighborhood, on the west side of town, that has been a significant residential community for blacks since the 1950s. The newest facility, Oak Manor, is located in one of the newer parts of town, a decidedly middle- and upper-middle-class community known colloquially as Eastover. Eastover is typical of the suburban neighborhoods that have grown up around the interchanges of the perimeter highway, which was completed in the late 1960s. Land in the area of Oak Manor, however, was sparsely developed before the whites who did live there moved farther out. Further development in the wider Eastover community has occurred largely in the past 20 years, and many of the nicest homes and businesses date only from the 1990s.

Characteristics of the Samples

The six homes we studied varied considerably by size, ownership, staffing, clientele, amenities, and, of course, cost. Although some variation was apparent among the small homes, the major difference was between the five smaller homes and the large facility, Oak Manor. All the five small homes had each been single-family homes before being converted to personal care use; their length of time in business ranges from one to 20 years. Each of them is owned by one person. Oak Manor, the large, purpose-built facility, is owned by a corporation that developed and manages it, along with several similar assisted living facilities in Georgia and other southeastern states. Befitting its size, Oak Manor has a typical staff (all shifts) of 35 full-time and 6 part-time employees, including an executive director, a business manger, and directors of marketing, resident service, activities, maintenance, and food service, in addition to various other office, care, housekeeping, and kitchen staff.

Three modes of administration and staffing are used in the five smaller homes. In the first model, employed in Rosie's and Peach Blossom, the owner lives in the home and carries out all administrative and management duties, as well as providing considerable hands-on care. Part-time staff are hired to help with cleaning and caregiving duties. In the second model, found in Greene's, the owner does not live in the home but provides day-to-day administration and some caregiving and hires an assortment of full-time and part-time staff to provide housekeeping, meal preparation, and resident care. In the third model, the owner does not live in the home and provides little daily management or regular caregiving. This is the case in both Blue Skies and Sunshine House, where the owners are regular visitors but leave most daily duties to paid staff. The owner of Blue Skies occasionally works there on weekends.

Fees charged by the homes vary within and across the five small facilities and range from $430 to $1,500 a month. Oak Manor uses a fairly standard industry practice of charging according to the level of care needed, with fees ranging from $2,095 to $3,645. Oak Manor's fees are published and ostensibly nonnegotiable, but the small-home owners tend to charge what they think residents can afford and use whatever higher fees they can obtain to "subsidize" lower-paying residents. Of the five smaller homes, only Peach Blossom, Greene's, and Blue Skies have any residents who pay $1,000 or more. Two of the homes (Rosie's and Blue Skies) participate in the Community Care Services Program, Georgia's home and community-based Medicaid waiver program. The Medicaid reimbursement rate, which averaged $14 a day per resident during the period of study, supplements what residents pay privately. Although all homes have at least one resident with a mental illness diagnosis, two homes (Sunshine House and Greene's) serve several mentally ill or mentally retarded residents. Table 2.1 summarizes some key characteristics and the fee structures of the six homes.

A total of 69 providers (owners and staff) worked in these six homes during the two studies, although we were able to obtain some social and demographic data for only 57 of them. The large majority (91%) are under the age

Table 2.1. Characteristics of Six Study Homes

Home	Date opened	Licensed capacity	Resident census	Ownership	Fee source	Fee range
Rosie's	1987	6	7–8	Individual	Private + CCSP	$500–800
Peach Blossom	1979	6	6	Individual	Private	$500–1,500
Blue Skies	1998	6	6	Individual	Private + CCSP	$850–1,000
Greene's	1983	13	15–18	Individual	Private	$430–1,050
Sunshine House	1986	13	7–11	Individual	Private	$500–?
Oak Manor	1999	75[a]	20–42[b]	Corporate	Private	$2,095–3,645

[a]Includes special care dementia unit.
[b]Only assisted living section.

of 65, but more than half are over 45. Nearly all are female (82%). Almost all providers also are African American (88%) or African Caribbean (9%); one is white, and one Latino. Three of the five African Caribbean providers work at Blue Skies, one of whom is the owner. Although most are at least high school graduates (83%), 6% have only an elementary education.

The 104 residents who lived in the six study homes are socially diverse. That only 77% of residents are 65 or older can be attributed to the number of younger residents with mental health problems, most of whom are in Greene's and Sunshine House. Except for Peach Blossom and Oak Manor, each of the homes has a combination of old and young residents. At one time, two residents aged 24 and 26 were in Blue Skies, and four residents were in their 70s, 80s, and 90s.

The large proportion of male residents (38%) also is notable for the population of assisted living facilities. Again, this percentage is skewed by the number of male residents with mental health problems who live in two of the homes. Seventy-two percent of residents at Greene's are male, while 47% are male in Sunshine House, where the gender distribution is in large part dictated by the physical segregation of males and females in the lower and upper levels. Most of the remaining males in our study resided at Oak Manor, where 30% of residents are male.

Not surprisingly, given our study goal, only 11% of all residents are white, all of whom live at either Blue Skies or Greene's. In fact, 44% of Greene's residents are white. The presence of white residents in these homes is, at least in part, related to the ways the owners typically recruit residents. Most of Greene's residents are referred by hospital discharge planners or social workers. Blue Skies gets some residents through the Community Care Services Program, and it is located in a racially integrated neighborhood, so it is known to white neighbors who are potentially future residents.

Residents' educational level is bimodal: most residents of the five smaller homes have quite limited education, while the residents of Oak Manor have much more. Only 54% of small-home residents are high school graduates, one-fourth have less than a high school education, and two have no formal education at all. Only four of those living in the smaller homes (10%) are college graduates, and three of those live at Peach Blossom (two have master's degrees). At Oak Manor, however, given its decidedly middle-class market, all residents have graduated high school, and 84% have at least a college degree.

Residents' most prevalent health conditions include incontinence, dementia, and hypertension (each found in 33% of residents), mental health problems, mainly schizophrenia (28%), heart problems (26%), arthritis (23%), and depression (21%), with a scattering of diabetes (except at Oak Manor, where almost one-third of residents are diabetic), stroke, and paralysis. (Sunshine House residents are not included in these data because the owner would not grant access to their files.) It might appear that, on the whole, this population is actually somewhat healthier than average for their age, but we are not certain of the accuracy and completeness of the medical records maintained by some of the homes, and, since about half of the residents in both Greene's and Sunshine House have a diagnosis of mental illness, the total sample appears somewhat less physically impaired.

Some differences in kinds of resident health problems exist among homes, and these differences tend to reflect the owners' admission policies. The large majority of residents need assistance with instrumental activities of daily living (IADLs)—for example, managing money (78%) and taking medications (86%). Fewer than half of the residents need help with each activity of daily living (ADL): bathing (45%), dressing (41%), toileting (29%), walking (16%), and eating (3%). We saw clear differences between the larger and smaller homes in the proportion of residents needing help with medications (100% of residents in the three smallest homes) and in the proportion needing help with bathing, dressing, grooming, and toileting—all activities requiring a significant amount of care time. Most of Peach Blossom's residents need assistance with all these activities.

Description of the Homes

Rosie's Loving Care

Rosie's house is like many other family homes in Atlanta: a red brick, bi-level, 1950s-era ranch. Situated on a large wooded lot in a quiet neighborhood, the house gives the same appearance as the middle-class, single-family residences surrounding it. On the main level are three bedrooms, two bathrooms, living room, dining room, kitchen, sunroom, and den. The basement level includes a double garage, used as a laundry room and food storage area, and one large room, where Rosie and two of her residents sleep. The interior of the house is in relatively good condition and is always kept neat and clean.

Entering through the front door, visitors step into a linoleum-floored entrance hall covered with a rug and brightened with artificial flowers on a small table. The living room is attractively and comfortably furnished. The red carpet and soft pink drapes lend a bright atmosphere, while a large picture window facing the street lets in a warm afternoon light. The numerous decorative figurines in the front window can be seen from the street. Two sofas, a recliner, and another comfortable chair are arranged to allow easy viewing of the television, ensconced in the large shelf unit that also holds an interesting array of family pictures, a small collection of cups and saucers, a few books, and, inexplicably, a large bottle of cognac standing next to a decorative doll. On one wall is a fireplace surmounted by a small print of "The Last Supper," while on the opposite wall sits a spinet piano.

In the adjacent dining room, with the same red carpet, stands a table and three or four chairs, often used by Rosie and her daughter for paperwork and sometimes for residents to eat. The buffet on the back wall is used to store residents' records, along with paper products and a variety of food items. The kitchen has just enough room for the appliances and a small table, shoved against a wall, where three residents eat. Rosie has a microwave but no dishwasher. Menus are taped to the refrigerator, and on a large bulletin board are posted phone numbers, appointments, citations from the state regulators, an activity calendar, and assorted notices. The linoleum floor is a high-traffic passageway between dining room and den, and some of its tiles have been replaced and mismatched. The kitchen opens to a sunroom, where four residents eat meals at a white round table. A long, plastic-covered sectional sofa runs nearly the length of the back wall, and on the opposite wall is a cot, where a staff person slept while living at Rosie's temporarily.

On the main level are three bedrooms, each of which sleeps two residents. The bedroom at the front of the house has a private bath, one dresser, and a double closet. One resident has taped family pictures over her bed. The second bedroom is attractively furnished with four-poster twin beds, a white double dresser between them, and two tall dressers, both cluttered with one resident's personal items. A wheelchair sitting next to the bed is filled with odds and ends. Two large pictures drawn with colored markers (one of Jesus) look down on the clutter. The final bedroom, shared by the two male residents, has a small black-and-white TV, a double dresser with mirror, and two straight chairs. To each room's door is taped a piece of white paper with the occupants' names lettered in black marker.

In front of the house, one tall pine tree provides little shade and shares space with a wobbly bench and four white plastic chairs, where residents frequently sit. Rosie's visiting children and grandchildren sometimes play in the yard. The street is rather busy, and Rosie's lies only a block from the even busier Old Canton Road, although no businesses are within walking distance.

Peach Blossom

Peach Blossom was bought by its 70-year-old owner, Esther Adams, 20 years ago to be operated as a care home. It is located on the fringes of a residential area in a low- to middle-class neighborhood in northwest Atlanta. Situated on a wooded corner lot, the white frame house, with a large glassed-in porch on two sides, faces a busy street with several nearby churches and businesses. A bus stop is right in front of the house. Peach Blossom is licensed for six residents and generally operates at capacity. Over the years, Ms. Adams has made various additions and renovations, and the entire house is neat, clean, and nicely furnished and has central heat and air conditioning.

Everyone enters Peach Blossom through the front porch, where residents often sit in warm weather. The porch opens onto the dining room, in which a square table, with seasonal centerpiece, is always set with tablecloth, mats, silverware, and napkins. Its six chairs provide space for all residents to dine together. The dining room opens with a Dutch door into the kitchen. Appliances are in good shape and are supplemented by a microwave. A kitchen table with two chairs is where Ms. Adams often eats or works. The living room has a comfortable sofa, a chair for each resident, and a color TV with cable access. Adding to its homey quality are several decorative items and a clock that chimes the hour with 12 different bird songs.

Three bedrooms are on the main level, each with twin beds, matching bedspreads and curtains, a dresser, and a ceiling fan. One bedroom opens with French doors off the living room. Two residents live in each of two rooms, while the third is shared by one regular and an occasional temporary resident. These five or six residents share one full bath. Ms. Adams lives in a fourth bedroom, upstairs, which is separated from the rest of the house by a door and a hall and has a private bath, TV, and telephone. A large downstairs area contains the laundry room, a very small bedroom and bath for the one male resident, and a more recently renovated portion, with bedroom, sitting room, and bath, which is occasionally used by temporary male residents.

Blue Skies

When the study began, Blue Skies had been open only about six months. Its owner, Clarice Hull, a Caribbean immigrant of African descent, had recently purchased the home and converted it to an assisted living facility for six residents. The house is a 1950s one-story brick ranch, located in a quiet, residential suburban neighborhood, which has been racially mixed since the late 1970s. It is situated on a wooded lot and has a large backyard and a covered carport furnished with a Formica table and several chairs. Although the street has no sidewalks, pedestrians are hardly troubled by residential traffic, and a bus stop and several businesses are within a mile.

The original house comprised living room, dining room, kitchen, two bedrooms, and one bath. In the conversion to a care home, Clarice added another wing with three small bedrooms, a den with skylight, a laundry room, and a fully handicapped-accessible, tiled bathroom. The original entrance to the house is up several steps into the living room, but a sign near the door directs callers to a side entrance with ramp access to the den. Because the addition was not built on the same level as the original house, a short, steep ramp connects the den and kitchen, making wheelchair passage difficult.

The interior of Blue Skies is attractive and well maintained, and the house is centrally heated and cooled. The living room is formally furnished with two red velvet Victorian sofas and a large chair, a coffee table, lace curtains, an ornate brass wall clock, and artificial flowers in matching sconces. This room also has a 20-inch TV and two file cabinets for storage of facility records and medications, and it is where the home's manager sleeps. The dining room, opening off the living room and kitchen, has a large table where residents dine together. Resident bedrooms are carpeted and newly painted; each has one small closet and curtains on the windows. Four are private, while one in the new wing is shared by two residents. For several months, until the owner's husband could hang proper doors, only curtains hung in the bedroom doorways in the new wing.

The den typically functions as the residents' common space, but its short sofa and three plastic lawn chairs do not accommodate everyone at the same time. Mounted on one wall is a small TV with grainy picture, while on the opposite wall is a portable telephone for resident use.

Sunshine House

Fronting on busy Old Canton Road, Sunshine House, like most of the other smaller homes in this study, is indistinguishable as a business, except for the home's name on a small metal sign in the front yard. The front of the house deceptively suggests a smaller house: entry is through a narrow white wooden door; there is no porch and no upper story. The small front yard has a paved-over area, used for parking, that extends to the curb. A glimpse down the steep, paved driveway alongside the house reveals that the home is actually built on two levels, one at ground level, visible from the front, and the lower one accessible from a large back yard.

Through the front door is a small foyer, its space limited even more by a magazine table holding, among other items, dated copies of the *New Yorker*. The living room is large, with a nonfunctioning tiled fireplace and a mantle, on which sits a bouquet of artificial flowers. Under the window is a large desk with a table lamp, phone, guest book, and, sometimes, fresh flowers donated by family members or friends. A television rests on a stand in the corner near the pipes attached to the indoor portion of a natural gas meter, which serves as a "ground" for a homemade antenna. Except for natural light coming through the picture window, the room is dim. The modest furnishings, arranged around the edges of the room, include three love seats (two faux leather and one cloth covered), an armchair, a lounge chair, three card-table chairs, a wooden bench, and a pole lamp. The room, devoid of wall decorations except for a picture of Martin Luther King Jr., is dominated by an array of industrial orange-painted sprinkler pipes that hang from the ceiling and around the perimeter of the room. The floor is covered with dark blue, low-pile carpet, and the room is clean and odor free.

Three sleeping rooms for the women open off the living room through a small doorway. Each has two single beds with floral, polyester bedspreads, windows with miniblinds and lacy, crocheted valances, and 1950s-style furniture in a tan "bamboo" design. Two of the rooms have a dresser with drawers, a night stand with a lamp, and two small chairs. One room has a small closet, and one has an extra dresser. A bathroom connects two of the bedrooms.

The dining room space is occupied almost entirely by a large, oblong table and a four-drawer lockable metal file cabinet where medications are stored. The kitchen opens off one end of the dining room, a den off the other. The den has been converted into an office for the owner. A sofa (usually piled with paper goods and boxes of packaged snacks), a large business desk, two metal file cabinets, and stacks of papers take up nearly all the available space. A cork bulletin board hangs on the wall and holds business cards, handwritten phone numbers, training certificates, and sticky notes.

The kitchen has older, white appliances and white cabinets, some with chipped paint. A large, black chain with a small padlock is draped through the handles of the cabinets above the stove to prevent residents from rummaging for snack foods. The countertops are worn, as is the linoleum floor. The back door leads out to the steps to the lower level and the back yard. The staff schedule, required postings of residents' rights and other policies, and notices regarding special instructions for residents are tacked to a bulletin board. A door marked Do Not Enter, which leads into one of the women's rooms, is kept locked.

A steep flight of stairs, painted yellow, leads from the kitchen to the lower level—the men's quarters. The full basement has a linoleum floor with a dimly lit sitting area containing a small sofa and end table, two lounge chairs, a card table with chairs, a small color TV, a soda-vending machine, and a nonworking snack vendor. The food freezer, washing machine, and dryer sit at the opposite end of the basement, near the back door. The three sleeping rooms are sparsely furnished. One has three beds, the others, two.

Greene's Personal Care Home

Greene's Personal Care Home, which is licensed for 13 residents but often has more, is a wood-frame, single-story bungalow characteristic of other houses built in the Ashby Grove area following World War II. One of the few signs of renovation is a wheelchair ramp that leads from the sidewalk up to the front porch.

Cora Greene's office, located immediately inside the front door, is furnished with a desk, two rickety chairs, a coffee table, a couch covered in cracked green vinyl, and an RCA color console television. To the left of the desk is a black-and-white surveillance camera that continuously monitors the long middle hallway and common area. The hallway leads to a sunporch in the back of the facility, furnished with a couch with ripped orange vinyl upholstery, two reclining chairs, a small black-and-white television set, and two vending machines filled with soft drinks, candy, and chips. The sunporch opens onto a wooden deck, the authorized smoking area for residents and staff. Two full bathrooms, a half bath, a kitchen, and a dining room are located on the left side of the hallway, and on the right are four bedrooms. Two smaller bedrooms are located in the front of the building, off the office. A 4×6 inch note card taped to each bedroom door lists in pencil the occupants' names. The rooms, furnished with twin beds and an eclectic mix of secondhand furniture, reflect few personal touches.

The kitchen, a large open room that has not been updated since the house was built in the 1940s, contains two refrigerators, an old microwave, an open pantry with wire racks filled with institutional-size canned goods, an old industrial-size oven, a sink, and wooden cabinets badly in need of paint. The large dining room, which also serves as the residents' common living area, is furnished with a crowded assortment of tables, chairs, bookshelves, a refrigerator, and a dresser and is decorated with plastic flowers and knickknacks. A large rectangular table that can accommodate 10 to 12 residents is located in the middle of the room, and two large green metal trash cans labeled with a fast-food restaurant logo stand in opposite corners. Chairs are arranged to face a small black-and-white television set. Connected to the dining room is a small laundry room, the walls of which are lined with wire racks filled with communal clothing, including underwear, socks, sweat pants, faded T-shirts illustrated with sports logos and pictures of cartoon characters; one shirt is labeled "Atlanta Department of Sanitation," and another, "Property of Fulton County Jail." The house has central heat and cooling but is almost always uncomfortably warm, both summer and winter.

Next door to Greene's is an unlicensed assisted living facility that Ms. Greene refers to as "the rental property." The house, which is occupied by Greene's staff members, local transients who pay room and board by the week or by the month, and some longtime residents who suffer from mental illness, sometimes is used as a temporary place for Greene's residents.

Oak Manor

Oak Manor is an upscale home targeted to middle-class and upper-middle-class African Americans. The assisted living unit has 42 suites with seven floor-plan options; a locked dementia area has 17 rooms. A few units in each area are shared. The home had been open less than a year when the study started and was only about half full. Oak Manor is located one block off a busy stretch of Old Canton Road, about three miles farther out from Rosie's. A large chain department store is nearby, and within half a mile are shopping areas with grocery stores, banks, laundries, restaurants, drug stores, other small commercial establishments, and a bus stop.

Outside the front door, on the right side of the building, stands a grouping of wicker furniture, white with brightly colored cushions. Hanging plants decorate the area, which also has a garden, fish pond, tables, and chairs. The front entrance and drive are covered, and a sidewalk encircles the building. The grounds are grassy and well manicured. Residents spend a lot of time outside—just to sit and watch the scene, to talk, to visit with family and friends, and to smoke. Occasionally, a picnic or other planned activity takes place in the side area.

Inside the glass double-door entrance are chairs on either side. The main lobby area, to the left, has a gas-log fireplace. Around this area are two love seats, three chairs, a coffee table, and smaller tables. Against the front wall is a table holding coffee, water, and pastries. The home is attractively decorated with traditional African colors and carpeted throughout. The lobby area decor includes artificial flowers, live plants, a mirror, several hanging light fixtures, and a large chandelier. An antique radio usually is playing jazz, occasionally rhythm and blues or gospel. The fireplace is a popular place to sit, especially in the winter. Other favorite spots are the chairs near the entrance, next to the telephone, and in front of the reception desk at the far end of the lobby. The receptionist is on duty from eight in the morning until eight at night.

Three offices (for the director, the business manager, and the marketing director) are located on a hall off the main lobby, and two others (for the resident services director and the maintenance director) are off the upstairs lounge. The downstairs hall leads to the elevator, the activity room, the beauty shop, the wellness center, and the dementia special care unit on one end and to the dining room and residents' rooms on the other. Two chairs across from the elevator are another popular place to sit. Nearby is a display board holding notices about residents' birthdays, activities, and photos of residents. The Oak Manor dining room is both attractive and cheerful. Twelve dark wood tables, each with four chairs, are covered with burgundy tablecloths and usually are adorned with fresh flowers. A small room for private dinners in the back can seat six to eight people. The beauty shop is small, with two sinks (over which hang ornate gold-framed mirrors), two dryers, and a manicure table.

The stairway from the lobby area to the second floor is carpeted and leads to an upstairs living room furnished with a sofa, comfortable chairs, two wooden game tables, a TV, a stereo system, and a shelf holding decorative items. A chess set sits on one table. Three hallways, each with hand rails on either side, lead from the lounge area to residents' rooms.

Residents' rooms vary in size and shape. Most are private, and several residents have two-room suites. Each unit has a kitchen area with upper and lower cabinets and a small standing refrigerator with a freezing compartment. Bathrooms are rather small, and all have modular showers. All windows have blinds, and residents can add curtains, but there are no ceiling lights. Bedrooms have only one medium-size closet, and except where adjustments have been made, closets are not wheelchair accessible. Each unit has a faux-metal nameplate and a small shelf for decorative items or personal artifacts next to the door.

The six assisted living homes that serve as the setting for this study represent a broad range of living spaces and management styles. Some are quite small and intimate, others are a bit larger and perhaps less personal, and one is significantly larger and projects a typical corporate, managed environment. Although the corporately owned assisted living community is attractive, comfortable, and hardly distinguishable from any of the thousands of upscale facilities built in every state over the past decade, the five smaller homes share a "limited resources" reality that marks each of them in one way or another. Yet the outward appearance of these places as older, worn, and sometimes even shabby is quite misleading. Beginning with little but ambition, instinct, and perhaps a calling, the owners of these small homes have carved out workable and supportive living environments for their clients. Clearly, each home's environment, both social and physical, shapes its residents' experiences and the quality of their lives.

Part II / Becoming a Resident

CHAPTER 3

Creating a Community

Residents' Life Stories

The African American elders profiled in the following pages are just five of the residents the reader will come to know in this book. Their life stories provide important insights into the differing social, economic, and cultural contexts surrounding residents' transitions into assisted living and lay the foundation for later chapters in which we explore in depth the overall resident experience. Like most of the African American participants in this study, these five residents were born in the early twentieth century and grew up in the South during the era of legal segregation. Because of racism, their opportunities for education, employment, housing, and health care were limited. Lifetimes of social disadvantage increased the likelihood that they would experience chronic disease and disability. For some residents, most of whom live at Oak Manor, social class mediated some of these adverse effects. For most of the residents living in the smaller homes, poverty compounded the disadvantages of racism.

Miss Fannie of Greene's Personal Care Home

Fannie Jo Morgan, "Miss Fannie" to her family and friends is, at the age of 92, the oldest resident of Greene's Personal Care Home. Miss Fannie was born into poverty, from which she never escaped, and her face portrays a lifetime of hardship. Her eyes are dull and bloodshot, all of her teeth are missing, and she often goes without her ill-fitting dentures, giving her heavily wrinkled face a hollowed look. Years of poor nutrition have contributed to Miss Fannie's immense size, and despite her obesity her body is frail. She is crippled from arthritis and struggles, with the aid of a walker, to support her weight on badly swollen legs. Miss Fannie also suffers from mild dementia, a heart condition, poor vision, and incontinence, the latter resulting in occasional embarrassing accidents. Although she receives a monthly income of only $564 and is severely impaired, Miss Fannie views her life positively: "I'm glad that the Lord let me live to get 92. Don't many people live that long."

Born in 1907 into a large African American family in rural south Georgia, Miss Fannie and her nine siblings began working in the fields as soon as they "got big enough." The long hours of backbreaking fieldwork stopped her education at the fifth grade, but Miss Fannie accepted that as her lot in life. After all, her own survival and the survival of her family required her to contribute to the family finances. When asked about her life, Miss Fannie recalled a past typical of many African American residents:

> My sisters and brothers and I worked in the field. Didn't have no job working making money like they do now. My papa made us stay home and work when we ought to been going to school. We had to chop cotton, hoe cotton, and hoe corn and cut grass and stuff like that. Papa wasn't mean to us, you know, like that. He treated us all very nicely. We had to obey, though. I come here to Atlanta 'way on down the road. I forgot what time. When I come to Atlanta, I went to work for some Jews for three dollars a week. The lady done all the cooking, and I did the washing and ironing, sweep the floors and mop the floors and like that. I worked there a long time. When I retired, I worked at County Hospital. They had the white cafeteria and the colored cafeteria. I worked in the white cafeteria and then I worked in the colored a little bit.

Despite her past, Miss Fannie expresses satisfaction and pride regarding her childhood, particularly about "Papa's" self-reliance. Papa did not depend on white people for work but earned the family money by farming, gambling, and selling his homemade liquor. Miss Fannie recalled that both "white and black folks" came from around the county to buy "Papa's whiskey." Miss Fannie also speaks highly of her "Mama," a deeply religious woman who instilled strong religious values in her children, though she admits that her own hot temper and tendency to curse, as well as her enjoyment of chewing tobacco and an occasional "nip" of whiskey, make her more like her father than her mother.

Miss Fannie lived on her parents' farm until she married at the age of 17; sometime in the late 1920s she and her husband moved to Atlanta to look for better-paying work. They settled in Reynoldstown, a bustling African American community only a half-hour's walk from downtown Atlanta. Fannie worked for a rabbi and his wife in nearby Summerhill (which included a small

Jewish population) until her early 50s, when she left to work in the cafeteria at County Hospital, a large, segregated, inner-city public hospital. By the time Miss Fannie retired from the hospital in 1978, all patient care facilities, including food service, had been desegregated as a result of the passage of the Civil Rights Act of 1964. After her husband died, Miss Fannie lived with her widowed 73-year-old sister, who owned a home in Reynoldstown, a historic working-class community that had undergone significant economic decline. Soon her nephew, unemployed and "on dope," also moved into her sister's house, and Miss Fannie moved to a Section 8 (public housing) high-rise near County Hospital. By now, few members of Miss Fannie's large tight-knit family remained. Her only child died as a baby, and her husband and most of her siblings were also deceased. Miss Fannie spoke on the phone to her elder sister every day but rarely saw her.

After a heart attack at age 90, Miss Fannie was hospitalized at County Hospital. Because she was too ill to return to her apartment and had no family members to care for her, a hospital discharge planner placed her in Greene's Personal Care Home. Miss Fannie recalled that she "didn't know nothing 'bout the place" and was "sent" there from County Hospital, where Greene's was "on record" as a placement option for indigent patients who needed rehabilitative care.

Alma Burgess of Oak Manor

Like Miss Fannie, Alma Burgess was born in Georgia in the early 1900s and struggled against racial oppression throughout her life. In contrast to Miss Fannie's rural background, though, Ms. Burgess grew up in Atlanta. As a child she lived with her parents and younger siblings in an affluent, predominantly African American neighborhood in southwest Atlanta. Her mother was a housewife and her father, an academic, was dean of a black college and later served as a college president.

Ms. Burgess described her parents as "exceptional people." They believed that education was necessary for success in a white-dominated society and paid the tuition for their children to attend private secondary schools, one of the few options for advanced education available to African American children at the time. They exposed their children to art and cultural events and provided them the opportunity to travel. Ms. Burgess recalls that, while traveling during summers, she "learned a lot about the United States and met black leaders all over the country."

Ms. Burgess's educational background and economic position allowed her to attend one of Atlanta's historically black colleges, where she received degrees in both English and education. She went on to complete a master's degree in English at another historically black institution, where she met her first husband. After teaching elementary school for a year, Ms. Burgess accepted a faculty position at her college alma mater and remained there for more than 25 years.

Ms. Burgess and her husband settled in a house that was "just three doors" down from her parents' home. They had three children, two boys and a girl. The first child, a girl, died from pneumonia soon after birth. Although busy teaching and raising her two boys, Ms. Burgess stayed active in the community. In addition to helping start a local chapter of the Jack and Jill Club, a program that provides African American children access to social and cultural activities, she actively participated in her church, Alpha Kappa Alpha sorority, and various other social organizations and civic groups.

Ms. Burgess's husband died when her oldest son was just seven years old, and, wanting her young boys to have a father figure, she soon remarried. Her second husband, 17 years her senior, abused her both physically and mentally, and that marriage ended after only five years. Ms. Burgess never remarried. She credits her first husband and her parents, who "were crazy about the boys," with helping her raise two "pretty well-rounded" children; like their mother, her two boys graduated from college and pursued professional careers.

Ms. Burgess remained in her home for "47-odd years," but at age 87, after two falls resulting in broken bones, she decided that moving to nearby Oak Manor was "probably the best thing" to do: "My children, my boys, were wanting me to get out, go somewhere else. I was looking for somewhere I could go, and I actually saw this building [Oak Manor] go up from the ground. When I knew what it was all about and the type of facility, the first of this type available to blacks, I decided that's what I would want to do."

Eugene Ellis of Oak Manor

Eugene Ellis is one of a small group of residents who did not grow up in the South. Like Alma Burgess, he is one of a number of middle- to upper-middle-class residents in our study. Despite growing up in a working-class family, Mr. Ellis earned a college degree and became upwardly mobile. He worked in state government and public education and dabbled in politics and in real estate. At 85, he recalled his life story:

I was born in the city of Columbus [Ohio]. My mom was a housewife and my daddy, prior to coming to Columbus, was a school teacher in North Carolina. Probably the kind of certification that was needed in North Carolina was certainly not acceptable in Columbus. In other words, I don't know if my dad had a degree or one year of college or two years of college. Nevertheless, he ended up being a chauffeur. He had two kids when he met my mom, and his wife had died. He had five with my mother, and I was the oldest. Two sisters and two brothers were younger than me. I would say that we might have been poor but didn't know it. We lived good and had good family relationships. I lived with them until I moved in 1937 [after leaving college].

I went to college from home, and my father subsidized me at [historically black] Wilberforce University. I only attended school about three semesters, and I dropped out and went to work. I worked for the state of Ohio as chief investigator for professional licensing. We would investigate illegal practice. A white guy got caught selling the exams for the pharmacy board for $2,000. So I guess those white folks in their wisdom said, "Let's get us a black guy." So they hired me.

I went back to school, back to Wilberforce, in 1955 and finished. Then I went with the public school system about 1959. I started out in elementary and got a double certification, elementary and special ed. Then, I went to junior high and then senior high and then went into a federal youth training program. I took the exam for a motivational coordinator, which was in a [grades] 9–12 high school, and then ended up with my own school. These were kids that might have difficulty in exams, but if properly motivated, [they could] succeed. We had a very unique program that would still be excellent today.

[I've been] married, almost all of my life, married 'way back in my college days. I had two wives. One [I] got a divorce [from] in '95, and the other one is still in Columbus and has her doctorate. That's my daughter's mother. We have a very good relationship. The other one was a schoolteacher, too. We have a beautiful relationship. Getting a divorce never made a difference with my relationship with my kids. My son, the oldest, passed at 50 in 1990. My daughter is 54. We're tight as wax.

I would be remiss if I did not mention that I joined a fraternity, Alpha Kappa Psi, in 1936, and stayed active. That is quite a heritage that I would belong to anything that long, over sixty years. Now, those brothers, or members of the fraternity, were very fond of me, gave me a lot of attention, [were] extensions of my family.

Aside from the many things I've done in life, I've done a lot of traveling. I've been around the world. I've been to London, I've been Paris, I've been to Spain, I've been to Portugal, I've been to Africa, I've been to most of the Islands. That would mean Puerto Rico, Freeport, Bermuda, most of the Islands, all of the United States, all sorts of resorts. Prior to downsizing and going to an apartment in 1995, I lived very comfortably in a house: a home with four bedrooms, two baths, two-car garage, and a corner property with a Jacuzzi. Every morning before I ate breakfast, I would run the water in the Jacuzzi and let the water just gush all over me. So I lived a good life. I've been blessed. I've lived a good life and I've enjoyed it and I still enjoy it.

Following "the trauma" of three heart attacks compounded by "a few handicaps," including diabetes, poor circulation, and swelling in his legs, Mr. Ellis entered Oak Manor at the age of 82. He looked for "assisted living quarters" in Ohio but "leaned away from it" when he found that the upscale facilities located in his community were predominately white. He decided to relocate to Oak Manor after visiting his grandsons who lived in Atlanta. Oak Manor, "a black facility" near his family, provides "beautiful surroundings, quality service," and an opportunity to interact with his African American "peers."

Thomas "Boss" Cook of Greene's Personal Care Home

Like Eugene Ellis, Thomas Cook ("Boss" to his friends and acquaintances) grew up in a working-class family in Ohio, but Boss had only a high school education and lived in poverty much of his adult life. Previously employed in menial labor and disabled by a stroke at age 50, he receives a monthly Social Security income of only $673.

Boss admits that his colorful past, "running in the street," has probably contributed to his poor health. Though he still considers himself "a ladies' man," he recognizes the changes time and hard living have brought: "When I was younger, I was real wild, tall and skinny. I had a lot of girlfriends, more than I can count on my fingers. Now I'm old and tore up and crippled, crazy, and everything else. I don't get out in the street now, you know. Well, it's a lot of things that I'm not doing, like maybe going to a nightclub or to a dance in the evening. I miss dancing. I miss going to the clubs, meeting all the girls."

Boss was born in Cleveland in 1939, the youngest of five children. At the age of 17, he married his 16-year-old sweetheart. They had two children but divorced before Boss turned twenty. Soon after that, Boss moved to Atlanta in search of work. Until then, he had "never known race issues." He described the world that he encountered: "[White people] picketed the counters in the cafes and things like that and didn't allow black [people] to drink out the water fountains. Like the water had 'colored' and 'white' on it, you know, so [race] was kinda a issue." Finding that being African American limited his employment opportunities, Boss did "cleaning work" at a country club.

Over the years, Boss lived with assorted female companions in various apartments, mostly located in low-income African American neighborhoods in southeast Atlanta. Boss, "a fun guy," involved himself in the area's active street culture, which included "the girls on the street," a street preacher named Earl, and his fictive "cousin," Junior, who, among other odd jobs, helped operate a neighborhood "chop shop" that dealt in stolen automobile parts.

When we met Boss at age 60, he had lived at Greene's for 10 years. In addition to partial paralysis from his stroke, he is limited by obesity, hypertension, and poor vision. Like Miss Fannie, Boss has no family support and was placed in Greene's by a social worker at County Hospital. Despite his lifestyle change, Boss is "still happy" and views Greene's as his best option: "I don't believe I can live no better."

Cleo Kellog of Rosie's Loving Care

Cleo Kellog, like almost a third of the residents (28%)* living in the smaller homes, has mental illness. Assessments of her cognitive functioning differ. Although Ms. Kellog has been diagnosed by physicians as paranoid schizophrenic, Rosie Samuels, the owner of Rosie's Loving Care, describes her as "retarded, [with the mind] of about a six-year-old child." Despite her high blood pressure, Ms. Kellog functions well physically.

Ms. Kellog receives Supplemental Security Income and is enrolled in the Community Care Services Program, Georgia's Medicaid waiver program. She

---

*As indicated in chapter 2, this percentage does not include mentally ill residents who resided at Sunshine House.

moved to Rosie's from another small assisted living facility (ALF) in 1997, at the age of 73. This move, facilitated by a Community Care Services Program caseworker, left Ms. Kellog feeling "blessed" because "the Lord took [me] away" from the other home, where the provider was "mean" and "it was lonesome." Living at Rosie's, in contrast, is "just like being at home," and Ms. Kellog finds solace in the kind attention provided by Rosie, whom she affectionately refers to as "Mama."

Although Ms. Kellog enjoys recounting her past, her mental illness interferes with her ability to recall certain facts, leaving gaps in her life story. Like Miss Fannie, she grew up in "a great big family" in rural Georgia. She cannot remember how much schooling she had but rues her illiteracy, which prevents her from reading the Bible.

In the 1940s, when in her early 20s, Ms. Kellog left her family farm and moved to New York City's Bronx area. How she got to New York or supported herself there is a mystery. Her most vivid memories are of Harlem club life and venturing out in "high-heeled shoes with hair curled" to see entertainment legends including Duke Ellington, Ella Fitzgerald, and Cab Calloway. Ms. Kellog revels in remembering this exciting era of her life, though painful memories of a boyfriend's physical abuse taint her recollections.

Ms. Kellog never married, and after leaving New York she spent some time in Iowa and South Dakota, where she lived with a close female friend. Eventually, because of physical problems requiring surgery, she moved to Atlanta, where she has "people" (an extended family that includes three nieces and their families). Although Ms. Kellog speaks proudly of her "big family," she rarely sees anyone and is grateful for Rosie, her new "Mama," who helps fill this void: "I am blessed. Mama takes care of me. I mean her and Jesus."

Recurrent Themes in African American Life Histories

The life histories of these five residents set the stage for a detailed examination of the social, economic, and cultural contexts surrounding their transitions into assisted living. Guided by life course theory, we use these stories and those of other participants to explore how particular life events and experiences have influenced residents' needs for care, their choice of assisted living, and their adaptation processes.

The life course perspective provides a useful framework for considering ways in which social forces, such as policies and social institutions, influence individuals' life experiences, including the movement through social roles and statuses over time (Settersten, 1999). According to this approach, life transitions, such as moves to assisted living, are viewed as part of an entire life process rather than as isolated life stages. A major focus is on how individuals adapt to changes in their lives based on knowledge gained from past experience and the use of personal resources (Clausen, 1986; Holstein & Gubrium, 2000).

Despite a lifelong struggle against racial oppression, common themes in residents' life stories include a sense of pride in their own lives, their families, their communities, and their race. African American community life (which includes residents' involvement in African American churches, schools, social clubs, and community organizations) and residents' families are key sources of these resiliency-promoting values. Some residents, such as Boss, developed their social networks "on the street." Often, these alternative settings became communities in their own right and served the same functions for marginal citizens as more traditional settings do for the mainstream.

Families: "They Were Able to Shore Us Up"

Coping with stressful life events, including those related to racial discrimination, requires great personal strength. For many of the residents, families were an important source of this strength. Alma Burgess recalled how her parents prepared her for the obstacles she would face as an African American living in the Jim Crow South: "I hear people talk about, you know, self-worth. I guess I had a superiority complex rather than an inferiority complex. But you'll have to understand, too, about black parents in the South, where they had such segregation. My parents went out of their way to see to it that we got certain advantages that compensated for being excluded. I've always said the one traumatic experience of black children was being told you were not acceptable or you were not as good, and that's a traumatic thing. It can make or break you. I was very glad that my parents were able to shore us up. I never felt other than I was a good person, a well-thinking person, and a person who mattered." In addition to self-esteem, other strengths instilled within the family included racial pride, close family and community ties, religious values, respect for hard work, and a focus on self-reliance.

Families also fostered the value for education. Growing up in a racist society, Alma Burgess and Eugene Ellis, among other residents, learned at an early age that education was critical to their economic security and social mobility. Without an education, African Americans had few employment options outside of domestic or menial labor. Alma Burgess summarized a common sentiment held by college-educated participants: "Blacks who accomplished anything at that time had to be better [surpass the standards set for whites]."

Despite racism, several residents excelled as scholars, professionals, and community leaders. Some even broke the "color barrier" in their fields. Calvert Hughes was the first African American to work as an electrician for the Pentagon, and Hattie Houseworth the first African American chemist employed by the federal government. Several residents, including Hattie Houseworth, credit their families for "always pushing" them to achieve.

Communities: "Black Meccas"

Close-knit communities often reinforced values learned at home. In areas of cities and towns where whites allowed them to settle, African Americans frequently established their own institutions and businesses. African Americans thereby minimized their interaction with whites and used these segregated spaces to build collective unity and resist oppression (Dorsey, 2004).

Atlanta, a previous home to most (81%) residents, boasts a rich chronicle of African American community life dating back more than 140 years. Beginning in the 1860s, many freed slaves moved to Atlanta. Restricted from settling within the city's core, they established neighborhoods in the southwest, southeast, and northwest quadrants of Atlanta, interspersed between white communities (Clarke, 1996). Often the races shared opposite ends of the same street, which typically bore different names denoting the "color line" (Barnes, 1985). In the late 1940s, many formerly all-white neighborhoods began the transition to African American as middle-class whites left the inner city. With this "white flight," living conditions steadily declined in black communities; Reynoldstown, where Miss Fannie settled, and Summerhill, where she worked, became poor and crime ridden. The urban renewal projects initiated during this period, including construction of new expressways to provide white residents of the North Side with easier access to downtown, exacerbated these conditions by pushing out existing African American businesses and contributing to overcrowding in residential areas (Harmon, 1996).

One of the best known of Atlanta's traditionally African American neighborhoods is the Sweet Auburn District, the birthplace of Martin Luther King

Jr. and a hub of the 1960s civil rights movement.* Many scholars consider the Sweet Auburn community one of the most significant centers of African American economic, social, and political development of the early twentieth century, alongside Harlem and Durham, North Carolina. By the 1920s, Sweet Auburn boasted more than 120 African American–owned businesses, including small businesses, restaurants, hotels, financial institutions, and several popular entertainment venues (Clarke, 1996). The Citizen's Trust Company Bank, which opened in 1925, was the first African American bank to affiliate with the Federal Reserve System. This bank financed most of the business operations in the Sweet Auburn District and also provided home loans for African American families, who undoubtedly would have been denied financing by white institutions (Harmon, 1996). The Sweet Auburn area, where several residents grew up and some worked, also was the site of the first African American church in Atlanta[†] and the first African American newspaper in the United States. Greene's resident Edgar Allgood, who once operated a shoe store in the area, often recounts his youthful experiences as a radio announcer at Sweet Auburn's WERD, the nation's first African American radio station. This historic community, like Reynoldstown and Summerhill, declined following the civil rights movement.

The Sweet Auburn District provided the focal point for African American community life in southeast Atlanta, while the Atlanta University District, a prestigious consortium of five historically black colleges,[‡] did so in the city's southwest quadrant. Many African American professionals, including business leaders and university faculty like Alma Burgess's father, settled near the college campuses. As living conditions in other inner-city areas deteriorated during the 1960s, more middle-class African Americans moved into this area,

---

*The larger residential area that encompasses the Sweet Auburn District is referred to as the Old Fourth Ward. During the first decades of the twentieth century, this area became predominately African American, as middle-class blacks settled to the east of the growing Auburn Business District and in the area where Georgia Baptist Hospital presently stands.

[†]The Big Bethel AME (African Methodist Episcopal) Church was founded on Auburn Avenue in 1865. It was the first established African American church building in Atlanta. During this era, many worshipers held services in makeshift tabernacles. Friendship Baptist Church, for example, initially held services in an abandoned boxcar (Clarke, 1996).

[‡]In 1929 three of Atlanta's historically black colleges (Atlanta University, Spelman, and Morehouse) affiliated to become known collectively as the Atlanta University System. As a result of this affiliation, Atlanta University had to relocate near the other two schools. That year, Morris Brown College also relocated to the Atlanta University District, followed by Clark College in 1941. These five institutions eventually reached a formal agreement of cooperation in 1957 (Cohen, 2000).

often referred to as the West End. No longer restricted to streets proximal to the Atlanta University District, many newcomers settled in heretofore all-white areas in southwest Atlanta or newly opened subdivisions farther out (Barnes, 1985; Harmon, 1996). Elsie Joiner, a resident of Oak Manor and a former school teacher, who grew up in Pittsburgh, a working-class neighborhood adjacent to Summerhill, spoke with pride about her ability to retire in the prestigious area near Clark College, her college alma mater: "Well, when I retired, I lived near Hunter and Ashby [Streets]. You know, that was the black mecca at that particular time. The nicer families tended to live in that section."*

Although African Americans from lower-income groups also occupied the West End, many areas became predominately middle to upper-middle class. Elsie Joiner settled there, and other residential areas, such as Mozely Park, which was opened to blacks in 1949, beckoned to other upwardly mobile African Americans. As economic conditions gradually improved for certain segments of the African American population, these middle-class residential areas expanded, and class distinctions within African American communities became more pronounced (Barnes, 1985; Harmon, 1996).

When referring to their former homes and communities, many middle- and upper-middle-class residents, including some who moved from areas outside Georgia, proudly noted the economic gains they had made during their lives. Eugene Ellis told us that his education and status as "a successful professional black man" enabled him to move from a low-income slum area into "the big house on the hill." Similarly, Malcolm Harding, a retired lawyer who considers himself a member of the Atlanta "black elite," recalled that he relocated from "the ghetto in northeast Atlanta" to the West End, where he set up a successful law practice.†

Regardless of where residents lived, lasting, close-knit relationships emerge as recurring themes in their stories about community life. Mr. Harding's words

---

*When Elsie Joiner and other residents attended Clark College, the institution was located in south Atlanta.

†Mr. Harding grew up in a middle-class enclave in the Old Fourth Ward area. Interspersed within that area were low-income African Americans, and adjacent to it were low-income white areas, including Cabbagetown, a community of millworkers. Another middle-class resident who also grew up in the Old Fourth Ward described the neighborhood as "rough." Fashionable middle- to upper-middle-class African American neighborhoods that developed on the west side stood in stark contrast to the "middle-class" neighborhoods that some residents remembered living in as children.

illustrated a common pattern: "I knew all the people in the neighborhood. I played with 'em, I grew up with 'em. So I know those people." In many cases, these close relationships continued as residents moved into ALFs and reacquainted themselves with old friends from their communities.

Religion: "Raised Up in the Church"

African American churches often serve as the primary center of group activity within communities. Indeed, many residents frame their life experiences within the context of "being raised up" or "reared up" in the church. The various denominational churches attended by our residents ranged from small one-room buildings, such as "the little small church" that Miss Fannie attended as a child, to elaborate structures, such as Wheat Street Baptist Church on Auburn Avenue, where Mr. Harding kept his membership. Some churches were not housed within any building. Boss Cook, for example, attended services conducted by a street preacher that were held at various locations, including people's backyards: "We go somewhere in the country and have meetings, church meetings, have revivals at certain places at certain times of the week."

Some residents and their families had connections to churches that extended back several generations. Carole Seymour, a 60-year-old resident of Rosie's, recalled her long-standing connection to Wheat Street Baptist Church: "I was born and raised at Wheat Street Church. Yeah, born and raised at Wheat Street. All my ancestors, my grandmother and them, joined Wheat Street back in 1800-something."

Class stratified churches as it did residential areas. One resident's family member described how social status affected where some residents worshiped: "Back in the day, there was some strict class and social division in blacks. There is a church in Atlanta, I don't know if you've ever heard about, it's around the corner from here. It attracted the cream of the crop in the black community. In addition to that, there was another church whereabouts the same thing occurred for years and years and years. If you weren't a member of the elite, don't come to our church." Besides location, another feature that distinguished churches by class was the level of emotionalism manifested during religious services, generally inversely related to the socioeconomic status of the congregation (Barnes, 1985; Dorsey, 2004). Carole Seymour, whose church boasted a large middle-class membership, described her aversion to certain forms of gospel music: "We were brought up to sing songs that have meaning. We sing gospel songs in our choir, but they're not the ooh-ah and all that hollering."

Many residents' weekly schedules had been structured around church activities. Alma Burgess recalled that church attendance was stressed in her home and later at college and describes her (mandatory) commitment to these activities: "As little children, we understood that we had to go to church. Growing up, we had to go to church. We went to Sunday school on Sunday; we went to church on Sunday, the church service and then we went to Upward League or whatever you called the various and the different churches on Sunday afternoon. We *stayed* in church on Sunday! When I went to college, Sunday vespers were compulsory, Sunday school was compulsory, prayer meeting on Wednesday night was compulsory. Everything, where religion was concerned, it was compulsory." Even families, such as Miss Fannie's, who could spare little time off from work devoted Sunday to church: "I was raised up in the church. Mama carried us to church when we was little bitty things 'bout that high. We went to church every Sunday and went to Sunday school every Sunday. We didn't miss that."

For many residents, being active in the church included participating in the choir, youth groups, and social clubs and holding church offices. Some residents indicated that church attendance and membership were important for maintaining respectable status in the community. For example, Viola Wheeler, a resident at Peach Blossom, believes that her status as a teacher and role model necessitated church participation: "I always thought it was very important that we take a part into church life in the community, because we will be working with students in the community in which we were teaching." Furthermore, church membership often linked members of the same denomination within a nationwide network. Although unwelcome in most hotels, Ms. Burgess and her family found themselves welcomed into the homes of fellow members of the CME (Christian Methodist Episcopal) Church during their travels across the country.

In addition to providing spiritual and social activities, churches and religious organizations aided communities by raising funds for college scholarships and charities. Faced with a total lack of governmental support, African American communities depended heavily on these religious institutions. Carole Seymour, for example, could not have attended college without her scholarship from Wheat Street Baptist Church. Miss Fannie recalled that a religious society to which her family belonged provided a safety net when community members became ill or died without money for burial: "The Home Missions Society, they help you along when you're sick. Then, when you die, they help bury you. [My family] didn't put no whole lot of money in there 'cause they didn't have no whole lot of money. Just like 25 cents a month, something like that."

Looking back, many residents deem their church membership and participation as key to their satisfactory, indeed successful, lives. George Kelner, a 68-year-old resident of Greene's, expressed a common feeling: "Well, being a member of my church over close to 40 years, I've enjoyed that more than I do anything else." In many cases, this religious training provides a source of strength for residents as they age. Frankie Johnson, a resident whose 13 children placed, then abandoned, her at Greene's, said, "The good Lord is taking care of me. I don't depend on my children to take care of me." Faith in God motivates Beatrice Dove, a fellow Greene's resident, to face each day: "I just try to live for the Lord."

Schools: "They Got Us Ready for the Real World— The White World"

Like families, communities, and churches, African American schools helped "raise up" African American children by providing them with the skills they would need to survive in white-dominated mainstream society. Malcolm Harding recalled how, despite low pay and armed only with inferior books and supplies, "dedicated" African American teachers contributed to the advancement of African American children during the Jim Crow years: "At that time, the black teachers, females, were making $199 dollars a year. Black male teachers were making $200. They were making one dollar more than the female. That was supposed to be a big deal. And these teachers had to carpool all the way across town. They would ride six in a car. And those were some of the most dedicated people I've ever met in my life, because they got us ready for the real world—the white world. We got our books from Boys High, Tech High, and Girls High [white schools]. Pages would be torn out of the books. The cover would be torn off the books."

Most African American residents, however, were denied an adequate education. Although 84% of the residents at Oak Manor hold college degrees, only 9% of residents living in the smaller homes graduated from college. Almost half (46%) of these residents did not finish high school, and 24% had only an elementary school education.

Like Miss Fannie and Cleo Kellog, many of the residents living in the smaller homes grew up in the rural South. Because their families needed their help to earn a living, most children in low-income farm communities spent their time laboring in the fields instead of in the classroom. Even those children who attended school seldom went beyond the elementary level.

Like other southern states, Georgia practiced strict segregation and provided little funding for black schools. Booker T. Washington High School, the first public high school for African Americans in Georgia, did not open until 1924. Until 1947, this school, established near the Atlanta University Center, was the only African American high school in Georgia. Before 1924, African Americans who wanted to attend high school paid tuition to attend private classes conducted in colleges at the Atlanta University Center. Several residents at Oak Manor attended Washington High School, which educated many prominent Atlanta citizens, including Martin Luther King Jr. A few residents, including Alma Burgess and Malcolm Harding, whose parents could afford the tuition attended classes at the Atlanta University Center. Mr. Harding described the typical educational pathway that many middle- to upper-middle-class African American Atlantans followed during legal segregation: "At that particular time, because of racism, segregation, institutional racism, you started off at Spelman's nursery. You left Spelman's nursery and you went to Oglethorpe Elementary School, which was the elementary school within the AU [Atlanta University] Center. You left Oglethorpe Elementary School and you went to Laboratory High. After Laboratory High you had a choice of branching to Morehouse, Spelman, Morris Brown, or Clark [all historically black colleges]. If you wanted to stay in the city, you could get a master's at AU."

Some residents, such as Eugene Ellis, attended schools outside Georgia, but most college-educated residents hail from Atlanta's black colleges. While providing training in the customary fields of teaching and ministry, these schools, which boasted a distinguished list of alumni, including W. E. B. DuBois, Henry O. Tanner, and Martin Luther King Jr., offered additional courses in the arts, sciences, business, and law. Mr. Harding accurately described the caliber of education that these schools provided during his student days and even now: "That system of education was the best that [the African American community] had to offer. In fact, if you came through the AU system, you could hold your own with anybody, black or white, anywhere."

As a result of having received good educations, a number of residents became successful professionals. Many became educators. Some achieved other professional status, as judge, physician, or college dean. Like having a college degree, status as a professional provides a source of pride for residents, some of whom described themselves as members of the "black elite" or as "successful professional black[s]." To complement that professional standing, some of these residents couched their identities in terms of college affiliation, describing themselves as a "Morehouse man" or a "Spelmanite."

Social Clubs and Community Organizations: "A Legacy" of Commitment

Many African American residents who had been able to go to college joined sororities or fraternities. Membership in these Greek social organizations often engendered lifelong friendships. Perhaps more important, residents gained an ongoing sense of pride in themselves and their new places in society. As members of these exclusive clubs, they became part of a nationwide constituency of African American scholars and professionals. Ms. Burgess, herself a sorority sister, recalled that her childhood association with her father's fraternity brothers contributed to her own personal growth and development. Her interaction with those "men who had accomplished and made a difference in society" inspired her to reach for, and achieve, her own goals.

Many residents, including Eugene Ellis and Alma Burgess, have stayed active over the years as alumni in these Greek social clubs. Mr. Ellis described his fraternity brothers as "extensions of family" and explained how his status as a fraternity member opened doors even after his move to Oak Manor: "Fraternity brothers learn that I'm a Kappa and they want to strike up a conversation. They come from all parts of the country to visit their own friends [fellow members]. One of the school principals here in one of the school districts happens to be from Ohio, happens to be from Wilberforce, and happens to be a Kappa. He came to visit."

In addition to Greek social clubs, many college-educated residents joined academic clubs, college alumnus groups, and professional organizations, such as teaching associations. For example, Julia Shields became a lifelong charter member of a nursing sorority soon after earning her nursing license. Some residents, like Ms. Burgess, who helped start a local chapter of the Jack and Jill Club, have stayed active in charitable groups and civic organizations.

Like other community factors we have discussed, membership in these groups bolster residents' positive self-image and promote racial pride. As residents age, they continue to value these associations, and their lifelong commitments demonstrate the crucial role these groups play in driving residents to define and fulfill their successful roles in society.

The Effects of Racism and Poverty over the Life Course

Despite the concerted efforts by African American families and communities to protect their youth from the ill effects of racism, all elderly African American residents, even members of the middle and upper-middle class, show evidence of racism's cumulative effects. For these residents, health status and retirement income are the most visible results of that lifelong oppression.

Lack of quality education and discrimination in employment hindered residents' chances for occupational mobility. Even those who had been able to acquire a college education found their career choices were narrowly defined, especially women. Usual career paths included teaching, nursing, social work, and clerical work. Of residents who went to college, 94% chose careers as educators. Some achieved master's and doctoral-level degrees. Although highly revered in their communities, professional status did not relieve residents from the economic effects of segregation. Salaries of African American professionals, like those of the African American population in general, were considerably lower than those of whites. Some residents (including Eugene Ellis, who accumulated his wealth through investments) enjoy substantial retirement incomes. Many college-educated participants, however, lack the financial security usually commensurate with their professional positions. This lack of funds affects residents' ability to stay in ALFs and to purchase services while there. Poor and uneducated residents who lack family support face even more limited choices. Having been relegated to lifetimes of low-paying work, often in jobs without Social Security benefits, many of these residents pay for their long-term care largely with Supplemental Security Income. Their poverty has defined not only their addresses but also their ability to satisfy care needs.

Independent of socioeconomic status, their race put all African American residents at high risk for chronic disease and disability, especially diabetes, heart disease, and high blood pressure (Gornick et al., 1996; U.S. Department of Health and Human Services, 2001). Most middle- and upper-middle-class residents had access to adequate health care as elders, but discrimination over the life course has left many with a legacy of poor health. In Atlanta, for example, most residents' only health care option as children and young adults was the understaffed public clinics at County Hospital, the city's only hospital serving African American clients. Mr. Harding recalls that it was not uncommon for County patients to wait an entire day before being seen. Many poor and uneducated residents, like Miss Fannie, never received adequate health care and suffered the consequences of poor nutrition throughout their lives. The risks of poor health were intensified for those residents. Lack of education, for example, increased the risks of cognitive impairment, and their low economic status added to the likelihood of mental illness. Independent of race, individuals in the lowest stratum of education, occupation, and income have been found to be two to three times more likely to suffer a mental disorder than individuals in the highest stratum (U.S. Department of Health and Human Services, 2001).

The Impact of Mental Illness

A large percentage of residents living in the small homes, like Cleo Kellog, have some form of mental illness.* Seven of the 12 residents in this category are white, and all live at Greene's. It is unclear from Ms. Kellog's case history when she was diagnosed with schizophrenia. No evidence exists that she ever spent time in a mental hospital or psychiatric treatment center; perhaps she received that diagnosis late in life. Persons she encountered over her lifetime, like Rosie, may have dismissed her cognitive impairment as "simplemindedness." Most mentally ill residents, in contrast, have long histories of treatment for their disease, often including frequent hospitalizations. Rosie's resident Sarah Eubanks has a history of mental illness spanning 48 years.

Other common themes in the life stories of residents with mental illness include dysfunctional and nonsupportive family relationships (including abuse in one case), homelessness, and histories of assisted living residence. Lack of family support often reflects the absence of close kin. Only 4 of the 12 mentally ill residents have been married or have children. Two of these are estranged from their immediate families. Even Ms. Eubanks, with her large network of supportive kin, has a history of family dysfunction. Judith, her youngest daughter, observed that her mother's absence during her childhood because

---

*A small number (4) of residents living in the small homes had developmental disabilities, including mental retardation, Down syndrome, and multiple sclerosis. Because they represent a small proportion of the resident population, we do not profile them in this chapter but discuss their experiences in later chapters as applicable.

of institutionalization affected their adult relationship: "I have only a couple of memories of her from when I was in kindergarten, but that's all. For some years, I had no mother, basically. I remember going to first grade and my teacher asking me who combed my hair, and I'd say, 'My big sister.' . . . We were raised by our stepmother. So, it gets a little complicated sometimes because I don't get caught up in the emotions." Although still involved in her mother's care, Judith admitted, "It's been real hard for me to deal with mental health kinds of issues and stuff." She recalled one of the times when her mother was hospitalized with severe depression: "I saw her go from being able to do everything [for herself] to being so low that they had her in diapers. She couldn't chew the food in her mouth, she couldn't feed herself, she couldn't do anything."

In some cases, drug abuse (either by the resident or family members) contributes to family dysfunction. One case involved drug and sexual abuse. As a young adult, Half-Pint, a 57-year-old African American resident of Greene's, was sexually abused by her father and an older brother, both of whom were addicted to drugs.

Half (6) of the mentally ill residents have lived in other ALFs. Of this group, Ms. Kellog is the only female and the only elderly African American. The other five are white males, three of whom have been homeless. These five Greene's residents are able to go out into the community independently, and they spend considerable time out of the home. Their extensive social networks include friends from their mental health programs, former ALFs, and street living. Burt Hatfield often spends time in a local park with homeless people he knows from his street days. In the absence of family, these tight-knit and often lasting relationships provide an important source of socioemotional support.

Similar to the African American residents who derive a sense of pride and identity from their participation in various social clubs and community organizations, all five of these white residents have gained considerable rewards from their participation in mental health programs over the years. In addition to pride and identity, these programs have fostered lasting relationships and provided grounding and a sense of normalcy for social misfits locked out of mainstream society.

Occasionally, when mentally ill residents venture out of their protective enclaves (the ALF, the mental health community, and "the street"), they are ill equipped to cope with the demands of mainstream culture. Edward Fitzsimmons's sister's attempts to include her brother in family holiday parties over-whelmed him so severely that he once fled the scene: "He would listen to my other brothers talk about their jobs, their cars, their this, their that," she re-called. "He would feel like he had to join in, and I think it just made him feel bad. It would increase his paranoia, and he would tell 'em about *his* jobs. One time, he walked out of my house in the suburbs—we couldn't catch him—with no money in his pockets. I have no idea how he got back to town. There's no buses out there." Like elderly African American residents, these white men with mental illness find themselves alienated from the dominant culture. Some residents, like Cleo Kellog, endure the double stigma—and disadvan-tage—of being both African American and mentally ill in a society that is pre-pared to accept neither.

Building Strength and Community in Assisted Living

These disenfranchised groups place considerable importance on their com-munities. Included in our definition of "community" are families and signif-icant others (Jesus for Cleo Kellog and homeless guys for Burt Hatfield) who help make up residents' social worlds. Bolstered (or "raised up") by their com-munities, residents gain strength to triumph over adversity. They reciprocate by helping to build community within their neighborhoods, churches, schools, social clubs, and "on the street." These concepts of community and commu-nity-building are important throughout the rest of the book as we examine how individuals adapt to their new lives and find meaning as assisted living residents. Harnessing resources developed over time, many residents have sought, and often found, meaning within their new roles as residents of ALFs. They have adapted to life there not as some isolated incident but as a part of their ongoing life stories.

A broad literature documents the individual and collective strengths that African Americans possess and exercise to resist oppression and succeed in so-ciety despite enormous odds (Hatchett & Jackson, 1993; Hill, 1999; Milburn & Bowman, 1991; Stack, 1974). In addition to cultural strengths passed down through generations, the importance of community is a recurring theme in this literature. Our findings show that other oppressed groups, such as men-tally ill individuals, also may gain strength from involvement in community life, including that developed inside an ALF. These findings have led us to adopt a strengths-based approach throughout our book. The strengths-based approach, an important trend in the study of at-risk populations, seeks to promote the successful (as opposed to pathological) aspects of aging and human development. We identify major problems and challenges faced by our residents. Yet we recognize, and praise, the tenacity of our residents in facing life's challenges. By focusing on the positive, we promote a positive image of this often marginalized population and identify important strengths at societal, community, and individual levels that can be drawn upon to enhance the assisted living environment. In the following chapter, our story of residents' transitions into assisted living begins with an in-depth examination of situations surrounding residents' decisions to move into the six unique care environments that make up this study.

CHAPTER 4

Moving to Assisted Living

Ethyl Burns, recalling her decision to move to Oak Manor, told us, "I won't say I wouldn't rather be in my own home, but I was going to be somewhere, because I found out I could no longer live by myself. I knew that I was in no condition and never would be. I faced facts." Her words reflect the sentiments and situations of many of the residents in these six communities. Ideally, she would have "aged in place" in the Atlanta home she had lived in her entire married life. Her deceased husband, an architect, had designed the home, which was across the street from the high school where she had been both student and teacher. But Ms. Burns's health and neighborhood both were declining, and when the nephew she helped raise "started talking about 'you don't need to be by yourself,'" she knew the time to move had come.

This chapter tells the story of moving to assisted living, beginning with how decisions to enter a home are made and ending with how residents settle into their new communities. How the moving process evolves for each resident has important consequences for the individual and for other members of the community. Multiple factors determine residents' unique pathways into assisted living, including where they lived before moving, the type of care they need, their resources for obtaining care, who makes the decision, and their options for moving. The following cases reflect the complexity of typical pathways.

Typical Pathways

Elsie Joiner of Oak Manor: "Nobody Was Pushing Me"

Elsie Joiner, at the age of 79, decided to leave her home, where she lived alone, and move to Oak Manor. She reached this decision gradually and rationally, considering not one but a combination of factors. First, she was lonely. She had wanted one of her three children to move in with her, but they "had their own households" and "didn't care to move back home." Although it had been more than 20 years since Ms. Joiner had divorced her husband and her last child had left home for good, she now was tied more to home owing to increasing symptoms from Parkinson disease, which left her unable to drive. In addition, she could no longer keep house in a way that met her standards: "I had gotten to the place where things needed to be done, and I wasn't able to do them. I couldn't keep my mind on 'em long enough to do them, and I didn't feel up to having someone come in to clean for me when I was there, you know, all day long. You see, I was from the old school. My mother, during the seasonal times of the year, would wash those curtains and wash the windows. My windows hadn't been washed in I don't know when. My draperies hadn't been cleaned. I was accustomed to doing all of those things, and I couldn't do them anymore, and it worried me."

Ms. Joiner, in fact, had always been a worrier, a trait that contributed to her inability to hold on in her current environment, given her declining health. So in November, soon after Oak Manor opened its doors, she made a deposit to hold a room, waiting until after Christmas, to allow her to prepare one more holiday meal, before leaving home. Her three children supported her decision to move, but, as she said, "It wasn't anything that nobody was pushing me. I wasn't the type that could be pushed anyway. Nobody tells me what to do or not do." She made this life-changing decision reluctantly but on her own terms.

Ethyl Burns of Oak Manor: "He's the Reason I Came So Fast"

As living alone became increasingly difficult, at the age of 84 Ethyl Burns had begun to think about doing "something," but she had not reached the point of moving. She described her early thoughts: "I had been ill. I just wasn't able to do anything much, and, by now, I had no family, I mean, no family that could come and be with me, and I was trying to decide what I was going to do." It was her nephew, Everett, who initiated the moving process. Everett lived in Alabama, and he worried about his aunt not getting enough to eat and living alone in a neighborhood with increasing crime. He even asked her friend Opal to bring her meals and help convince her to move. Ms. Burns recalled:

[Opal] did start mentioning to me that "maybe you need to find somewhere to go," and I said, "Why should I leave my home?" You know how stubborn we can get. But anyway, Everett came up one weekend, and he didn't say anything to me about talking to her, but when he got back to, I think he was living in Birmingham by this time, he called me, and said, "I went out to Oak Manor when I was there on the weekend." And I said, "Oak who?" I'd never heard of it. And he said, "Oak Manor. It's an assisted living place, and I think you would like it, and I think it's just the place for you." And I said, "Well, I'll think about it once I've seen it, you know." I didn't know a thing about it. So he called the next weekend, and he couldn't make it up here, but he said, "I'm thinking, Sylvia"—that's his wife—"will be in Atlanta over the weekend, and she's going to take you out to Oak Manor. I just want you to see it. I know you'll like it. I just can't stand to see you there by yourself." Now that's the way he put it, that was it. I said, "OK" 'cause usually I do almost anything he says.

Ms. Burns liked what she saw at Oak Manor and even found she already knew some of the longtime Atlantans who were residents, but it was because of her love for Everett that she "went so fast":

Really, the reason I had decided that I was going to leave was because I did not wish to interfere with Everett and Sylvia's lives. I said, "Well, now he's worried, and he's going to get on Sylvia to move to Atlanta." And I didn't mind her moving to Atlanta, but I didn't want her to move to Atlanta because of me. I didn't want to move into a house with them. I never believed in that, you know, moving in with a young married couple. And I didn't think they'd be satisfied in my house, 'cause it's not their kind of style of a house. So, he's the reason I came so fast. I don't have any regrets. My hope is that as long as I'm living, I will not have to do anything that will hurt Everett. And I have to tell you the truth, if somebody else had brought that idea to me, I probably would still be thinking of it.

Lily Porter of Blue Skies: "I Don't Have the Money or Time Now" (Lily's Daughter)

Lily Porter had hoped to escape her two greatest fears—living alone in a high-rise where "someone would find me dead" or "just kind of dwindl[ing] away" in a nursing home where "no one cared about me." Her first choice was to remain in her daughter Sharon's home. Lily had left her own home in Cleveland less than a year earlier to move with Sharon to Georgia after a stroke left her wheelchair bound and no longer able to care for herself. Sharon was the youngest of her four daughters and, as Lily said, "the only one who stuck by me." But Lily's care had become overwhelming. Sharon described her struggle: "I asked for help from my sisters and brothers. Everyone either ignored me or said they couldn't afford it. They couldn't give me anything to help out. For six months, I was trying to work a part-time job and care for her, so there were periods of time when I would leave her at home, you know, watching TV. I had to fix her meal, and it had to be a cold meal for lunch, like a sandwich or something, and leave it where she could get it, and then I would fix a hot meal in the evening."

In the end, Sharon had to break the news to Lily that she no longer could keep her at home: "I'm going to have to find a place for you to be, because I don't have the money or time now. I can't find any state assistance to help me while you're in the house, so that's our only choice." Sharon visited three family model homes and picked Blue Skies because it best met her mother's needs. Although neither Lily nor Sharon was happy about the decision, Blue Skies seemed more homelike and was "not a nursing home." "When I walked into Blue Skies," Sharon recalled, "it had a feeling of home. My mother was a collector who had a lot of stuff all over her house, just like Clarice [the owner] does, and I said, 'This is the place.'"

Harold Stamps of Rosie's Loving Care: "I Was Getting Very, Very, Very Tired" (Harold's Daughter)

At the age of 95, Harold Stamps was in good physical health, but because of the progression of his Alzheimer disease he was no longer able to manage even his basic needs. By the time he moved to Rosie's Loving Care, he needed help with bathing, dressing, and toileting. His daughter Lola, unlike Lily's daughter Sharon, had other family members to help care for her father, but still the burden was more than she could handle:

> He was by himself for a long time, but then we found out that he no longer could stay by himself. My sister-in-law, my husband's sister, stayed with him from 11 to 7 every night. My daughter was with him during the day. My sister-in-law Mavis came in to help out when Daisy needed to rest. Then I was there for the weekend. So it was killing me. I mean, every weekend. Then there was Daddy going to the bathroom. He went at two and four, and I'm on the sofa and I'm hearing Daddy getting up. I said, "Daddy, use the pot. Don't try to walk in the bathroom." "Oh, no, oh, no, I can make it." Halfway down the hall, I hear the urine coming down, and I'm saying, "Oh my God, he didn't make it." I get up, change his pajamas, mop, get back on the couch, and four o'clock this whole thing starts all over again, and I was getting very, very, very tired.

Lola had wanted her father to stay in his own apartment, but his care, on top of her full-time job as a nanny, had worn her down. When she saw her friend Rosie Samuels at a church banquet one night, she asked about placing her father in her home: "I said, 'Rosie, do you have a space?' She said, 'Who is it for?' I said, 'My daddy.' She said, 'Oh, I'll make a space for him,' and I felt so much better. So, I called her later, and in about, I bet it was less than two weeks, we had placed him. But I never wanted him to go into a nursing home. Not that I feel that those people are neglected or anything, but I just felt better that he was with somebody that he knew, and I knew that it would be better on all of us."

Burt Hatfield of Greene's: "It's Better Than Outdoors"

Burt Hatfield's pathway to assisted living (AL) began in his youth. Burt had been a troubled, drug-addicted boy who moved out of his mother's house as a teenager. He migrated to Texas, Florida, and then back to Atlanta, where his life became a series of moves in and out of homeless shelters and small assisted living homes, interspersed with street living. In addition to ongoing problems with alcoholism, Burt has schizophrenia. The move to Greene's—from an assisted living facility (ALF) where he had lived for 12 years—was the result of the home's closure by the state agency that regulates assisted living. Now, at the age of 40, Burt defines Greene's as home: "Home to me means you got something free to yourself. You got a bed and you got wood around you. You're warm, you got your clothes. It's better than outdoors. I been outdoors." Although estranged from his mother in his earlier life, in recent years they have become closer, and it was she who helped him find Greene's.

Former Homes

The places residents moved from when entering these six communities influenced the overall moving process, as well on the outcomes of their move to assisted living. The largest group (39%) in our study was made up of residents who had been living alone in their own homes or apartments. Some, like Ethyl Burns and Elsie Joiner, gave up homes they had owned and lived in for many years. Almost all of the former home owners in our study are residents of Oak Manor, Peach Blossom, and Blue Skies, ALFs with at least some residents of higher economic status. Most residents of other homes have never been home owners, having lived instead in a series of apartments over the course of their lives. Still others, like Eugene Ellis, had made earlier transitions from former homes into apartments.

The next largest group (36%) includes those residents who had left their own homes at an earlier time and were living in a primary caregiver's home at the time of their move to assisted living. Almost half of these, like Lily Porter, had been living with an adult child. Others shared the homes of siblings, spouses, nieces or nephews, parents, and, in one case, a cousin. One resident of Blue Skies moved from the home of a friend. Two sisters who had shared a home and two married couples moved together into Oak Manor.

Almost a fifth of residents moved from other assisted living homes. Because of mental health problems, a number of these, like Burt Hatfield, had lived in small, low-income homes during most of their adult lives. Three such residents of Greene's moved with Burt from the same unlicensed ALF when it closed. Three Oak Manor residents had lived together in a large, upscale, majority-white facility that closed for financial reasons, and another had left a similar one in South Carolina to be closer to her nieces. A few residents had moved from independent senior housing, one from a skilled nursing facility, and one, a resident of Sunshine House, from a psychiatric hospital.

Although most residents of these six homes had lived previously in the Atlanta area, one-fifth (19%) had moved from out of state—all of them Oak Manor residents who migrated from various places in the United States to be nearer to family members. The two sisters, Elizabeth Bell and Dorothea Buffington, came from Chattanooga to be near Ms. Buffington's son, the only child between them. Mr. Ellis left his daughter and longtime friends in Columbus, Ohio, to join his grandsons and great-grandsons. Hattie Houseworth moved away from Louisiana and her only sister to be closer to her younger daughter. All these residents who relocated to Atlanta, or their families, had the financial resources that made a long-distance move possible. A number of elders, like Lily Porter, who had left their homes earlier to live with adult children, also moved from out of state or from other parts of Georgia. Much like leaving a longtime home, abandoning geographic roots affected the outcomes of the move to assisted living.

Deciding to Move

Although sometimes sudden, decisions to move to these six communities typically evolved over a period of time, sometimes years. They began with recognition by someone, often not the resident, that the current situation was not working—either for the resident, for persons involved in the resident's care, or for both. Decision making was complex and often wrenching. In most cases, no one event was critical. Multiple factors determined how, why, when, and by whom decisions were made. How each situation evolved depended on a variety of factors, and, for most residents and their caregivers, decision making involved a cost-benefit analysis of staying where they were or moving to assisted living.

The Context of Decision Making

All decisions to move into these homes originated with some type of disability that generated a need for care. For slightly more than one-third of residents, care needs were related primarily to physical disability, stemming mainly from chronic diseases common in old age. Decline typically was gradual, but in cases of an acute event, such as a heart attack or stroke (less than 10% of the total), it was abrupt. Only Hannah Tilly, a 64-year-old resident of Blue Skies, had a lifelong physical disability, caused by a congenital arthritic condition. For the remaining two-thirds of residents, mental disability precipitated their need for care. Slightly more than half of these residents had some type of dementia, and 42% had other mental conditions, mainly schizophrenia. Mental retardation was the primary disabling condition in two cases, and severe depression in two others.

Both the type and level of disability determined care needs and influenced moving decisions. Many residents with long-term mental illness, like Burt Hatfield, moved to these ALFs as young adults or in middle age and needed only food and shelter, watchful oversight, and medication management. Among residents with cognitive impairment and physical disabilities, care needs were wide ranging. When Elsie Joiner moved to Oak Manor, the only "care" she received was her meals and weekly housekeeping services. In contrast, when he moved to Rosie's Loving Care, 95-year-old Harold Stamps was unable to bathe, dress, or toilet himself. Although disability of some level and type was prerequisite for making the decision to move to assisted living, disability was only part of each resident's story.

Essential for deciding to move to AL was the perception that a move was necessary, or at least optimal, for the health and well-being of the prospective resident. Generally speaking, the person who perceived the need also made the decision. In a minority of cases, it was the resident who recognized the need for moving and was the primary decision maker. For most residents, another person, typically a family member, first perceived the need and ultimately made the decision to move, either unilaterally or jointly with the resident. The length of time between perception of need and deciding to move was variable. The gravity of the situation and the options for moving were two key factors affecting the timing of decisions.

Control of Decision Making

Control of decision making was on a continuum. On one end, the resident exerted primary control, and on the other, the resident had none. Between these extremes, the resident shared, to varying degrees, the decision-making process with another person, typically a family member. Slightly fewer than a quarter of residents (22%) were primary decision makers, and most of these were residents of Oak Manor. Although a few residents of Greene's "decided" to move there on their own, in reality, they had little choice. All had experienced acute health crises and had neither the financial nor family resources for other options. In contrast, Oak Manor residents who controlled moving decisions had greater options, as they had throughout their lives, and they made their decisions while they still had the physical and mental ability to exercise control.

For the remaining residents (more than three-fourths), control, in varying degrees, was in the hands of others—children (53%), other family members (32%), friends (4%), and social workers (11%). The residents in this group either were no longer able to make decisions independently or acquiesced to the decisions of others. Most accepted the inevitable and complied gracefully, knowing they had little power. Many even ultimately agreed the decision was for the best. Others, though, accepted neither the need for nor the reality of the move. Individuals who made moving decisions for residents (either with or without a resident's blessings) believed they had no other choice. Most also believed they were acting in the resident's best interests. Yet for many residents, their actual or perceived control over the decision to move affected their satisfaction with both the decision and their experiences in these communities.

Decision-Making Scenarios

Although each resident's situation was both unique and complex, we identified three common decision-making scenarios among residents: those in which acute health crises triggered moving; those in which residents made moving decisions independently and over a period of time; and those in which residents were pressured by others to move. These scenarios reflect differences in residents' disabilities, prior living situations, family support, and control of decision making.

An acute physical or mental health crisis precipitated the decision to move to AL for about 15% of all residents.* All residents in this category had been living alone at the time of the critical event, and most moved directly from either a hospital or nursing home. For residents like Boss Cook, a resident of Greene's, who had experienced no disability before his stroke at the age of 50, the move signaled an abrupt end to a former way of life. Some, like Rosie's resident Sarah Eubanks, had lived with mental illness for most of their adult lives, and others, like Greene's resident Miss Fannie, had suffered previous age-related physical or cognitive decline.

Common to all of these residents was the absence of family support that might have helped them avoid the move to assisted living. Boss Cook was divorced from his wife and estranged from his children. In other cases, family members had neither the resources nor the inclination to assume a primary caregiving role, particularly when the person needing care was especially challenging. Although five of Ms. Eubanks's nine children lived in Atlanta, her long-term mental illness had taken its toll on their ability to provide care. Miss Fannie's only available caregiver was her 96-year-old elder sister. Although some individuals, like Boss and Miss Fannie, were the primary decision makers, the decision in each case derived, in effect, from the critical nature of the triggering health event.

A small group of residents made independent, considered decisions to leave their homes and move to assisted living. All were mentally competent elders who, with the exception of sisters Elizabeth Bell and Dorothea Buffington, lived alone and moved to Oak Manor. Although these elders had differing needs and resources for care, they had all felt overburdened in their former environments. Certain stressors were common, including uncertainty about the course of disability, loneliness, fear, and the demands of housekeeping. Elsie Joiner's increasing decline from Parkinson's was perceptible and worrisome. She was lonely and no longer able to drive or keep house as she once had. Alma Burgess's circumstances were similar. Growing awareness of her need to move was set in motion by a car accident and a series of falls: "Well, it took certain

---

*Sunshine House residents are not included in these calculations owing to lack of information about reasons for moving for most residents of that facility.

experiences at home to get me out. For instance, the falling, and I began to be fearful of being there by myself, afraid of going to the door and maybe someone pushing and coming into the house. There were these apprehensions, you know, what might happen to me as a lone person, old woman, in a house."

Also common among these elders was a desire to relieve, or at least not increase, the care burden of their families. They were proud of the achievements of their upwardly mobile children and understood the pressures in their lives. A key reason for Eugene Ellis's decision to leave his life in Ohio and move to Oak Manor was his desire to minimize his family's care responsibilities: "Here, if I pick Oak Manor, my daughter and my grandkids would not have to give me any daily attention. They could come whenever time would permit them, but, during the interval, they would know that I was in a facility where I was secure, where I had attention, where if I had any emergencies, [staff] would respond. Therefore, I didn't hesitate to entertain the idea of coming back and making Oak Manor my permanent home." Alma Burgess's goal of lessening dependency on her family was bolstered by a desire to preserve her own independence: "I decided that the best thing for me to do was to find somewhere to go where I would still have my independence, would not have to live with either my daughter-in-law or my other son, with either of the families, you know. I felt that I didn't want to put that on them because they'd had enough already."

None of these elders making their own decisions to move to AL reached this point quickly or easily, and none left their homes and communities without some regret. They knew in their hearts they would miss much about their former lives—for Elsie Joiner it was hosting her family for holiday dinners, for Alma Burgess, having her friends just "drop by." But they also felt relief at relinquishing responsibility for meeting their needs. As Alma Burgess said, "Well, there's no place like home, but I feel comfortable here."

Most residents were, in essence, told they had to move. Some of these residents ultimately agreed that a move was necessary and went peacefully. Others resisted to the bitter end and were forced to comply. About half of the residents were elders who had been living alone. The rest, including a few young or middle-aged adults, had lived with a caregiver. Decision makers were typically residents' children, and the reasons for their decisions were much like those given by elders who decided for themselves—worry about the health, safety, and well-being of the resident and the burden on themselves of providing care.

Most of those elders still living alone had given no thought to leaving their homes. Many of their caregivers had little involvement in day-to-day care, and, in quite a few cases, the elders and caregivers lived some distance apart. A typical example was Hattie Houseworth, whose children and grandchildren decided to move her to Oak Manor from her home in Louisiana. Ms. Houseworth's daughter Phoebe described the scenario leading to the family decision: "My mother was not doing well in Louisiana, although I don't know if she will admit that at all. She does sometimes, but sometimes she doesn't. She wasn't eating well, she was losing a lot of weight, she was getting somewhat confused about what was going on in the house. My sister's family went down and packed her up over Thanksgiving. My mother was not opposed to it in any way. I think she knew that this was the best bet." Clearly, Ms. Houseworth's family believed they were acting in her best interests, and no doubt they were. She was 81, had Parkinson disease and congestive heart failure, had fired the cleaning lady hired by her daughter, and frequently "burned up" her dinner. Ms. Houseworth admitted she "liked" Oak Manor, but about the decision to move she said, "They decided for me. They came down there and picked me up. I did what they told me to do." She knew the choice was not hers.

Although some elders, like Hattie Houseworth and Ethyl Burns, complied gracefully with the wishes of their family members, others fought harder. One was Annette Freeman, a longtime Atlanta resident whose only child, Ike, lived in Connecticut. One day Ike took her to Oak Manor, ostensibly "just for the weekend," and there she stayed. Ms. Freeman felt that she had been, literally, "put" in the home by her son: "The way I got here, my son, as I said, read about this place, and, out of the clear blue sky and before I know anything, he had me out here. I made no preparation for coming or anything. He raked this [clothing] out of my closet and raked this out, threw it in the suitcase, and he brought me over here." Unlike Hattie Houseworth, Annette Freeman cannot make her peace with the move. A year later, she has moved none of her furniture and few of her clothes and continues to talk about returning home. For Ms. Freeman, her home represents her identity and her life: "I don't care what anyone says, our little treasures that we have are in our homes, whatever the treasures are, they are in your home."

In these situations—much like those in which elders made their own decisions to leave home—crisis lay dormant. For other elders, circumstances had become more critical. Ninety-two-year-old Viola Wheeler, though increasingly confused, had lived alone in the house she once shared with her now-deceased elder sister. Ms. Wheeler had two paid housekeepers, one in the morning and another in the evening, and a neighbor who helped with banking, grocery shopping, and doctors' appointments. Her only family, a nephew, was recuperating from heart surgery. Despite her tenuous situation, Ms. Wheeler remained adamant in her refusal to move, and only when she wandered from her home one night, looking for her sister, and fell did her caregivers take charge. Enlisting the help of her physician, they told Ms. Wheeler she was moving and took her from his office straight to Peach Blossom. For weeks after moving, Ms. Wheeler routinely grabbed her pocketbook and headed for the front door, stating she had "enjoyed her visit" but was now going "home."

In other situations, family members had gone to great lengths to keep elders at home but over time had reached their own physical, emotional, and financial limits. Harold Stamps's family had moved into his home and provided round-the-clock care until they found Rosie's. Michael Waldman's daughter Bernadette drove weekly to Alabama for more than two years trying to keep him at home with full-time sitters before giving up and moving him to Oak Manor. Although these two elders had significant dementia and offered no resistance to the move, Bernadette admitted that, had she "tried [to move him] two years ago, it would not have occurred, because Daddy would have said no."

Even with intense opposition from elders, some caregivers prevailed, simply to preserve their personal well-being. Hassie Hicks's daughter Ernestine explained how the burden of caring for her mother with Alzheimer disease forced her decision, despite her mother's protests:

I'm a worrier, so that's why I got sick and that's why I had to make the decision to do something with Mom. I do know now I could not keep her. Even if I didn't have work or a busy life, I couldn't do it because of my nature. I mean, because when I'm with her, it's just too depressing. God bless anybody that can take care of their parents in this state [Alzheimer disease]. I have ulcers, and that was one of the reasons I decided to move her, too, 'cause I've passed out, and the only way they brought me back was two pints of blood. My doctor told me that I had to change some things. I've always been a worrier, but that really worried me with my mom, because I knew she didn't want to move from home. What am I gonna do? I'm the only child left, and I knew I couldn't take care of her. . . . But, then, after her doctor suggested it was time to move her, she said, "I am not leaving my home." She told the lady next door that if I tried to move her, she would burn the house down. So then I said, "Now, if you say that again, I'm gonna go tell your doctor and"—she always used to recollect Milledgeville [a state mental institution]—"they will institutionalize you, because they know that you're a danger to yourself." And then she said she would chain herself to the house and all this stuff, but she knew it was time to go. She was afraid to stay there.

Although Ernestine feels remorse over not being able to let her mother stay at home or move her into her own home, she further justified her actions: "I don't feel like children should give up the days that God give them to devote to a elder parent like that. I think you should make sure that they're okay." Ultimately, Hassie Hicks was "okay" at Peach Blossom and even admits she had been afraid staying alone in her "big old stone house."

Similar scenarios evolved for residents who had been living in the homes of their caregivers. Many of these caregivers were employed away from home, and the care receiver, typically an older person, was left at home alone for long periods of time, creating problems similar to those experienced by elders living in their own homes. Sharon's worries that her mother, Lily Porter, might fall, not have a hot meal, or feel lonely were all factors in her decision.

For elders who were cognitively impaired, additional problems arose. Irene Garrett had lived most of her life in south Georgia, where she had been an elementary school teacher. Her only child, Elva, lived in Atlanta, and when Ms. Garrett's behavior became erratic owing to the progression of Alzheimer's, Elva moved her mother into her own home. Elva was married, with a teenage daughter and two adult sons still at home. She hoped to keep her mother with her until she could retire. Initially, the plan seemed to be working, but an event characteristic of other situations precipitated a change: "She loves outside, and that's why my husband brought her rocking chair from home. As long as she could sit outside, she would be happy, but we started getting a little concerned about her here at the house. My husband came home one day, and she had let someone in the home, and we thought that was not good for her, because it could be the wrong person. And so, I said, okay, during the day what I'll do is find somewhere for her to go."

Elva began taking her mother to Peach Blossom for a few hours a day, but from the beginning her mother was unhappy. Elva attempted again to keep her at home, but in the end the stress of trying to balance work and multiple caregiving roles became too much, particularly after Ms. Garrett became incontinent. Similar to other situations in which physicians played pivotal roles, Ms. Garrett's doctor helped Elva make, and finally accept, her decision: "Dr. Sanders, he felt that if I continued the way I was going, eventually I would break, and he said, 'You cause problems on yourself. If you get sick, then [your mother] has no one.' So after, you know, talking with everyone and all, then I decided just to go ahead and place her in."

Elva's decision—much like decisions of other family members—was fraught with uncertainty and pain. The comment by Eleanor Winfrey's daughter Joyce could have come from any of the decision makers: "I felt really guilty. I promised her I would never put her in a home, that I would let her stay home. I tried, and it just didn't work."

Preparing to Move

For all residents, preparations for moving begin with selecting a facility. For some, preparations also involve selecting rooms, sorting through possessions and deciding what to take with them, and selling former homes. Most residents in these communities had little control over these preparations.

Choosing a Home

Home selection typically follows on the heels of the decision to move. At the outset, selection options are limited by residents' financial resources, type and level of disability, age, and care needs, which have to be compatible with the fees and admission criteria of their prospective homes. Low-income residents can consider only the small homes. Those who are young or have a history of mental health problems are further constrained. Selection also varies with how quickly a decision must be made and who makes the decision.

For about one-fifth of the residents of the small homes—all admitted from hospitals or connected to the mental health system, the Veterans Administration, or the Medicaid waiver Community Care Services Program—homes were located by a social worker. Three who moved to Greene's were "found" in County Hospital by the owner, Cora Greene, who regularly locates new clients through the hospital discharge planner. Most residents in this group were presented with a "choice" of one facility, and they had no opportunity to visit before moving in.

In most cases, the small homes were located largely through personal relationships and word of mouth in the African American community. The way Estelle Washington's daughter Elaine found Peach Blossom was typical of how these homes were located: "Ms. Adams lived right around the corner here next to my girlfriend, and she told me, 'She'll be ideal for your mom.'" Although Elaine looked at "several places" and "went out as far as Stone Mountain,"

Peach Blossom best fit her criteria: "I didn't like the way some of 'em looked, and once we got with Ms. Adams and went in, I liked the cleanliness. It didn't smell like a personal care home, and it was airy looking, and they were sitting on the front porch, and they had so much going around on the outside . . . and [Ms. Adams] seemed to be a person that was concerned about the people that was in her care and then she came highly recommended . . . and, then, another thing, it was just so convenient. Ten minutes, you know, she's right here."

Most family members selecting these small homes named similar traits: clean, convenient location, and good reputation. Many also emphasized the importance of "homelike" qualities that distinguished these small ALFs from nursing homes, a distinction that made the decision more palatable for both family members and residents. As Ms. Washington's daughter said, "I didn't want her to feel that we were giving her away, 'cause I didn't want to put her in a nursing home. A personal care home, it was still just like family away from home." Hassie Hicks's daughter, who screened homes before taking her mother to visit them, was relieved at her mother's reaction to Peach Blossom: "She thought she was going to a nursing home. I never took Mother any place until I found the place that I thought would be right for her. So once I found Ms. Adams's, I carried her over there, showed her, and she was very excited." Families also liked the less restrictive nature of the small ALFs. Slick's sister Iola chose Greene's because she did not want to "put him in a complete care home [nursing home]" but preferred somewhere he "could have access of getting out and going places." Among small homes, only Blue Skies has some private rooms, a key criterion for Lily Porter's daughter Sharon, who maintains that finding the "proper" home helps ease African American families' anxieties over AL placement: "I think it is a good solution for African Americans, because it helps relieve you of that burden of guilt because you're putting your loved one outside of your home, but it also allows you to have some comfort level, because you know they're being cared for, if it's the proper home."

The low-income status of most residents of these small homes placed significant restrictions on their choice of home. Although participation in the Community Care Services Program, the Medicaid waiver program available in ALFs, increased the options of some, access is limited, and reimbursement rates are low. Homes specializing in the care of individuals with mental retardation and mental illness are especially scarce.

The selection process for Oak Manor has some important differences from the selection for the small, lower-income homes. First, the higher socioeconomic status of both residents and their families provides more options. Second is the unique character of the home and the importance of race and culture in the selection process. Third is the greater involvement of residents in the decision-making process.

Although, as with the small homes, Oak Manor was located in most cases through word of mouth in the black community, people heard about it not so much because of its reputation for care as for its unique status as a high-income facility targeted to African Americans and its location in a predominantly African American neighborhood. Oak Manor had a reputation long before its doors opened. Even the few who discovered Oak Manor just "driving by" probably would not have noticed it had it not been an anomaly in their neighborhood.

Race for both families and residents was a key selection criterion. Alma Burgess was clear: "I wanted to be, you know, in a predominantly black facility." "Comfort" was a reason commonly given by family members, referring to the preference of their parents' generation, particularly in the South, for racially segregated settings. Michael Waldman's daughter Bernadette said, "Because Daddy's from the old school, not saying that he would not be able to get along with other races, he's just more comfortable, I think, with his own." Hattie Houseworth's daughter Phoebe, who moved to Atlanta from the Northeast, expressed a similar view: "I would not have liked it if she were, especially in the state of Georgia, in a facility where there were only a few African Americans. You are not too sure what you are going to run into." For Eugene Ellis, commonality based both on race and class was important: "I was not all comfortable staying in a facility that was predominately of the other race. I would like the comradeship, the friendship, the shaking the hand, the patting on the back that you get in a black facility. Here, I was coming to a facility where the folks were more or less my peers. They're black, they can afford this living style, the food would be cooked by blacks, the activities would be around the black culture, I would be around retired school teachers, retired social workers, retired college professors. I could eat three meals a day with people that I could sit with comfortably and just talk about life."

Although several residents and family members stated that race was not the reason they had chosen Oak Manor, they are proud the facility is available in their community and believe its presence reflects the improving status of African Americans. One family member said, "What excited me was when I started asking about it and learned it was one of the few in the country in an African American community. We always want things to be able to go [be profitable] in your own neighborhood. That really did make me want to say, 'I know this can go.' It also helped me to recognize that [white people] do recognize that we do have pensions, we do have persons who are hopefully able to sustain a facility like that in our neighborhood."

Residents moving from out of town to Oak Manor typically did not participate in the selection process, and most did not even visit the facility before moving in. Those who were Atlanta residents had greater involvement in selection, although selection usually meant saying yes to Oak Manor. Only a few residents or families considered other facilities once they discovered Oak Manor, and some most likely would not have decided to move from their former homes had it not been an option.

Choosing and Furnishing a Room

Choosing and furnishing the room where they would spend the next years of their lives was a luxury the majority of residents did not have. Constraints mainly revolved around a facility's size, design, and bed availability and a resident's financial resources and gender. Most residents moving to the small homes had no choice of rooms but simply were offered whatever bed was vacant. At Sunshine House, men are restricted to the basement and women to the main floor. Four of the five bedrooms at Blue Skies are private, but selecting one depends on availability and the ability to afford the extra fee. Three of the small homes (Greene's, Rosie's, and Peach Blossom) usually operate at or over capacity, making room choice a rarity.

Small homes also offer little opportunity for residents to "furnish" their rooms with more than their clothes and a few decorative items. Blue Skies residents can bring one or two pieces of furniture, a favorite chair or TV, for instance. Lily Porter brought her bed. Some small-home residents had nothing to bring, such as Greene's resident Beatrice Dove, who had lost all of her possessions in a fire, and others, like Burt Hatfield, who had for years lived in AL homes or on the streets.

Again, Oak Manor differs from the small homes. All bedrooms are private, and all, except for a few companion suites, have private baths. Because our study began the first year the home opened and the facility was far from full, most residents could choose from a number of rooms and were restricted chiefly by what they could afford to pay.

Only a few residents made their own room choices. One was Lula Merriwether, whose niece Georgiana took her to visit Oak Manor. It was, in fact, the availability of a two-room suite, and Georgiana's understanding of its importance to her aunt, that clinched the decision to move: "What I knew was that Aunt Lula's things are very important to her. I think a lot of that has to do with the fact that she doesn't have any children [and that] her husband is gone. Everything she has, all of her things, helps her to be who she is. She's real attached to her things. So then they showed me the two-room suite, and I thought, 'Okay, this is perfect. Don't let this go. I'm going to go get her [and] bring her out here.'" As soon as Ms. Merriwether saw the room, she was ready to put down her deposit. Family members made room choices for most residents, and some took great care to abide by what they believed were residents' own preferences. This decision-making responsibility, though, as Hattie Houseworth's daughter Phoebe stated, could be a challenge: "Picking out her room was a nightmare. I kept trying to think about what she would like. I ended up picking out the room with the most windows and closet space, which I think was right."

Oak Manor residents are allowed to bring whatever furniture and personal belongings they can cram into their rooms, and cram some do. Most brought furnishings from their former homes, except for a few who moved from out of town or who, like Annette Freeman, had not accepted the permanence of their move. Being able to participate in the sorting and distributing of their possessions gave some residents a greater sense of control over the entire moving process. Eugene Ellis, who was "in charge" of his own move, described his central role: "Frankly, when I moved out of the house, I made most of the furniture that I could not take to the apartment available to my grandchildren. That was in '95. The sofa, I brought to the apartment, and the love seat. My computer, I made it more convenient by buying a computer table with file drawers and all the accessories. The lamps you see, I brought with me, the valet, to hang my current clothes on. The bed was a bed from my home and [from] the apartment, which is a king-size bed. That dresser is older than you. I bought that back in the '40s. These chairs and whatnot came from the apartment." Mr. Ellis valued not only having control over what he took to his new home but also having the power over distribution of belongings to his grandchildren. Ethyl Burns's experience was quite different. Although her nephew chose "just about" what she would have chosen herself, not being a full participant in the selection process upset her:

> They chose what to bring from the house. They wouldn't let me move. I couldn't supervise. I just could see what they decided to take, but they just insisted that I just sit. They brought what they thought I should have out here. And Sylvia and Opal and them chose, you know, clothes for me to come out here with. And they left me and Opal at home, and the rest of them came out here about five o'clock. They came back and said, "We ready now, we ready." I said, "You ready [for] what?" They said, "We ready to take you out to your new home." I said, "I am not going out there tonight. No one said anything to me about going to leave my house tonight. What's wrong with y'all?" They said, "No, you have to go tonight. You better go, 'cause we're going home. We're coming back, but I don't want to leave you here anymore by yourself." So, I said, "Yes sir," and then we came here, and, when I walked in here, this room looked almost like it does now. All of the furniture came from that house, except that lamp. And they chose everything, yeah, just about what I would've chosen.

Having furnishings and other personal effects from their former homes helps some residents create a feeling of home in their new surroundings. Even though Ethyl Burns did not control when to move or what to take, she admitted, "I really do feel at home. I guess 'cause I got so much home around me, with the furniture and everything." Alma Burgess shares this view but makes it clear that "home" does not extend beyond her "little room": "One thing about it is, having my own bed here, some of my own furniture, being able to have things that I'm familiar with as a part of my everyday living, I sort of have that at-home feeling right in this room. . . . Right here in this little room, it's somewhat similar to my own home." But furnishings cannot create home for all. Although Hamilton Brewton takes pride in the many photographs documenting his rich African American heritage, his grandmother's antique bed with the hand-carved headboard, and his chest from the Crimean War, to him Oak Manor feels more akin to a "dormitory" or a "hotel" than a home.

Eugene Ellis's furnishings allow him to continue many of his favorite activities: "I like my room. As you can see I am able to do a lot of things. I was able to bring my computer, which is quite extensive. I can stay in touch with the outside world, both by fax, by e-mail, Internet, and various programs, such as a scanner and video photography. I can go to my grandson's for Thanksgiving dinner, I can take pictures with my digital camera, come back and hopefully load it on to my computer, print the pictures up, and show it to him. I brought my music machine, which I have CDs [for]. I have the radio, which they call the receiver. I have the videotapes that I can play."

Settling In

When asked if he felt "at home" at Oak Manor, Eugene Ellis replied, "Yes, yes. As a person, I didn't find it difficult to settle in, because, aside from the many things I've done in life, I've done a lot of traveling, so I've been used to being in different locations." Of all the residents who moved into these six homes during our study, Mr. Ellis seems to have settled in with the greatest ease. His ability to feel at home in a variety of places is only one of the reasons. Also contributing to his relatively seamless adjustment are his control over the moving process (from beginning to end), his familiarity with the facility before moving, his compatibility with the culture of Oak Manor, and his ability to continue many of his favorite pastimes. Many of these outcomes are possible because of Mr. Ellis's own resources—his physical and mental abilities, his financial assets, his family support, and his positive approach to life. Facility features also are important—the opportunity to have a private room and bring his own furnishings, the amenities, and the African American culture.

Participation in the Moving Process

Generally speaking, the more residents were prepared for and involved in the moving process, the easier time they had settling in. Those who had visited these homes, or other ALFs, were better equipped, because they had some notion of what to expect. Since Alma Burgess had visited other family members in ALFs, she "knew what assisted living was like" and felt it was an environment she "probably could adjust to." Visiting Peach Blossom before moving there lessened Hassie Hicks's anxiety, which helped her accept leaving her home. Residents who had little or no participation in decision making, particularly those who were taken to their new homes without prior visits, had the most difficulty settling in. Because moving is a process consisting of discrete stages, control is a matter of degree. Each opportunity for control—from the initial decision to the move itself—helped residents accept, and even embrace, the decision to move, which facilitated settling in.

The Physical Environment

The physical environment affects residents' abilities to adjust in a number of ways. Size, design, and location are important. Small size makes it easier for residents to learn their way around, particularly if they have cognitive impairment. Having private space allows greater personalization, which helps some residents feel more at home. Feeling at home, though, depends both on residents' definitions of home and on how well the new environment fits those definitions. A resident like Annette Freeman, whose connotation of home is tied to just one physical place, finds it more difficult to achieve that "at-home" feeling. For other residents with few personal belongings and numerous past "homes," the physical setting is less important.

Remaining close to former neighborhoods and communities aids adjustment for some residents. Quite a few Oak Manor residents found they already knew one another, and these connections eased the stress of moving. Even Annette Freeman, a longtime Atlantan and a graduate of one of its historically black colleges, admitted, "I know a lot of people here. I guess that's one thing that makes me as contented as I am." When Ethyl Burns moved in, she received cards and flowers from her Atlanta friends, whose "kindness and interest" made her "feel better." The noise from the nearby freeway reminds Calvin Soames of his home in Cleveland.

Family and Friends

Families can help ease residents' transitions to their new homes. Their most common tactic is to visit frequently during the days and weeks following the move. Some, like the daughters of Oak Manor residents Michael Waldman and Hattie Houseworth, visit daily and often accompany residents to activities and meals. Such support helps new residents, particularly in the large home, learn how to navigate the facility and enter into the new social scene. It also reduces feelings of abandonment. Some family members choose not to help, diminishing or even barring contact. Annette Freeman's son, who forced her to move to Oak Manor, blocked her calls to his home in Connecticut when she first moved, adding to her already considerable stress.

Sometimes it is ties with other residents that promote settling in. Some connections had been formed in earlier lives, and others soon after moving in. Madonna McDowell's transition to Rosie's was relatively smooth because some of her fellow residents attended her adult day rehabilitation center. Her daughter Sybil described the meaning of these prior relationships for both herself and her mother: "I took her to visit before we decided, and what was so good about it was that she knew people there prior to going there. So, when we walked through the door, everybody said, 'Hey, I know you,' and, so, I mean, you have to understand how overwhelmed I was to know that she was in a place where people liked her, you know, prior to her coming. She saw her people there and said, 'Okay, this is where I'm gonna be.'" Eleanor Winfrey, who adamantly opposed full-time residency at Oak Manor (initially, she was only a day-time resident), quickly reversed her course once Watkins Orr moved in and she "fell in love."

Mental Status and Attitudes

The effect of residents' cognitive impairment was variable. Some residents with dementia have difficulty fully understanding where they are or how they got there and, like Viola Wheeler, want only to go home. For others, like Harold Stamps and Hassie Hicks, the fog of dementia seems to ease their transition. Confused residents generally have a harder time learning new routines and environments. Depression also impedes adjustment. The transition for Florida Franklin, whose daughter moved her to Oak Manor against her will, has been extremely difficult. "Breaking up housekeeping turned me around," she said. "I feel like my world has fallen apart." Her depression over giving up her home in North Carolina is aggravated by anxiety over her increasing confusion: "I have lost my memories, and I'm scared to death."

Individuals with a positive attitude toward moving on the whole settle in more quickly, as do those with a personality that encourages "making the best" of a situation. Rozena Banks, who cried her first night at Oak Manor because she felt her daughters "threw me away," said she was able to adjust in just two weeks: "I said, 'I need to get it together, because this is where I am going to be. Stop crying and go on and meet other people and go on about your business. This is where you pay your rent, so come up here [her room] and get your butt and put it in the bed.'" According to Madonna McDowell, liking yourself and others also helps: "Well, you can adjust yourself to [group living] if you want to. And I try to get along with everyone, and, then, I like people, and, when one likes people, it's easy to adjust. . . . And if you like yourself, you could adjust to other people."

Facility Role

Oak Manor has several formal mechanisms designed to help residents adjust to moving in, which include welcome signs in the lobby, name plates on residents' doors, and a "buddy" system matching a director with each new resident. None of these procedures, however, seems to be particularly effective. The welcome signs are quite small, nameplates often do not arrive until months after residents move in, and we observed no "buddy" activities. New residents are not routinely introduced in settings in which all residents gather, for example, the dining room. Hamilton Brewton's suggestion to allay the bewilderment of new residents was to assign a new resident to a current resident to "show them the works." In his view, "A person coming in does not know what is going on, what they are up against. An older person knows the problems of other older people."

In the small homes, residents typically are "shown the works" by the owner or manager. In homes with more structured routines, instruction is more specific. Sometimes one of the residents assumes the provider's indoctrination role. At Peach Blossom, Hassie Hicks frequently tells the confused new residents that they are "in a personal care home" and that Ms. Adams will "take care" of them. At Greene's, Boss Cook, who has been there the longest, instructs residents on both formal and informal rules. Miss Fannie attested to his invaluable role in her transition: "When I first moved here, me and him was friends like that. He [was] the only one would talk to me when I first come in this place, keep me company, talk to me and tell me, you know, different things, about the place, what's going on and what's happening, what to do and how to do this and that and the other, and things like that."

The Importance of Decision Making

In this chapter, we have told the story of residents moving to these six assisted living communities. Moving is a process with discrete stages, and our story follows those stages. It starts with a perception of the need to make a move, followed by the actual decision to move. Next comes finding a place to move to, selecting and furnishing a room, and, finally, getting settled in the new community. The stages we identify parallel those described by Young (1998) in her qualitative study of elders moving into retirement housing. Each stage in the moving process involves important decisions, and decision making is complex.

Residents' unique pathways into these communities were determined by multiple factors, including their prior living arrangements, type and level of disability, degree of family support, and attitudes and personalities. But these pathways to AL began long before the decisions we describe here were made, and underlying these more immediate factors are the circumstances of residents' earlier lives. As we have observed in this and preceding chapters, residents' moving stories reflect their status as African Americans and their experiences and opportunities throughout the course of their lives. Because residents experienced the moving process in many different ways, there are multiple stories to be told.

Despite the complexity of residents' situations, we identify three common decision-making scenarios. Control of decision making is a critical component of each. In the first scenario, decisions are precipitated by acute health crises, and it is the critical nature of the event that exerts the primary control. The second scenario, whereby residents decide on their own to move, is the only one in which residents have any meaningful control. In scenario three, the most common, other people, typically residents' children, are the decision makers.

Other studies have also found that most AL residents have little control over decisions to move and that family members, usually children, are the primary decision makers (Ball et al., 2000; Hawes & Phillips, 2000). Although a study of AL decision making in Oregon (Reinardy & Kane, 2003) finds that 63% of residents reported having complete or almost complete control over the decision to enter assisted living, little information was available about the context of their decisions, and it is possible that residents overrated their involvement. In our study, some residents stated they had made their own decisions, though circumstances surrounding the decision making indicated the decision was not theirs alone.

Residents who decided on their own to move perceived their need primarily in terms of increasing disability, which impeded their ability to manage in their current environments. Lawton and Nahemow (1973) propose that individuals adapt better to the problems of aging when they maintain a congruence between environmental press and competence, that is, when the demands of their home environments closely match their own abilities. These elders chose to move to AL because they no longer could maintain that steady state in their own homes. They all sought a better fit between their own needs and the demands of the environment (Lawton, 1980; Moos & Lemke, 1994).

Young (1998) finds that white elders deciding to move to retirement housing were also looking for a better fit with their environment.

Another factor guiding decisions of these African American elders to move to AL was a desire to reduce the burden on their caregivers, as well as their own costs associated with this dependency. Studies of elders moving to retirement housing (Young, 1998) and nursing homes (Groger, 1994) similarly find that reducing caregiver burden was a factor in elder decision making. In her qualitative study exploring decisions of African American elders to enter a nursing home or receive home care services, Groger (1994) has found that personality accounted for some of the variation in outcomes. The home care clients demonstrated a greater determination to remain "independent" despite their disabilities. These elders resembled those described in other studies of low-income, African American home care clients (Ball & Whittington, 1995) in the strong value they placed on independence. Although many of the elders moving to these six AL communities seem to have had no other choice, it is possible that, had some of those with fewer impairments (particularly in cognitive status) been more fiercely independent, they might have extended their stay at home. A similar qualitative study (Forbes & Hoffart, 1998) portrays the experience of disabled elders as a "precarious balance," and decision making (on whether to stay home or enter a nursing home) as a process of adjusting the scale for a better balance. The degree of imbalance that individuals could tolerate was shaped by their personalities, needs, values, attitudes, and beliefs.

Even though family members controlled most decisions to move, many had expended considerable effort to delay moves and keep residents at home. Most also expressed a strong value for family, as opposed to institutional, care and believed they had done the best they could. Residents' cognitive impairment and incontinence were major factors contributing to both their stress and their decision making. Economic factors were also significant. Almost all caregivers worked full-time, and, with the exception of several residents who attended senior centers or adult day rehabilitation programs, no residents or family members received any formal long-term care services before moving. None of these elders or their caregivers was able to pay for the full-time assistance or oversight many required for them to stay at home.

Groger's (1994) study of African American elders reveals that those who entered a nursing home had reached the limits of their informal support. Primary limiting factors related to caregivers' family, work, and health. Similar to our

findings, for Groger's entrants it was not a decline in support but rather sup-
porters' inability either to increase their aid or to find additional helpers that
was critical. Compared with the home care clients, those entering a nursing
home also had fewer children to provide care, either because of childlessness,
lack of relationships with their children, or geographic distance from them.

As with deciding to move, little research has addressed how ALF residents
select homes. A few studies (in all of which the large majority of residents were
white) that examine facility features valued by residents reveal that having a
private room was a high priority (Kane et al., 1998; Reinardy & Kane, 2003).
We also found that the availability of private space at Oak Manor and for a few
residents at Blue Skies was a key selection criteria. But driving the decisions of
most elders selecting Oak Manor was the opportunity to choose a high-end
home that had it all: services and amenities long available in the white community; residents of like race, culture, and class; and location in an African
American community. Until Oak Manor opened its doors, ALFs with this set
of features had not been available to African Americans in Atlanta, or possibly anywhere in the United States. Mutran and colleagues (2001) suggest that
African Americans' stronger preference for care at home reflects the absence
of acceptable alternatives. We are sure that, without the option of Oak Manor,
some of its residents might have delayed their decision to move, maybe in-
definitely. Recent news reports indicate that immigrant elders moving to nursing homes and assisted living homes are choosing facilities that cater to their
cultural traditions and in which residents are of like race and ethnicity (Associated Press, "Ethnic nursing homes grow in Chicago," October 12, 2004;
S. Kershaw, "Immigrants now embrace homes for the elderly," *New York Times*,
October 20, 2003).

Research on AL shows that most Americans, both black and white, find this
new model of assisted living unaffordable (Hawes & Phillips, 2000; Herd,
2001). As noted in chapter 1, most ALF residents are white (Hawes et al.,
1995), and most African Americans in AL are in small homes (Morgan, Eckert,
& Lyon, 1995; Mutran et al., 2001). Certainly, the residents in our study who
"selected" the small homes could not have considered Oak Manor. Most simply took what was available and what they could afford. Yet despite their limited options, most residents and their families found these smaller ALFs far
superior to nursing homes and valued their homelike traits.

Frank (2002, 17) suggests that ALF residents experience an "incomplete"
rite of passage (Van Gennep, 1960) because they often are suspended in the

transitional, or liminal, stage, where they have no defined roles. A number of factors have been found to affect, either positively or negatively, this state of liminality. A significant one is involvement in decision making, and other research supports our finding that control over the decision making affects both adjustment and satisfaction with placement. Young (1998) finds that residents who initiated their moves to retirement housing had the highest levels of satisfaction with both the decision and the overall moving process and felt more at home in their new surroundings, whereas those who felt "placed" by family members described feelings of hopelessness and did not view their residences as home. Numerous studies of nursing home placement also demonstrate a positive relationship between control of decision making and resident well-being (Davidson & O'Connor, 1990; Forbes & Hoffart, 1998; Mikhail, 1992; Rossen & Knafl, 2003).

Another nursing home study (Holzapfel et al., 1992) has found that the greater the number of choices residents had in the moving process (for example, selecting a facility, choosing a room), the more predictable the new environment became. Involvement in decision making before the relocation reduced residents' anxiety over moving and had a direct impact on their quality of life. We also found that residents who had greater knowledge of the new setting and of what to expect had an easier time settling in. Thornton and Nardi's (1975) theory of role acquisition has bearing here. These authors suggest that acquiring a new role is a developmental process with four stages—anticipatory, formal, informal, and personal. Adjustment, which is both social and psychological, depends on the degree of accuracy and congruence between what a person anticipates and what is actually experienced. Our findings show that for these African American elders, increased participation at any stage of the moving process facilitated role acquisition and increased overall satisfaction.

Other studies emphasize the importance of acceptance, or what Young (1998, 160) calls "reconciling life's changes," in the adjustment to moving. Davidson and O'Connor (1990) discover that, although perceived control over decision making had short-term benefits, acceptance of the move had more positive long-term effects and was a separate and important coping mechanism. Forbes and Hoffart (1998) also find that the attitude of acceptance, both passive and active, helped elders cope with increasing dependency and lifestyle changes. Among residents in our study, those who accepted the need to move seemed better able to settle in.

Our findings have shown that a facility's physical environment helped some residents adjust. Important aspects included having private space, bringing furnishings and other possessions from former homes, and geographic location. The importance of personalizing one's space lay partly in its contribution to making the care home feel more "homelike." Young (1998) finds similar effects of personalization among residents moving to retirement housing. However, a qualitative study by Hersch, Spencer, and Kapoor (2003) of the relocation experiences of low-income African American and white elders reveals that most elders did not consider physical setting or personal belongings important to creating a sense of place. These authors attribute their findings partly to cultural and economic circumstances that led these older persons to place relatively little emphasis on material things. While most residents in the small homes had little opportunity to bring personal effects, our data also indicate that not all found this aspect of moving important. Other studies have suggested that furnishings and physical environment are more critical for those individuals whose sense of self is developed through attachment to place (Eckert, Zimmerman, & Morgan, 2001; Rowles, 1993). We found that, for other residents, the significance of environment lay in the effect it had on their ability to continue valued activities and stay connected to former neighborhoods, cultures, and relationships.

The decision to move to assisted living is a watershed event for most African American residents and their families. When and how the process of moving comes to pass has a significant effect on residents' satisfaction with the move and their ability to settle in. Much depends on residents' control over the process. Much also depends on how well the new environment "fits" with the needs of the resident. Resident-facility fit is a key factor in residents' ability to find meaning in their new lives and to "age in place" in their new communities.

Part III / The World of Care

CHAPTER 5

The Business of Caring

Rosie Samuels: "Born to Do This Kinda Work"

Ten years ago, Rosie Samuels, who has just a 10th-grade education, quit her full-time job as an aide at a convalescent home to serve as a live-in caregiver for her cousin, who was suffering from Alzheimer disease. Rosie's Loving Care, which she continues to operate from her cousin's home, began out of necessity as a means of caring for her ill family member and making ends meet. Since then, Rosie has never approached her work as a profit-making venture. She treats her low-income residents, who live with her, as extensions of her family, often dipping into her own pocket to provide needed clothing and toiletry items for them when their family members fall short of their obligations. Like her residents themselves, most of their family members have limited resources, and though Rosie sometimes complains about them, she understands their limitations and tries to fill in for them as best she can.

Rosie herself struggles financially. Because of her residents' low income, she must keep her fees low. Even though she participates in the Community Care Services Program (CCSP), she receives only $14 a day for each participating resident, and her monthly income from the program and residents' fees often falls short of her expenses. Rosie's own medical bills compound her burden. Because her health insurance allows only three doctor visits a year, she often postpones seeking medical care, which contributes to her current poor health. At the age of 62, Rosie's health problems include obesity, diabetes, and hypertension. Recently, her diabetes caused her left eye to hemorrhage, resulting in costly laser treatments to save her eyesight.

Rosie's generous nature often causes her to overextend her resources, contributing to her financial and physical strain. She sometimes keeps residents whose care needs exceed the level of care mandated by state regulations, increasing her workload and putting herself at risk of regulatory sanctions. "I never have the heart to put out somebody," Rosie said. "If I take you when you in good shape and, then when you get in bad shape, I put you out, that makes me feel bad. So I try to keep the people until they pass. I kept a lady here that was bedridden. She couldn't even get up out of bed. She couldn't do anything, and I kept her here until she passed away. Thank God the state [regulators] didn't come out, 'cause they would'a made me put her out."

Her home is licensed for six residents, but Rosie often cares for one or two more. This practice provides her with a little extra income but increases her risk for regulatory penalties. Currently, three residents have significant dementia and need help with bathing, dressing, and toileting, and their frequent urinary accidents lead to extra bed changes, laundry, and mopping. Rosie estimates that she uses 16 to 20 gallons of Clorox a month in addition to regular $65 carpet shampooings.

Because most of Rosie's residents have some degree of mental impairment, she often must contend with problem behaviors, usually having to do with resisting care. Occasionally, Sarah Eubanks, who has schizophrenia, and Cleo Kellog, who is mentally retarded, display aggressive behavior, sometimes toward each other. Tracey Williams, a younger resident with a neurological disorder caused by advanced syphilis, sometimes wanders outside the facility and tries to pick up men on the street, occasionally succeeding. Residents' problem behaviors not only compound Rosie's physical and emotional burden, they also cost her money. Related expenses include repair bills for a clogged toilet and sink, a broken kitchen faucet, and damaged floor tiles, draperies, and furnishings.

Rosie also is generous with her staff, friends, and family members. When one daughter and her husband needed $3,000 for a down payment on a home, Rosie borrowed the money to help them out, and they are not likely to repay the debt. Before the couple moved into their new home, Rosie let them and their infant daughter live with her in exchange for help with chores and resident care. In the early months of the study, two adult grandsons slept on her living room floor. Virginia, a part-time staff person who cannot afford an apartment or transportation to work, sleeps on a cot in the sunroom and keeps her belongings in the medicine cabinet.

Finding dependable help is one of Rosie's biggest frustrations. Because she cannot pay more than minimum wage or offer benefits, her pool of quality personnel is limited. Scarce resources restrict the number of staff she can hire, which means she must perform many tasks herself. Typically, she relies on her own family members, and although three daughters have worked for her, none have felt "called" to the work. Rosie's most recent disappointment came when her oldest daughter, Marilyn, who now works part-time, confessed that her future plans do not include running Rosie's when her mother retires.

Unlike her daughters, Rosie does feel called to her work and often says, "I love taking care of peoples." Her soft, caring voice and the kind, gentle way she interacts with residents, two of whom call her Mama, are testament to Rosie's belief that she was "born to do this kinda work." Her home, she believes, becomes their home: "This is like home. Everybody that has came here to live, they feel at home here." Rosie has few house rules, and her relaxed approach to care contributes, in her view, to the family-like environment: "I don't make it like a production line, like I gotta bathe three people in 15 minutes, and I gotta have breakfast in 15 minutes, and rushing everybody through the house to do this and do that and get ready."

Because of residents' limited family support, Rosie transports all but two of them to their medical appointments (some see as many as four doctors); for residents with mental impairments or speech difficulties, this task includes staying with them and communicating with their physicians. Six residents participate in the CCSP, which requires that residents visit a physician every three months. Although it would be easier to take all the residents to the same clinic, Rosie takes them to their former doctors out of respect for their preferences.

Rosie cannot afford the annual $4,000 liability insurance premium required for transporting residents in her van, which causes her ongoing worry: "Every time I have to take them in my car, I'm praying all the way, don't nothing happen. Even just taking them to a doctor, you are taking a chance." Rosie sometimes relies on a Medicaid-funded nonemergency transportation program to take more-able residents to medical appointments, but recent funding cuts have created additional eligibility requirements. Now, she must schedule transportation three days before the appointment, and recipients must use the nearest qualified health care provider. In addition, Rosie is not comfortable sending residents with cognitive impairment to medical appointments on their own. Rosie's other transportation tasks include picking up medications, buying groceries, and taking residents to senior center programs.

In the face of these challenges, Rosie most values the care she provides for residents: "The most satisfying is when everything is clean, everybody is nutritionally fed, their clothes and the house is upright, and the people are happy. Nobody's wet, everybody's happy watching TV. That's the most satisfying. . . .

I'm doing this because I like it, because it's no money to be made and stacked up in the bank for me."

Although Rosie works hard to provide good care to residents on limited resources, she does not feel supported by the regulatory system. She has been cited by the state Office of Regulatory Services several times for record-keeping deficiencies, including failure to have evidence of training in home evacuation procedures or a signed copy of facility policies and procedures in each resident's file. A particular frustration is the apparent focus of regulators on record keeping rather than on the quality of care she provides: "Some of the things that I have to report and document, it just doesn't make sense. When you come in my home, you can tell from the time you enter the door that I am doing a good job with them. When you look at my patients, you can tell if they're not fed 'cause their ribs gonna be showing or their skin is gonna not look good. It's just a lot of little things that they're asking us to document. You shouldn't have all of this stuff and try to take care of the people, too. I feel it's just too much paperwork."

Rosie's participation in the CCSP provides some extra income, but it comes with additional burdens, including record keeping, and to Rosie, the costs of the program rival the benefits. Officials from the CCSP also have cited Rosie for record-keeping violations and recently insulted her with their concerns about the unkempt appearance of one resident, Joseph Render, a Supplemental Security Income recipient with little family support. Rosie regularly cuts Mr. Render's hair, but owing to her heavy care responsibilities and inadequate help, on this occasion other tasks had taken priority. Moreover, frequent delays in reimbursement from the CCSP make it difficult for Rosie to budget, and her repeated complaints have failed to rectify this problem.

A chief grievance of Rosie's is the failure of the CCSP and other agencies that monitor her home to provide useful training or help in addressing her problems, even those they identify. Because state regulations require that residents have access to "sufficient" planned recreational activities both inside the home and out in the community, a particular need is training in activities for residents with dementia: "What would be useful to me is if the state could provide activities for people that [they] are really able to do. We're not trained in the activity field on how to adjust to the needs of Altimer's patients."

Although Rosie loves caring for her residents, she is having increasing difficulty coping with the many challenges of running her business: "It takes all my time. It's just like I work seven days and seven nights a week." In the summer of 1999, a For Sale sign suddenly appeared in the front yard of Rosie's Loving Care, five months after we gained access to her facility. After 10 years of caring for residents, Rosie had begun the process of closing her home.

Providing Assisted Living for African Americans: Negotiating Risks

Like Rosie Samuels, many small homes providing assisted living (AL) to low-income clients are having difficulty staying in business. As a result, the supply of assisted living facilities (ALFs) serving low-income residents is steadily decreasing. Recent studies show that major factors responsible for this decline include stringent and expensive regulatory requirements, inadequate public support, and neighborhood gentrification (Eckert, Cox, & Morgan, 1999; Morgan, Eckert, & Lyon, 1995; Perkins et al., 2004). Our findings support these earlier studies. Rosie and the other four small-home operators express high levels of commitment and generally provide good care to residents. At the same time, they are subject to considerable physical, emotional, and financial stress owing to the combination of heavy care and administrative responsibilities and low financial compensation, coupled with inadequate support from residents' families and others in the wider community.

The inability of low-income providers to take advantage of economies of scale reduces their profitability (Eckert & Morgan, 2001; Morgan, Eckert, & Lyon, 1995; Stearns & Morgan, 2001), and some operators, like Rosie, barely break even each month or operate at a deficit (Morgan, Eckert, & Lyon, 1995; Perkins et al., 2004). Many residents of these homes pay for their care largely with Supplemental Security Income. In Georgia, one of six states that does not provide a supplement for Supplemental Security Income recipients, these residents live below the established federal poverty level, currently defined as an annual income of $9,310 for an individual. The only state funds available to ALF residents are from the CCSP and allocations to the Georgia Department of Human Resources Division of Mental Health/Mental Retardation/Substance Abuse (MH/MR/SA), and funding from these sources is limited. In 2003 only 15% of CCSP funds were allocated for ALFs (Community Care Services Program, 2003). Funding provided by the Georgia Division of MH/MR/SA varies by region and is limited to facilities that serve individuals with mental illness and mental retardation. Recent fiscal crises threaten both of these programs (Manisses Communications Group, 1999).

Providers' financial burden is intensified by expensive regulatory requirements (for example, structural requirements for fire safety) that do not necessarily result in improvements (Eckert & Morgan, 2001; Morgan, Eckert, &
Lyon, 1995; Perkins et al., 2004; Regnier & Scott, 2001). In Georgia, as in many
other states, small homes must abide by the same regulations and licensing
requirements as larger facilities (Lyon, 1997; Morgan, Eckert, & Lyon, 1995),
and many operators lack sufficient resources to comply. Particular problems
include extensive record-keeping requirements, inadequate training of regulators, and fragmentation of agency responsibility, resulting in inconsisten-
cies between state and county requirements (Morgan, Eckert, & Lyon, 1995;
Reschovsky & Ruchlin, 1993). Navigating this system is especially challenging
for small-home operators, who, like Rosie Samuels, tend to have limited education and may have difficulty dealing with government agencies (Morgan,
Eckert, & Lyon, 1995; Perkins et al., 2004).

The current provider reimbursement rate for the CCSP fails to provide sufficient support for low-income ALF operators. Because they must share the
payment with a provider agency, operators who are licensed for six residents
or fewer are particularly disadvantaged. State reimbursement rates are low
(approximately $14 a day for homes with 6 or fewer beds and $31 a day for
homes with 7 to 15 beds), and participants expressed frustration regarding the
small payments. Blue Skies owner, Clarice Hull, said, "They get all the money,
and I do all the work." Before deciding to sell her home, Rosie planned to
leave the CCSP because of the lack of meaningful benefit, and Esther Adams,
the owner of Peach Blossom, who earlier had abandoned the program, also
felt underpaid: "I don't know why they think small providers should work for
nothing."

Many small ALFs, including Greene's, are located in low-income communities. Municipal services in these areas, such as sanitation services, street
lighting, and public safety, often are substandard, and crime rates tend to be
high. These conditions pose safety risks for residents and providers and limit
prospective clientele. Providers serving low-income residents do not generate
sufficient revenue to upgrade their homes or services. Louis Ashley, the owner
of Sunshine House, described this conundrum: "We're kinda low on the totem
pole in field resources. Therefore, we're able to do less than if this home was
sitting in Buckhead [an affluent, predominately white area located in north
Atlanta] with the same beds. They're able to command $2,000 per resident. If
I could get $2,000 for a resident, I can think of a lot of things that I could do

to improve the physical structure here, to improve our programming, to improve quality of care and all of that. But when you're getting a fourth of that, it makes it much more difficult to run and operate. You know, the problems of the community tend to be the problems of the home. Do we receive the same services from the government, from the city that somewhere up north receives? I don't think so."

Homes located in low- to moderate-income areas also are at risk as neighborhoods gentrify; in some cases, neighborhood groups have forced facilities to close or relocate (Morgan, Eckert, & Lyon, 1995). As property values increased in her area, Greene's owner, Cora Greene, experienced ongoing problems with her local neighborhood association: "Within the last two years when the area start[ed] to develop for the better, I think [the neighborhood association] was questionable about my being here and sent peoples out to do the inspection of my home, you know, the zoning department men, because [my neighbors] wanted me to leave." Increases in property values also have resulted in higher property taxes. During the course of the study period, Ms. Greene's property taxes doubled.

In the face of such overwhelming barriers, small-home providers have devised creative strategies to manage residents' care needs and maintain their businesses. We have labeled this survival process "negotiating risks" (Perkins, 2002; Perkins et al., 2004). This process, which sometimes requires risking regulatory sanctions, involves continuing negotiation (or compromise) to meet facility resource needs and manage the care needs of residents. Paradoxically, this survival process sometimes results in risks that compromise residents' care and threaten providers' ability to stay in business.

Even Oak Manor, a facility with an affluent clientele, must negotiate risks because of its pioneer status in the untapped (and untested) market of upscale AL care for African Americans. Jordan Taylor, a corporate representative, said that since Oak Manor is "very new to the African American community," fees are set lower than in other facilities owned by the same corporation. Although low relative to comparable facilities, fees still are high ($2,095 to $3,645) relative to the population served because the financial status of many elderly African Americans does not match that of their white counterparts. According to executive director Kathy Wall, many family members who help pay fees struggle with multiple financial obligations, including children's college tuition. Attracting and retaining African American residents who can afford the high fees, therefore, is a challenge.

Compared with the five small homes in this study, a principal difference in the survival process at Oak Manor is the emphasis on regulatory compliance. Most residents and their family members expect services to be commensurate with the high fees. These consumers, who generally are more educated and knowledgeable about regulations than those in small homes, are more likely to file complaints when they feel that standards are not being met. These same savvy consumers may be less likely to choose or remain in a facility that has received excessive citations and more likely to file a lawsuit when they perceive negligence. Ironically, emphasis on regulatory compliance and concerns about liability limit the types of residents that providers can admit or retain. At the beginning of the study period, Oak Manor was only one-third occupied.

As pioneers seeking to stake out a niche in the competitive AL market, providers at Oak Manor, like those in the small homes, must continually balance facility resources with the needs of residents, staff, and residents' family members. Many factors, including hiring and retaining quality staff, influence its survival, which ultimately depends on the ability to make and sustain a profit. According to one facility administrator, "Like any business, it's all about the bottom line."

Although the small-home owners are most vulnerable, providers in all six facilities face considerable risk. Admission and discharge polices, staffing, administrative procedures, and service provision reflect the strategies they use to manage risks. Paradoxically, these risk-managing strategies often incur risks of their own. In all homes, the meanings that providers' attach to their roles form the context of this negotiation process. Each home's unique care environment reflects both the meaning of roles for providers (including not only those who provide direct care but those who provide funding and corporate direction as well) and the strategies they use to negotiate risks.

Communities of Care: Six Unique Care Environments

On the basis of the results of our study, we discuss the six unique care environments in terms of three general models of operation: the family model, the small-business model, and the corporate model. Rosie's and Peach Blossom, where the owners live in their facilities and provide substantial hands-on care, represent the family model. In these homes, part-time workers help with cleaning and caregiving duties. Blue Skies, Greene's, and Sunshine House represent the small-business model. The owners of these homes do not live on-site; instead, they rely heavily on managers who run the home in their absence. In both models, the personalities and management style of owners and managers shape the home's care environment. Another important influence is the presence of providers' family members. Oak Manor represents the corporate model, in which individuals at the corporate level set policies, including those regarding care and service provision. In addition to a large team of full- and part-time direct care staff, the facility employs a variety of specialized upper-level staff.

The Family Model: "The Residents Become Family"

Rosie's Loving Care and Peach Blossom typify the small, family-based homes described in the literature on small board-and-care homes (Eckert, Cox, & Morgan, 1999; Morgan, Eckert, & Lyon, 1995; Namazi et al., 1989). These homes represent a long tradition of care in the United States that dates back to the early nineteenth century, when dependent and displaced people were housed in the private homes of charity-minded members of the community (Morgan, Eckert, & Lyon, 1995; Namazi & Chafetz, 2001). In response to inadequate public funding for community-based care, home-based caregivers, who often were poor themselves, offered these services. Recent studies describe the typical modern version of this family model home as small in scale and characterized by intimate and lasting bonds between caregivers and care recipients (Eckert, Cox, & Morgan, 1999). Instead of being motivated solely by financial gain, many of these caregivers view their work as an important contribution to their communities (Eckert, Cox, & Morgan, 1999; Morgan, Eckert, & Lyon, 1995).

Although Rosie's and Peach Blossom fit many characteristics of the family-based board-and-care model described in the literature, the care environments of these two homes vary significantly. Rosie Samuels and Esther Adams both attach altruistic meaning to their roles as care providers and view their residents as extended family, yet their methods of providing care and running their businesses differ substantially. Just as families differ, the family-like environment of these homes differs.

Rosie's Care Home: "Everybody Is Not Born and Built for This Kinda Job"

Unlike some providers who are more business oriented, Rosie is not motivated by the need for profit. Her goal is to live comfortably in her own home and provide adequately for her residents and others, including staff and her own family members who rely on her for support. In an effort to fulfill her caregiving role, though, Rosie often overextends her resources, putting her own health and financial security at risk.

Rosie's decision to admit residents with heavier care needs is influenced by her participation in the CCSP, which mandates that clients be deemed eligible for nursing home care. Rosie describes her policy in this way: "I take ambulatory [residents] and people that can go to the toilet, that I can assist to the bathroom. As long as they can tell me they got to go to the bathroom. But as they grow older here, they [may] not say, 'I got to go to the bathroom.'" Because Rosie keeps residents as they decline, she has "had as many as three or four people using a diaper." Another strategy Rosie uses to maximize her income is to operate above her licensed capacity. During the study, she had two "extra" residents, originally introduced as friends, "just visiting." The downside of this strategy is the increased workload and the danger of regulatory penalties.

An important resource for Rosie is her own large, tight-knit family. Her family members often spend time in the facility, socializing with Rosie and her residents and helping with chores. In addition to her three daughters who have worked for her, several other family members regularly involve themselves in the home. Her two adult grandsons, while they lived in the facility, helped with cooking, cleaning, yard work, and resident oversight; her brother frequently stops by and sometimes conducts Bible study; and numerous younger grandchildren often can be found at the home. Rosie likes having children around, and their presence adds to the home's family-like atmosphere. Some even help with household chores, such as vacuuming and raking leaves.

During the past year, Rosie's most valuable source of support has been her daughter Marilyn, who assumed operation of the home while Rosie was hospitalized for an infection in her foot caused by diabetes and now works part-time. Unlike Rosie, Marilyn has an eye for business and helps Rosie manage her books and maintain required records. She also takes residents to medical appointments, cleans, and cooks. Marilyn's recent decision to change professions has been an important factor in Rosie's decision to close her home. According to Rosie, some people, like Marilyn, are "not born and built for this kinda job." Although she was willing to care for her mother when Rosie "got sick and down-and-out" and provides competent care, Marilyn "don't care too much for old people." She does not enjoy spending time with the residents, nor does she have her mother's warm approach. The different meanings the two women attribute to caregiving are reflected in their varying care strategies. Marilyn's more regimented way of caregiving contrasts sharply with her mother's relaxed approach. Rosie's casual nature, though, may be the root of her financial failure.

Esther Adams: "A House Is Not a Home without Rules"

At the age of 70, Esther Adams has been in the AL business for 20 years. Like Rosie, she felt called to care for elders. When she was a child, her family members instilled in her values to help elderly neighbors and relatives. Before starting her business, Ms. Adams worked first as a home health aide, where she developed caregiving skills and expertise. Later, when her own children were young, she cared for foster children.

Ms. Adams views her residents at Peach Blossom as "extended family," and like Rosie, she tends to keep her residents a long time. Bobby Bailey, a 78-year-old resident with mental retardation, has lived with her since she opened her home. Although Ms. Adams develops close bonds with residents and is willing to keep those with significant impairments, she prefers residents who adhere to her care "system:" "I don't mind hands-on [care]. What I need is a little cooperation." She is quick to discharge residents who challenge her authority or refuse to follow house rules.

During the admissions process, Ms. Adams screens residents carefully to make sure they are a good match for her home and "fit in" with her family: "I screen. I don't take everybody. I want people who are compatible, can sit quietly watching TV, and don't create a fuss." Ms. Adams tries to admit residents who are docile and easy to control, and they must be at least 60 years of age: because her home is located near an area with liquor stores, she is afraid that younger residents might get into drugs and alcohol, and she wants to avoid worrying about "people in the streets." She tries to visit prospective residents and their families in their homes and have residents spend time in her facility before moving in, so that "by the time they come here, we are not total strangers."

Ms. Adams also requires that "families have a role," and rarely does she admit residents who do not have significant support from family or friends. Her attitude toward families is this: "You are paying me, but I can't do it all." She expects them to assume all health care responsibilities, including taking residents to medical appointments, and to supply clothing, toiletries, and incontinence supplies. After residents move in, she has no qualms about asking their family members for needed items, and she strongly encourages them to visit regularly and take residents home on holidays.

When a resident's condition deteriorates, Ms. Adams negotiates with the family for a higher fee: "I just tell them what it would cost, based on the level of care. I don't ask what they have, because I found that was not the way to do it. I just tell them what [the fee] is, and the family member that's in charge find[s] a way to do it." Although Ms. Adams's residents have higher incomes than residents in the other small homes, their resources are limited, and her strategy is not always successful. This economic limitation, she says, goes with the territory: "I suppose when we decide we want to do a certain business, we know there are certain ramifications. One of the things in this business is the economic situation. I decided that I wanted to provide a service, and, along with providing a service, sometimes you're not always satisfied with the results." Another strategy Ms. Adams uses to increase her income is to keep residents on a temporary basis and provide respite for families, a service for which she charges five dollars an hour. During the study, she cared for four respite residents (from 2 to 12 days). Only occasionally has this practice caused her to operate above licensed capacity.

Ms. Adams opened her home just before Georgia adopted AL regulations in 1981. Although she contends fairly well with compliance, she complains that regulators do not consider the problems faced in most small homes: residents' low income and heavy care needs, she believes, make it difficult for small-home providers to "do all these extra things" that regulations require. Occasionally, Ms. Adams breaks the rules, such as when she used a bed rail in an attempt to keep Viola Wheeler from falling at night. Her strategy is to follow "the golden rule first and then the state rules next."

Ms. Adams's authoritarian manner, like Rosie's more relaxed way, is not unlike the one she assumed in raising her own children. Although she depends on part-time help, she performs much of the ADL care herself. Since most of her residents are incontinent and half require constant supervision and direction performing ADLs, having "a system" or "structured environment" makes her job manageable. Like Rosie, she encourages residents' participation in day programs, which provides her with needed respite and gives her residents regular access to recreational and spiritual activities. Another important resource is her own family, especially three daughters who live in Atlanta. Ms. Adams has instilled a strong sense of family loyalty in her daughters, and they are a constant source of both instrumental and emotional support.

Both Ms. Adams and Rosie belong to an association for small-home providers, which gives them an opportunity to network. Currently, this group is working with the Assisted Living Association of Georgia, a state provider association, to change AL regulations for small homes. Ms. Adams complains that the "big people" (providers at large homes) manipulate the system, and "we [small-home providers] are not given credit for the job we do."

Looking back over her 20-year career as an assisted living provider, Ms. Adams feels that the "the ups outweigh the downs": "I've accomplished what I wanted, a home away from home. A business should progress. My goal is to provide quality service. I feel I've met these goals because I get referrals. Even those I've discharged refer me. I feel I have rendered a service, that people have confidence their loved ones are taken care of."

The Small-Business Model: "I Bought This House for a Reason"

The three small-business model providers in this study represent a long tradition of ethnic entrepreneurship in the United States, defined by some researchers as "bootstrap capitalism" (Basu & Werbner, 2001). Faced with few opportunities for employment in the mainstream labor market, many African Americans and immigrants have achieved social mobility and economic success through self-employment. Like these small-home owners, ethnic entrepreneurs often serve their own communities and recruit members of their own ethnic groups, including family members, into their businesses (Basu & Werbner, 2001; House, 2000; Logan, Alba, & Stulus, 2003). Frequently, these small businesses expand within particular industries, like AL, creating entrepreneurial chains or enclaves (Basu & Werbner, 2001). Several social and cultural factors contribute to their success, including support from kinship networks and members of one's own community, the availability of entrepreneurial role models, development of support networks for mutual benefit, and a strong achievement orientation (House, 2000). Successful economic development through these small businesses strengthens ethnic communities by providing career paths and job opportunities and creating funds for education and home ownership.

In contrast to operators of the family model homes, operators of the three small-business model homes are strongly motivated by the desire for financial gain. Cora Greene, the owner of Greene's, and Clarice Hull, the owner of Blue Skies, are both ambitious entrepreneurs who hope to expand their businesses and one day own a chain of homes. Louis Ashley, the owner of Sunshine

House, has a professional career outside of assisted living, and he operates his ALF on the side for investment purposes. Because they do not share living space with residents, all three of these providers maintain some degree of separation between their roles as AL provider and their private lives. Of the three, Ms. Greene is the most involved in the day-to-day operation of her home. She spends time in the home every weekday and performs a wide range of tasks, including direct care. Clarice, who works full-time as a nanny, fills in at her facility on weekends when part-time staff are unavailable. Mr. Ashley does the weekly grocery shopping and stops by his facility almost daily to check on residents and staff, but he provides no direct care.

Although their primary focus is on business, these providers also have altruistic motives. Mr. Ashley believes that his role as an ALF owner is to "give something back to the community." Ms. Greene strives to be the "caring person" that her parents raised her to be. Clarice "need[s] to give back the love to someone, even though I am getting paid for it." She believes that in pursuing a caregiving career, she is honoring the memory of her deceased grandmother, who raised her in Jamaica. As with the family model providers, common themes in the narratives of these small-business model providers include the importance of family and community.

Blue Skies: "I Was Here for Five Months with No Residents"

Clarice Hull came to New York from her native Jamaica as a young adult. After working in a nursing home for 11 years and saving money, she moved to Atlanta, where she has connections among a large community of Jamaican immigrants, many of whom work in the AL industry. Two years later, Clarice bought Blue Skies, a residential home, and applied for a license to operate it as an ALF; it is now licensed for six residents. Since then, she has purchased a second small ALF, licensed for four residents, and is in the process of buying a third. Although Clarice is considered successful among her peers in the Jamaican community, her homes are not yet profitable.

When the study began, Blue Skies had been open for only six months and had remained empty for the first five. At the suggestion of another Jamaican AL operator, Clarice applied to participate in the CCSP in order to have a ready source of residents. She soon recruited four CCSP residents. Although Clarice relies on the CCSP to fill beds, she prefers the higher private-pay fees and reserves one private room, the largest and nicest room in the house, for such residents. Like Esther Adams, Clarice bases private-pay fees on care needs. Mamie

Hoover, aged 97, who needs help with all ADLs and has frequent bowel accidents, pays the highest rate ($1,000 a month). On occasion, Clarice has charged her an extra "cleaning" fee for accidents. During the study, three of the eight Blue Skies residents were private-pay clients. Clarice struggles to keep her beds full, and at different times during the study, her census dropped to only four or five residents.

Clarice's participation in the CCSP has produced a diverse group of residents who vary in age (from 24 to 97 years), race (three are white), and disability. Gary Cotter, a 24-year-old, has Down syndrome, and Terry Prospect, age 26, has multiple sclerosis. Although this heterogeneity sometimes leads to conflict, some residents have developed close ties. Clarice compares the situation in her small home with that of families: "Residents don't always get along, but that's just like families." Because she values a family-like environment, Clarice is more likely to discharge residents who disrupt the social balance of her home than those with heavy care needs, and she often uses threats of discharge to control problem behaviors. When this strategy did not work with Gary, Clarice raised his fees. Now Gary's mother works in the home on weekends to offset the fee increase and helps Clarice with her son's discipline, effectively preventing his discharge. Like Esther Adams, Clarice expects family members to provide most IADL care, including transportation to medical appointments, though her interactions with them are not always positive. One problem has been language and culture barriers between family members and the Jamaican staff.

With the exception of Gary's mother and one African American who worked only for a short while, Clarice has employed only Jamaicans recruited through the Jamaican community and pays staff "under the table" to avoid Social Security taxes. Since becoming a U.S. citizen, Inez Sawyer, a 40-year-old Jamaican woman who served as the facility's on-site manager for most of the study, has expressed concern about working in an "undocumented" job and even threatened to quit. Inez's employment options, however, are limited by lack of proficiency with English and her inability to drive a car or operate a computer.

Inez lives in the facility each week from Monday morning until Friday night and with her daughter on weekends. She is a responsible manager who prides herself on keeping the home clean and organized, but she has a controlling manner. More submissive residents get along best with Inez, and some of these "pets" receive more individualized care. Although some Blue Skies workers are not as strict, their casual mode of operation verges on neglect. Angel, a 23-year-old Jamaican who works on the weekends, often leaves the facility and residents unattended to spend time with her boyfriend, Clarice's brother-in-law. Other workers, because of language difficulties, are unable to record medications correctly, a failure that has led to a citation from the Office of Regulatory Services.

Clarice herself is quite competent and relates well to residents, but the limited time she has to devote to Blue Skies and her lack of attention to regulations has resulted in several citations. Despite problems with regulators and representatives of the Long-Term Care Ombudsman Program, Clarice receives invaluable support from the county fire marshal, who regularly visits her home and helps her correct deficiencies. Her family members also help. Her husband performs yard work and all household maintenance, and her sister often fills in as staff. Despite this support, Clarice finds operating a small ALF stressful. Her biggest frustrations are problems with residents' families and keeping beds occupied: "No one knows how hard this [job] is and how many hours we work."

Greene's Personal Care Home: "I Balance It Any Way I Can"

Fifteen years ago, Cora Greene inherited her business from its elderly owner, her employer and AL mentor. Before this, she worked in an older sister's ALF and as an outreach worker for a county mental health program, experience that gave her valuable skills for dealing with residents with mental illness.

Since her home opened, Ms. Greene's family has been very involved in its operation. Her husband takes care of all household maintenance and yard work and sometimes helps care for residents. Several siblings have been staff persons, including a younger brother, who sometimes picks up residents' medication and takes them shopping or to the doctor. Three of her most supportive siblings have opened their own homes and now are available to help only in emergencies.

Ms. Greene views staffing as one of her biggest frustrations. Her pool of quality staff is limited, and she continually deals with problems such as theft, drug abuse, and absenteeism. One strategy she uses is employing older workers and people with disabilities who lack other employment options. Recently, she hired Mandy, an older woman who attends the same senior center as her residents, to fill in as on-site manager and help with cooking. Other strategies include employing people who need room and board and allowing some residents to serve as staff. By supplementing their wages with food and shelter, Ms. Greene is able to pay live-in staff less than minimum wage. Generally, she pays such workers in cash, does not list them in official facility records, and schedules them at night and on weekends, when regulators and other officials are less likely to visit. During the study period, we identified two "residents" who appeared to be staff. Both had histories of mental illness, and neither was listed as a resident in facility records. Using these strategies, Ms. Greene avoids the radar of government authorities.

Ms. Greene believes that she can operate efficiently during regular business hours with at least one responsible staff person to act as on-site manager, administer medications, handle emergencies, and deal with regulators and other outside authorities when she is away from the facility (for example, when she is transporting residents to medical appointments or the senior center). Maintaining even this level of efficiency often proves difficult, however. Finding a responsible night manager is almost impossible. The current night manager, though dependable, lacks competence to dispense medications. Because Ms. Greene doubts his ability to care for residents, she remains in the facility until her residents have taken their evening medication and gone to bed, and she is therefore thankful for "early bedders." Maintaining adequate staff is even more challenging on weekends, when family responsibilities keep her at home.

Because of staffing limitations, Ms. Greene typically admits only elders with minimal physical and mental impairments or higher-functioning middle-aged adults with mental illness. These admission policies have produced a "very mixed group" whose common denominator is a minimal need for hands-on care. Ms. Greene's primary source of residents is County Hospital, where the home is known to discharge planners. Recently, she recruited several residents from an unlicensed ALF that was closed by the state, and she occasionally receives a new resident "through word of mouth."

Ms. Greene also bases admission decisions and fees on residents' ability to pay and their care needs: "Basically, I look at what their earnings is. I look at what I have to do for them, you know, that type thing. That's why I keep 'em on a scale. Suppose I had everybody here that couldn't pay nothing, [for example] $334 a month. None of us would be here. So, therefore, if I got a person that is receiving $1,200, $1,400 a month, $900 is not too much to ask. Family members not gonna come out of their pocket with no more money. Ain't no family members, you know, so I just charge accordingly to what they're receiving."

Discharge of residents usually results from a decline in function. Rarely does Ms. Greene tolerate incontinence or the inability to perform ADLs, though when she has accommodating workers, she is more lax. Over the course of the study, discharge policies evolved from lenient to strict along with staff unwillingness to assist with ADL care. Sometimes Ms. Greene negotiates with a resident, a strategy hinging on factors such as a resident's tenure, income, and compliance with care regimens.

Ms. Greene's primary goals are succeeding in business, creating a better life for her family, and securing her retirement. To meet these goals, she engages in certain unauthorized activities, primarily operating her home over the licensed capacity and admitting temporary residents for rehabilitation following a hospital stay. To hide these additional residents, Ms. Greene routinely shifts various permanent residents between an unlicensed home she operates on an adjacent lot and her own family home, though she risks having her facility shut down by state regulators by using this creative strategy.

Despite serious regulatory infractions, Ms. Greene has to date received few citations. Regulators typically focus on facility records, which Ms. Greene keeps current and matched with the "official" residents. Her residents, many of whom have been homeless or lived in worse conditions, are by and large happy with their care and view Greene's as their best available option, even though they are routinely moved to accommodate temporary residents and do not always receive adequate care.

Although Ms. Greene's tactics are questionable, her willingness to dip into her own pocket to give residents (most of whom have no family support) necessities such as clothing and toiletry items reflects her value for providing good care. This value also is evident in the extra time she spends searching for bargains so that she can provide nutritious meals. Her full schedule (which includes record keeping, transporting most of her residents to medical appointments, and picking up medication) means she often is unavailable to fulfill all resident care needs. Residents have their own strategies to compensate for this lack. Others receive assistance (for example, with haircuts and other grooming needs) at local community programs.

Sunshine House: "There Are Lots of Things We Could Improve If We Had the Resources"

Louis Ashley opened Sunshine House 15 years ago, and managing it requires far more work than he envisioned. Like Cora Greene, he considers staffing one of the most difficult tasks, and like Clarice Hull, he struggles to keep his beds occupied. Although Mr. Ashley maintains that he is not in the AL business "for the profit," he is often concerned about losing money: "When the owner walks through and sees empty beds, he starts to think about the dollars that aren't there. It's not to be inhumane, but you have to think about it. I have to protect my investment."

For years, most of Mr. Ashley's residents were elders recruited from the facility's low- to moderate-income African American community. Now, his residents resemble those at Greene's—a mix of elderly residents with minimal disability and younger residents with mental illness. Because he is "kinda hard pressed for residents," Mr. Ashley has begun recruiting residents from a public psychiatric facility, but this strategy creates new problems because discharge planners, pushed to place patients, often fail to provide accurate patient information. Recently, Mr. Ashley unknowingly admitted a resident with a history of violence, who subsequently assaulted a staff person and had to be discharged.

As an absentee owner, Mr. Ashley relies heavily on Kay Hughes, his manager and "right hand." In addition to providing direct care, Kay helps manage staff, participates in admission and discharge decisions, conducts weekly inventories of food and supplies, and handles record keeping. Kay regularly works from seven at night until seven in the morning, and she is also on call during the day to answer questions and handle emergencies. Unlike the other staff, who receive minimum wage, Kay is paid a weekly salary, which nonetheless amounts to little more, and she receives no health benefits. Kay often works extra shifts, and these increased responsibilities have taken a toll on her health.

When Kay is not at Sunshine House, other staff sometimes fail to follow directions and complete required tasks. A recurring problem has been their failure to adhere to the posted menu, which has resulted in regulatory citations. Mr. Ashley tries to visit the home at least daily to check on residents and monitor staff, but his primary job and family responsibilities limit his involvement. In an effort to find reliable staff, Mr. Ashley, like Cora Greene, often hires "mature" women, but because many of these older workers are not physically able to do heavy care work, he does not admit or retain residents with heavy care needs. Although four elderly female residents receive some assistance with bathing and dressing, none of the younger male residents needs any help with ADLs. Mr. Ashley expects residents' family members or mental health caseworkers to provide all IADL care, including transportation to medical appointments.

Given the home's limited budget, Mr. Ashley considers his "good relationships" with the community central to the management of the home. A friend of Mr. Ashley's, who is a minister, provides part-time home maintenance, and neighbors help keep tabs on his male residents, who spend most of their time out in the community: "If they see 'em in the street and they think they're doing something they're not supposed to be doing, they'll come and report it to us."

Mr. Ashley acknowledges that lack of revenue limits the services he can provide, but he still derives a sense of satisfaction from the important contribution he makes to his community as an AL operator: "Well you know, it provides me with a good sense of self-satisfaction, even though I'm doing things on a small scale. There are benefits to the community in small ways. We're providing a base of employment for some people. We're providing [a personal care place for] residents who can't afford high fees. We try to make sure that we do the best we can in terms of the quality of what they receive. It has to correlate with the kind of monies that we receive. We think we do a pretty good job that way."

The Corporate Model: "Our Mission Is to Provide the Highest Quality Care"

Oak Manor belongs to a rapidly growing industry that caters to an affluent clientele. In contrast to the small owner-operated homes, this upscale, contemporary AL model generally is represented by new construction and has gained increasing popularity among owners and developers in the real estate and hotel industries (Kalymun, 1992; Regnier, Hamilton, and Yatabe, 1995). A common theme in this industry, particularly among homes in the corporate sector, is a philosophy that emphasizes consumer choice and independence, and Oak Manor subscribes to this principle. This large, corporate model home—built with the specific purpose of providing assisted living—offers a broad array of personal care and supportive services aimed at upholding its ideology. Other characteristics that distinguish Oak Manor from the small homes in this study are its physical and social environment, the type of resident served, the number and type of staff employed, and the staff's overall training and education level.

Oak Manor was the first African American ALF of its kind in Atlanta and possibly the nation, but it would not be the only one for long. When it opened in the fall of 1999, administrators and corporate executives acknowledged that "competition was right around the corner, literally": another upscale African American ALF was being built in the same affluent African American community, and soon Oak Manor would lose its monopoly in this market.

From the beginning, Oak Manor has engaged in an intense marketing campaign. An on-site marketing director, as well as other Oak Manor administrators and corporate representatives, actively participate in this campaign. To facilitate these efforts, the corporate office hired a "marketing guru," who provides training and is heavily involved in making the facility well known to Atlanta's African American community. In addition to inviting interested parties to the facility and giving on-site tours, the marketing director and other administrators make presentations in the community once or twice a week, often using a "lunch and learn" format. Groups they target include churches, health care professionals, hospital discharge planners, and senior groups. Initially, the focus was the neighboring affluent African American community, but now corporate officials have recognized the need to "spread marketing efforts all over Atlanta."

Oak Manor, like other upscale ALFs, offers a broad range of personal care services, including help with ADLs, scheduled weekly shopping trips and medical transportation, individualized care plans, daily planned social and recreational activities, "restaurant-style" meals, and access to a "wellness program" supervised by a licensed nurse. The facility also partners with a university geriatric hospital that provides regular on-site consultations regarding residents' care. Because of the prevalence of diabetes in the African American community, the facility, unlike others in its corporate chain, offers a diabetes management program.

Residents at Oak Manor pay a basic monthly fee determined by the floor plan of their units. Weekly housekeeping and laundering of bed linens and towels are included in this basic rate, but personal laundry services are an additional $50 a month. "To ensure continuity of care," the facility offers three levels of ADL care in addition to a separate dementia care program. Additional fees for care are based on need. Regular medication management charges are $150 a month, and residents who take more than nine medications a day or have complex medication needs (such as daily injections or special measurements of medications) pay an additional $100 a month. Residents also pay additional fees for incontinence and diabetes management. At least in theory, this method of pricing allows the facility to staff according to residents' care needs.

Admission policies are set by the corporate office and are based on state AL regulations, as explained by Kathy Wall, the home's executive director: "As far as the personal care guidelines for assisted living, they must be able either to ambulate by walker, wheelchair, cane, etc. They must be able to transfer with the minimum [assistance] of one person. If it takes two people to do it, they are not appropriate for assisted living." Oak Manor also does not admit potentially combative residents. Discharge policies reflect the criteria for admission. Although ALFs can obtain waivers to retain hospice residents, Kathy indicated that her facility is unwilling to consider this alternative because of possible liability.

To determine residents' appropriateness for assisted living, the resident services director conducts an assessment of residents' functional abilities before admission. This evaluation, which includes a mental status exam, supplements the state-required physician's assessment and, for residents who are admitted, guides care plans. Residents are reassessed 30 days after moving in and thereafter at three-month intervals and after changes in health status or a hospitalization. According to an administrator, this comprehensive assessment process is based on the facility's "philosophy about individualizing."

To build a good reputation in the community and keep beds occupied, administrators and owners recognize the importance of customer satisfaction. To corporate representative Jordan Taylor, it is key: "If people aren't happy, they're going to move down the street . . . or cross town to the competition." Although hiring and retaining high-quality staff are integral to this effort, high staff turnover has been a significant problem at Oak Manor. The facility offers health benefits and bases its pay scale on averages in the Atlanta market, but that pay, beginning at seven dollars an hour, is low.

Oak Manor's emphasis on customer satisfaction has paid off. The facility is not yet full, but only one of the 26 residents who have moved out did so because of dissatisfaction with services. The facility also has successfully met regulatory standards. According to an administrator, "When [the Office of Regulatory Services] came in and did the annual survey, we were deficiency free." Although regulators have returned twice since their last annual inspection to investigate anonymous complaints, they decided the complaints, attributed to a disgruntled former employee, were unfounded.

Despite Oak Manor's success, employees are "under tremendous pressure from corporate to fill beds." "In a home that is not full," says Taylor, "obviously there is an operating deficit. The goal is not to be putting money into it anymore, because it should be creating a positive cash flow. It is a business. It is not a nonprofit, and we have promised investors a specific return on their investment, and we've got to provide that to them." With regard to Oak Manor's target population, he says, "It is an all–African American home today. It might not be tomorrow"—implying that, if it became necessary, they would market to the white community.

Communities of Care: The Role of Race, Class, and Culture

Throughout this book, we draw upon the life course perspective to examine how participants adapt to stressful life events based on knowledge from past experience and the use of personal resources (Clausen, 1986; Holstein & Gubrium, 2000). The five small-home operators in this study, like their residents, have a history of disadvantage. Although they represent different cultural and class backgrounds, all have experienced racism and have acquired skills necessary to survive in an oppressive system.

To manage the care needs of residents and survive economically, these small-home owners employ a variety of adaptive and risk-managing strategies, sometimes involving illicit activities. Ironically, these strategies, which we call "negotiating risks," often compromise resident care and jeopardize this very survival. Our findings support previous research demonstrating that poor people, when confronted with few legitimate sources for subsistence, engage in unauthorized activities to cope (Edin & Lein, 1997; Fine & Weis, 1998; Newman, 1999; Valentine, 1978). Such activities often demonstrate innovation and involve considerable labor, dispelling the popular myth that people are poor because they are ignorant and unwilling to work. Furthermore, our study confirms findings from recent research (Hill, 1999) showing that African Americans and black persons of Caribbean origin share important cultural strengths, including a strong work ethic and a high achievement motivation. The small-home providers in this study draw upon these strengths to maintain their businesses against overwhelming odds. Other important resources they share include close family ties, strong religious values, and supportive social and community networks.

Although these small-home owners have commonalities, each is unique. Important distinguishing features include individual traits, such as personality and temperament, and the personal meanings they attach to caregiving.

These attributes form the context in which providers negotiate risks. Rosie, who is highly religious, believes that she has been "called" to her work by God. Besides caring for residents, she has cared for various family and fictive kin throughout her life. Her facility's family-like environment reflects her spiritual commitment to caregiving, and her strategies for negotiating risks focus on fulfilling residents' needs, often at her own expense and to the detriment of her business. Although Esther Adams has much in common with Rosie Samuels, her superior business skills and regimented care system enable her to provide quality care without overextending her resources. In contrast, Cora Greene struggles endlessly to be (and be considered) a "caring person," but her strategies to "balance it" often tip the scales in favor of maintaining profitability. Her foremost goal, to provide a better life for her family, often compromises resident care. Similarly, despite Clarice Hull's efforts to provide a family-like environment at Blue Skies, her strategies often favor economic success, sometimes at the expense of residents and staff. Because Louis Ashley has a professional career outside of the AL industry, he assumes less economic risk than the other four small-home providers. Although, like Ms. Greene and Clarice, he is primarily motivated by profit, he is less willing than they to risk regulatory sanctions.

Administrators and corporate employees responsible for running Oak Manor face major challenges in securing a niche in the competitive AL market. They recognize that the facility's staying power ultimately depends on making and sustaining a profit by keeping beds occupied, and they consider customer satisfaction the key to achieving this goal. Because these providers believe that keeping customers happy includes upholding high regulatory standards, they emphasize regulatory compliance. Ironically, this emphasis, together with concerns about liability, leads to increased restrictions on admission and retention, which ultimately impede the facility's ability to fill beds.

Each facility's unique care environment reflects both the meanings providers attach to their roles and the strategies they use to negotiate risks. Race, class, and culture also play an important part in shaping these communities. At Oak Manor, these variables are selling points. In the small ALFs, they serve as protective factors in providers' ability to adapt and thrive.

CHAPTER 6

The Soul of Self-Care

For Madonna McDowell, a resident of Rosie's Loving Care, "It's important to be able to do things for yourself, rather than to depend on someone to do it for you." Her words echo the strong value for independence shared by most people with disabilities and most residents of the six care communities in our study. Yet the reality for Ms. McDowell and other assisted living residents is one of at least some dependence. The inevitable clashes between value and reality have been termed the "dilemmas of dependency" (Lustbader, 1991). Central to these dilemmas is the loss of control over one's life that accompanies the loss of ability to "do for oneself," which remains a basic value of older persons with disabling chronic conditions. Studies of disabled elders still living in their own homes (Ball & Whittington, 1995; Lustbader, 1991), as well as of those who have moved to assisted living facilities (Ball et al., 2000; Ball et al., 2004b; Carder & Hernandez, 2004; Mitchell & Kemp, 2000) or nursing homes (Wieland, Rubenstein, & Hirsch, 1995), demonstrate that even individuals with considerable disability struggle to take care of their own daily needs and resist dependence on others.

In this chapter, we continue our strengths-based approach and focus not on dependence and the care residents receive but rather on residents' remaining independence and their own roles in care (self-care). We see residents' best efforts, however small, as the soul of self-care.

Concepts of Independence and Self-Care

According to Hofland (1990), independence represents the physical dimension of the broader concept, autonomy. This physical dimension concerns freedom of mobility, physical independence, and the restrictiveness of the environment. It is separate from the psychological dimension, which involves control over one's environment and choice of options, and from the spiritual, relating to a continuity in the sense of personal identity over time and decision making consistent with an individual's long-term values and life meaning. Although the logical association between the ability to perform daily tasks independently and autonomy makes it easy to "glide into" equating the two concepts, such merging has been called "conceptual error," since some autonomy can be maintained even by people with substantial disability (Kane, 1991). Yet separating the concepts is not so simple. Collopy (1990) distinguishes decisional autonomy from autonomy of execution. As the labels imply, decisional autonomy refers to the capacity to make decisions about one's life, and autonomy of execution entails the freedom and ability to carry them out. Collopy's distinction reminds us that for physical independence to have meaning it must be accompanied by autonomy, that is, the freedom to act independently. In this chapter we focus on independence as captured by Hofland's physical dimension of autonomy. We address autonomy, the psychological and spiritual dimensions, in chapter 9.

The term *self-care* also has received varying conceptualizations in the literature. Viewed narrowly, *self-care* denotes responding to and coping with illness or a medical problem (Hickey, 1980). When applied to older adults, self-care frequently is defined to include a broad range of behaviors undertaken by individuals, often with support from others, to maintain or promote health and functional independence and to cope with chronic illness (Mockenhaupt, 1993; Ory, DeFriese, & Duncker, 1998). In discussing self-care in institutional settings, Small (1993) broadens the definition still more to include ADLs. In this book, we use *self-care* to refer to the ways that residents take care of themselves in these communities, including daily living (both ADL and IADL) and health care activities. Residents' independence is closely connected to their self-care roles, and the soul of self-care is the essence for these impaired residents of maintaining a whole identity and the crux of their quality of life.

Doing Self-Care

Two Profiles

At the age of 85, Eugene Ellis, like many elderly residents, has multiple disabling chronic problems. His feet swell, his joints ache, and his vision is deteriorating. He walks slowly and only with the aid of a walker. Much of his day at Oak Manor revolves around self-care:

A typical day for me in this facility would be, starting out in the morning: I have a clock radio that comes on at 6:30 and it plays for an hour. During that hour I take a shower and clean my teeth, I put my underwear on. The one assistance that I get is they prick my finger for my [blood] sugar [test] once a day. Coupled with that, I take my own medicine every day. They do not furnish my medicine, nor do they give it to me. I take it on my own, with the assistance of my grandson and my daughter, in working with the doctor, who prescribes what I take. The lady that comes in to take my sugar and prick my finger would give me a little assistance. The assistance that I get from that person is that, the last two weeks, I wear elastic stockings, called hospital stockings. They go up to my knee, and, for convenience, I have her put them on. After that she would leave, and I would get dressed. Because now, I have my stockings on, I've had my shower, I have my underwear on, and it's a case for me [of] picking out a shirt. Like this T-shirt, I went to the closet and picked it out and put these pants on. Slide these pants over these socks and put my shoes on, get my medicine, put it in my pocket, and I'm ready to go down for breakfast.

My breakfast is almost the same every day. If they have a banana, I'll take it. I have a little oatmeal, one poached egg on an English muffin, and a couple of pieces of bacon, orange juice. I might have hot chocolate, or decaf coffee. I might come up here maybe and look at my e-mail about ten [o'clock]. I might take a nap with my legs propped up. I have a problem with accumulating fluid. I am a diabetic, and I have to be very careful about salty foods. And I need to keep my legs propped up so that my blood runs toward my heart. Other than that, the chances are great that I might develop fluid on my lungs, fluid on my heart, which makes it difficult for me to breathe. Maybe a month ago I had that problem. Since then I wear these stockings, and I try to keep my legs propped up in the afternoon and most certainly at night.

I might follow the same routine after lunch and then in turn go down for dinner at five o'clock. I don't get any assistance for any of that. Now later in the night, going to bed, to a degree I have a custom of getting a snack, and I used to take their snack, which would be orange juice and graham crackers. My daughter, in turn, has bought snacks like Jell-O, applesauce, Snapple diet iced tea, things with less sugar. So if [the staff] don't come about nine, I call them to get the snack out of my refrigerator.

Miss Fannie, at the age of 92, has some of the same health problems as Eugene Ellis, including heart disease, arthritis, and poor vision. She also has mild dementia and is beginning to have trouble "holding her water." Her portrayal of daily self-care reveals a much-abridged role:

> When I get up, they have somebody bring the water and sit it right down here, and I take me a bath and [a staff person] bring my clothes, lay 'em here on the bed, and I put [on] clean clothes. I put [on] my own clothes. I sit down and put 'em on. Now sometime, 'bout every month, I go back yonder in the shower, but my condition, standing up, you know. See, I can't stand up, [so] she'll let me sit here. I have arthritis in my knees, arthritis what I caught when I was young. Didn't have on enough clothes, caught the arthritis in my bones. Arthritis settle in your bones. This left knee be so stiff, I can't make it. Sometime I can't hardly walk. I bought me some Ben Gay. I got it in the drawer there now, put it on my knee. Honey, that stuff penetrate. . . .
>
> They give me my medications. They give me pills, and they put that patch on me everyday and give me them pills in my hand. There be a whole handful of pills. Yeah, I take all them pills, and all make me pee all the time and stuff like that. Then I eat breakfast, and then I sit down and watch TV till I get sleepy, you know, if it's a good baseball game or football game or something's on. Other than that, I can lay down until it's time to get up again. That's it. I don't go anywhere, because I'm, I would say, handicapped really. I'm old, too. You know, when you get old, you can't do like you did when you was young. So I just look at it like that and go on do the best I can. I'm 92 years old and happy to tell anybody.

The Reality of Self-Care

We observed a wide range of self-care in these six communities. On one end of the spectrum is James Higgins, a resident at Oak Manor who still drives his car and leaves the home daily on his own. Because of tremors associated with Parkinson disease, he needs help removing his prepackaged medications from their containers, but he is able to perform all ADLs independently, manage his own money, take himself to medical appointments, and do his own shopping. In contrast to Mr. Higgins is Harold Stamps, a resident of Rosie's, whose remaining independence includes minimal participation in bathing, dressing, and toileting, walking, rather unsteadily, and eating unassisted. Most residents, including Eugene Ellis and Miss Fannie, fall somewhere in the middle.

Basic ADLs include bathing, dressing, toileting, grooming, eating, walking, and transferring. According to AL regulations in Georgia (and in most states), residents of AL homes must be able to transfer and ambulate independently; all of the residents in our study are able to do these two tasks, with varying degrees of competence and speed, but some only with support from wheelchairs, walkers, and canes. All residents can eat unassisted, although a few need cueing (encouraging or reminding how) and help cutting up their food. Most perform at least one of the remaining ADLs independently, and approximately one-third manage them all. Even the most dependent have at least a minimal role in most of these basic tasks.

Although the inability to carry out IADLs—shopping, money management, doing laundry, meal preparation, and housekeeping—figured into most decisions to move to AL, some residents continue to perform such tasks. Only James Higgins and Greene's resident Slick still drive (and Slick's driving ability is questionable), but 13 residents leave their communities independently, either walking or using public transportation. All in this group are relatively younger men who, because of mental illness or problems with addiction, live at either Greene's or Sunshine House. These men are able to shop for themselves when they have money. Other residents can shop if they have access to transportation or someone to accompany them. Approximately one-fifth of residents manage their money themselves. Others "manage" only a small allowance. More than one-third of residents at Oak Manor write their own checks to pay their monthly fees.

Some residents participate in meal preparation and serving, along with laundry and housekeeping tasks. At Oak Manor, these tasks as a rule are carried out in residents' private apartments. Only Gwen Runnels prepares full meals, and she often eats one meal a day in her apartment. A few others prepare simple foods, either occasionally or on a regular basis. Hattie Houseworth, while still able, cooked oatmeal every morning for her breakfast. Some residents regularly dust their furniture, make their own beds, and do their personal laundry. Elsie Joiner does all of these and even launders her sheets and towels. On occasion, residents help set the table in the common dining room, and one resident, Lula Merriwether, has the job of watering the plants on the terrace.

In the small homes, participation in IADL tasks usually benefits the entire community. The extent of resident participation varies across homes. At Rosie's, Carole Seymour washes dishes and sometimes prepares resident snacks;

Cleo Kellog and Sarah Eubanks set and clear the table; and Tracey Williams, the one young resident, makes frequent trips downstairs to fetch food items from the storage room. Bobby Bailey's job at Peach Blossom is to take out the trash. At Sunshine House, Mayetta Stewart helps the manager "straighten up" at night after most residents are in bed, and Matilda Anderson often mops the floor in her room. Three residents at Blue Skies have regular duties: Marlena Morton folds clothes, mops the bathroom floor, and clears the table after meals; Terry Prospect sets the table, helps serve meals, vacuums the living and dining rooms, does laundry, and gets the mail; and Gary Cotter sweeps the driveway. A number of Greene's residents also have housekeeping and meal-related responsibilities: Half-Pint cleans and helps with cooking, laundry, and serving meals; Hoagy does some house cleaning and yard work; Frankie Johnson folds laundry; and all residents who are able make their beds, change their sheets, and clear their own plates from the table—though some of these tasks are more voluntary than others.

Residents also participate in their own health care. Although only a few can obtain medications on their own, approximately one-fifth keep up with and administer them independently. Still others manage medications with aid from a "daily pill container" and someone to fill it. Estelle Washington, a resident at Peach Blossom, checks her own blood sugar daily. Oak Manor resident Elizabeth Bell both monitors her blood sugar and administers her insulin. Several Greene's residents walk or take public transportation to their day programs and health clinics. A number of residents at Oak Manor arrange their own medical appointments and transportation. Most engage in some form of health promotion.

Self-Care Strategies

Residents in these communities have developed various strategies to cope with their disabling conditions and continue to perform self-care. Some strategies are relatively universal. Others are unique. The primary strategy of most residents is to try to do as much as they can. "I try to do for myself" is a frequently heard refrain among residents. Since almost all residents need some kind of help, a complementary strategy is to ask for help only when needed. This is Mr. Ellis's standard: "When I need it I want it, but I don't need help for everything. I do most things on my own." Mr. Ellis "likes" his independence but acknowledges his "handicaps." He knows he cannot put on his support hose by himself, and he does not mind asking for, and sometimes demanding, help. He also has found that he can feel independent, even when being helped, as long as he is in charge: "I like to be as independent as I can. In fact, even on the computer, when I get people to do things, I can direct them, and that gives me a sense of independence. I remember when I could do it myself." Mr. Ellis is able to perceive himself as independent both by performing a task on his own and by telling someone how to help him. In effect, by managing care from others, Mr. Ellis further enhances his self-care role.

Some residents resist help to preserve their sense of independence and self-care ability. Julia Shields, aged 92, retains control of her care at Oak Manor by flatly refusing offers of help. When asked what kind of assistance she needs in managing her daily life, her indignant answer was, "I don't need anybody to help me. I am my own boss. Ain't nobody got nothing to do with me and my business and my affairs. Nothing!" Annette Freeman's response to staff members who try to assist with her bath was less dogmatic but still clear: "If I needed help, I'd ask for it." Although Alma Burgess, at the age of 86, is mostly confined to her wheelchair and can walk only short distances using her walker, she too rarely asks for help: "What I try to do is keep from calling, to do for myself, because I hate to feel I am infringing on somebody's else's time whose need might be greater than mine, but I do feel that sometimes that I need help, but I don't call for it. I try to do for myself." Some residents are even more assertive. The director of resident services at Oak Manor reported that "some of them will tell you, 'Don't make my bed. I want to make my own bed.' If you make their bed, they're mad."

Many residents use assistive devices to optimize self-care. These supports go beyond the canes, walkers, and wheelchairs used for mobility, although these are critical. Mr. Ellis has a rolling desk chair in his bathroom, which he uses while washing and grooming himself. A hanging "valet" with a mirror at eye level and pockets for his comb, brush, and razor hangs on the back of the door. His hospital bed and a recliner permit him to elevate his feet throughout the day. Alma Burgess uses a portable toilet by her bed to increase her independence. Hattie Houseworth has a rolling laundry basket with a belt attached to it to pull her clothes to the laundry room. Gwen Runnels bought a microwave and installed florescent lights above the kitchen counter to facilitate meal preparation.

Residents also devise new ways of doing old tasks to compensate for disabilities. Several have found alternatives for tub or shower bathing. Miss Fannie's strategy is to have someone "bring the water" to her. Beatrice Dove, another Greene's resident, also uses a wash pan for bathing, but she fills and carries the tub herself. Half-Pint and Julia Shields wash at the bathroom sink. Others find adaptive ways of dressing. Eugene Ellis changed from suspenders (once his signature clothing style) to belts, Alma Burgess gave up her more stylish shoes for a pair with special orthotics, and Campbell Jenkins now wears a moccasin-type shoe instead of the lace-up ones he no longer can tie.

Just spending more time performing self-care tasks is a common strategy. Elizabeth Bell and Dorothea Buffington, the two sisters who live together at Oak Manor, get up early to be ready for breakfast at eight. Ms. Bell, the younger of the two at 91, has arthritis, diabetes, neuropathy in her legs, and poor circulation. Although her legs "hurt most all the time," she can walk "a little tiny bit." She described her morning care routine thus: "I get up about five-thirty and go to the bath and wash myself up the best I can. As long as I am holding on to something I can move. I can't walk, but I can move. Then about six o'clock, you know they have these night girls, the night girl comes in and she puts my shoes and socks on and combs my hair. Then about seven o'clock, I am ready to put my clothes on. I have already got my underclothes on when the girl comes in. I try to lay my clothes out at night so I don't have to do much but just pick them up. You finish dressing and go to breakfast about eight o'clock."

Ms. Buffington has additional strategies to compensate for her limited vision. One is arranging her clothes in a precise manner "so I know exactly where my blouse, my underwear, my pants are. I can put my hands on it. I know where I have placed things." She also has learned the geography of her room: "Your sense of touch increases. In other words, I know to come to just about this point when I want to get up and hold the door. I know just about where to reach out. I keep my eyes closed most of the time, because I can almost visualize in my mind where I am. Now, sometimes I will get lost in that bathroom, turned around and maybe go in the wrong door, and all you got to tell me is move a little bit to the right or left and I will have an idea. I don't know how I would be if they put me in a new place." By learning how each container top feels, Ms. Buffington also is able to self-administer her three glaucoma medications.

Engaging in activities to maintain or even improve health and functional status is an approach used by residents in all homes. These strategies include following prescribed treatment regimens, making healthy lifestyle choices, and educating themselves about their conditions and how to promote their own health. Trying to eat a wholesome diet and exercising are common. Carole Seymour, describing her approach at Rosie's, said, "I try to eat properly. I like wheat bread. I like the white bread, but I think the wheat bread is more healthy for you. I try to drink more water, 'cause, see, I wasn't too much drinking water, so I at least try to get three glasses in. . . . When I go outside, I do a little motional exercise and then walk around. I don't go too far, but I walk out the front door, go around, come around this way or something like that. I get a little exercise." Hassie Hicks drinks the water the owner of Peach Blossom regularly serves her because "if you don't drink water, you can't pee." Mose Rogers, who "feel[s] better when I'm walking," claims he would miss his daily walks in the neighborhood around Blue Skies only if he were "dead." Eugene Ellis does leg extensions before getting out of bed each morning. More than half of the residents at Oak Manor, including Ms. Bell and Ms. Buffington, attend the daily exercise program. Quite a few regularly walk around the building at least once a day. For some residents, continuing to perform ADLs and IADLs is their only exercise. Lily Porter propels her own wheelchair because she knows that "if you stop, then you won't be able to do for yourself."

A key strategy for many residents, and maybe the most important, is acceptance of their limitations. Dorothea Buffington put it most eloquently: "I am trying to accept it with grace. When I listen to a man who is blind climbing Mt. Everest, I say, 'Well, if he has the nerve to climb a mountain, then I ought to have the nerve to do the little bit I do around here.'" Acceptance helps residents focus on their remaining abilities and adapt to their deficiencies. As Jane Smithers, whose competence has been compromised by her stroke, said about helping with household tasks at Blue Skies, "Anything I see that needed to be done, I'll try anyway, whether I can do a perfect job or not."

Determinants of Resident Self-Care

The fundamental determinants of residents' self-care roles and the strategies they employ are the level and type of their disabilities. But many other factors shape self-care. These factors relate both to the personal characteristics and attitudes of residents and to their surrounding social and physical environment, and, as with the decision to move, the influence of some factors was set in motion long ago. These resident and facility factors affect not only residents' independence (that is, their ability to perform self-care activities) but also their autonomy (that is, the freedom to carry them out).

Resident Factors

Attitudes and values are key factors in shaping self-care. At the core of self-care is a strong value for self-reliance. The words of Madonna McDowell that open this chapter express her own independent attitude and embody the values of most residents: "It's important to be able to do things for yourself rather than to depend on someone to do it for you." For many residents, this self-reliance is a lifelong value. Lily Porter's daughter Sharon recalled that her mother's independence was "always" there: "She's always been independent, always been able to take care of her family, always did domestic work, always provided on meager earnings. We were very poor but never on any type of public assistance or anything like that. She always managed to make ends meet, and she continued to work until she was 82."

Closely connected to the value for self-reliance is that of not being a burden on others. Jane Smithers at Blue Skies expressed this motive for her self-care efforts: "I try not to be a burden to anybody else, but that's the best I can do at this point." As noted earlier, the desire to avoid burdening family was a factor in some residents' moving decisions, and once they are in the facility, residents try to avoid burdening facility workers.

Some self-care is prompted by altruism. Carole Seymour, who helps daily with household tasks at Rosie's, stated what she believes should be the norm for residents: "Yeah, I feel this way if you staying at a place with persons—if you see what need to be done, you get off of your rump and do it, too." Hassie Hicks expressed a similar attitude about helping at Peach Blossom: "You fix the food, and I can't sit there too lazy to bring my plate." The small-home environment seems to reinforce this attitude toward helping.

The value of maintaining former roles and identities and feeling useful also promotes self-care. Women tend to value housekeeping roles more than men. Carole relishes her dish-washing responsibilities at Rosie's. Hamilton Brewton, however, is happy to let Oak Manor workers take care of such tasks: "They do my laundry. I never did it before. I don't miss any household chores. Always had someone to do it for me, and I don't want to get started." An exception is Watkins Orr, another Oak Manor resident, who misses the exercise he got from cleaning his former home, where he lived with his son. Unlike Mr. Brewton, who as a professional in Chicago had always hired someone to clean house, Mr. Orr, with lesser economic means, took over those chores after his wife died.

For many residents, the desire to stay in these AL communities rather than move to a nursing home reinforces the importance of caring for themselves. Most are aware of the dependency limits in their respective homes and understand that increased care needs beyond those limits may lead to discharge. Boss Cook, for one, knows that to stay at Greene's he must adhere to a strict diet in order to lose weight and improve his mobility, and Blue Skies resident Mamie Hoover, who has considerable difficulty walking, spends the mornings sitting outside the bathroom door to avoid bowel accidents, a sure path to discharge.

Self-care requires knowledge and skills. Although residents have performed activities of daily living and instrumental activities of daily living throughout their lives, some with dementia have forgotten how to do them or why they need to be done. Sometimes residents need to learn how to do tasks in a new way or how to use an assistive device. Obtaining support for self-care often entails knowing what their needs are and being able to communicate them effectively to others. Self-care also depends on understanding chronic diseases and how to manage them. Residents like Eugene Ellis and Dorothea Buffington, both college educated, understand their health conditions and the crucial treatment regimens. Others, like Miss Fannie, with less formal education, are both less knowledgeable and less motivated to engage in activities to promote their health.

Money is a key support for self-care. It afforded Mr. Ellis a college education, and in later years it provided him ready access to skilled cardiac-care physicians and allowed him to acquire his hospital bed, computer, and hanging valet. Money makes it possible for Alma Burgess to purchase incontinence pads. Money, on a smaller scale, lets Greene's resident George Kelner catch the bus to Kroger to buy the food he wants. An incentive to save money encourages self-care at Oak Manor, where fees are based on the level and type of care provided. Fiscal concern motivates Alma Burgess to handle her own personal care, laundry, and medications.

The degree to which residents struggle to be independent in the face of infirmity also is influenced by their personalities. Some simply are more determined, their independence more ingrained. According to her sister Maude, Julia Shields gets her independent streak from her father: "There was a lot of things she couldn't do, but she didn't want you to do those things for her. She wants to still try to do them herself. Anything you say, she's going to resist, she's going to always have her rebuttal. She'll argue about anything. She's always been like that." Other strategies, such as acceptance and assertiveness, also are rooted in long-standing personality traits.

Families add considerable "value" to these communities of care, and, for some residents, family support is a critical component of their self-care roles. Family members who assume this role understand the importance of resident self-care, and their support takes several forms. Hattie Houseworth's daughter Phoebe visits her mother daily at Oak Manor and assists her with daily bathing and dressing, mostly through encouragement. Her goals match those of her mother: "I am hoping that she can retain as much of her independence and ability to function as possible. I think that most of what I do is try to support that. She is really a very independent person." Other family members support ADL self-care in different ways, such as arranging matched outfits in closets and supplying assistive devices and incontinence pads.

Family support for IADL self-care also is common. Some weekends, Maude brings Julia Shields to her home, where she can continue her housekeeping roles: "Sister was used to doing things, and there are some of the things that she learned to do when she was younger that she can do real well. When she's here I let her iron and wash dishes, and she likes to sweep and empty the garbage. She doesn't have as much trouble with her arthritis as I do, and she can go up and down the steps." This support allows Ms. Shields, who has been diagnosed with Alzheimer's, to perform tasks not available to her at Oak Manor and help her sister, fulfilling her values for both self-reliance and altruism. Before Rose Bowman was moved to the dementia unit at Oak Manor, her daughter Daphne helped her continue to do her own laundry in the facility: "Those are the things she likes to do. She did that fine. She would wash clothes and fold them and what not. She liked to do that. That took up time, and she felt she was accomplishing something by doing that."

Family members support residents' financial independence in numerous ways, such as providing monthly allowances, writing checks, balancing accounts, and taking residents to the bank. Although Hamilton Brewton was happy to relinquish financial control to his son because he was "goofing up" with his money, his son enables him to retain a modified fiscal role: "Anytime he buys anything he uses his [debit] card, and I mean he uses the card, [even] if it's a 25-cent purchase. . . . We put an account at Sun Trust, and anytime he wants cash, he can get what he wants. The account has enough money in it for spending change and to get anything that he needs, you know, within reason."

Families also facilitate shopping. Irene Garrett, a resident of Peach Blossom, has moderate dementia, but her daughter Elva helps her shop, an activity she has always loved: "I take her shopping and everything. So even if she goes grocery shopping, she loves to push the basket and things like that. And when I buy things for her, I say, 'What do you think about this? Do you like it?' And then I say, 'Well, if you don't like it, look and see if [you like] something else,' and she might pick up something that maybe she like."

Families contribute to residents' physical and mental health through emotional support and various health care roles, such as monitoring conditions and transporting them to medical appointments. Several manage residents' medication regimens through weekly visits to fill pill containers. They also support health promotion. Sarah Eubanks's son encourages her to walk at Rosie's and brings puzzles and craft activities to promote mental activity, and Estelle Washington's daughter urges her mother to walk when she brings her home from Peach Blossom on the weekends. Others buy dietary supplements and encourage healthy eating. Oak Manor families attend meetings and lobby for less salt in food and the use of more fresh vegetables.

In some cases, family members advocate for residents' rights to independence. Lula Merriwether's niece understands her aunt's value for self-care and has intervened on her behalf: "I try to allow Aunt Lula to be as independent as she possibly can. There was a recommendation around the first of the year that at that time [the facility staff] thought she needed to go to a different level [of care], and I did not go along with that. I wouldn't sign it, and the reason why was because I told them, 'You know, she is like anybody else, and I know you all know this 'cause you are people who work with the elderly all the time, but she needs to feel like she is in control of her life as much as she can be, for as long as she can be. And until there is a reason to take her to another level, I refuse to go along with it.'"

In each of these communities, residents support one another's self-care. In the sisters' symbiotic relationship at Oak Manor, Elizabeth Bell provides the eyes and Dorothea Buffington the feet. Mary Overton checks daily on her neighbor Corrine Wallace, who otherwise forgets to go to meals. Residents who are able to go shopping make purchases for others who cannot. At Rosie's, Cleo Kellog is able to dress herself, with help from Carole Seymour in finding her clothes. Harold Stamps can go to the senior center because Carole assists him with toileting. Female residents at Greene's and Blue Skies also help one another with bathing. Oftentimes, through mutual support, close ties are formed. Although helping between residents is not encouraged at Oak Manor, the director recognizes such support as "how we become family." A staff person noted, "I think they do a lot of taking care of each other. A lot of them feel as if their families have abandoned them, and so they basically take on some of the other residents as their family. Like, for instance, Ms. Overton and Ms. Wallace live next door to each other. Ms. Overton feels as if she's Ms. Wallace's mother, and if anything is wrong with Ms. Wallace, it's almost like we don't have to find out. Ms. Overton is gonna let us know. So they, I think, basically attach to each other and find alternate families here in Oak Manor."

Facility Factors

The physical and social environments of these six homes play a significant role in shaping residents' self-care. The individuals who own and work in these homes constitute a key component of the facility influence through their personal strategies aimed at promoting resident self-care. As with residents and families, their strategies are influenced by individual traits, including attitudes, values, knowledge, skills, and health status. Other facility factors, such as financial resources, policies, physical environment, and resident profile, also affect residents' self-care roles.

Provider Strategies to Promote Self-Care

Providers in each of these homes profess to promote resident self-care. Their key strategy is to allow residents to do what they can for themselves and provide only care that is needed. This strategy parallels the principal resident strategies of doing the best they can and accepting only needed help. Cora Greene, the owner of Greene's, explained, "As long as a resident can do, I agree to let them do what they can do, and my thing is I try to fill in if I see that they need assistance." A staff person at Oak Manor expressed a similar view: "When they get to the place where they cannot do it for themselves, you step in, you do what needs to be done. But on the whole, try and do as much as you can for yourself."

Often, allowing residents to "do for themselves" is all that is needed, but some residents need encouragement or assistance, usually owing to mental impairment. Kay, the manager at Sunshine House, explained her tactics for helping two residents with dementia bathe themselves: "When Ms. Hortense bathe, you have to actually talk her through her bath, and Ms. Mayetta. They're basically like children. They would get in the water and get out of it if you don't stay. With Ms. Mayetta, when she get in there, I basically just get the washcloth, I wet it 'cause she don't like soap on her face. I let her do her face, and then I do her back, and I tell her, you know, do under her arms and stuff like that. The same with Ms. Hortense."

Support for residents with dementia typically consists of cueing them to carry out tasks they have long been accustomed to doing. For some residents, stronger "encouragement" is required. One caregiver at Oak Manor described her efforts to coax Janie Benton to get up from a chair on her own: "You have to encourage them. For instance, today, Ms. Benton, I usually help her up, but some days I have to be like, 'No, Ms. Benton, I am not going to help you up. Today you have to help yourself up. Get up on your own, because you be lazy and just sit there always wanting somebody to help you.' I try my hardest to help and encourage them to do better." Even stronger measures are needed for other residents. Cora Greene has creative strategies for reluctant residents, such as threatening to withhold Slick's check until he agrees to bathe and bribing Frankie Johnson with a walk.

In some cases, for residents who are mentally impaired, providers teach new self-care skills. Esther Adams, the owner of Peach Blossom, has taught Bobby Bailey (her one resident with mental retardation) how to manage his own ADL care: "I've learned a lot working with him, and I still would say, for any person like that today, you need to teach them how to help themselves. Mr. Bailey does his own personal hygiene every morning. I usually leave his clothes lying out at night, and then he'll get up and he get dressed."

Although providers generally believe that most residents want to be independent, as the resident services director at Oak Manor said, "Some think it's not important to do anything." Eva, a caregiver there, believes that unnecessary helping of residents encourages dependency: "If you have somebody that's doing for them, they're prone to depend on it. A lot of them who know how to do things will not do it, because they're used to depending on us to do it for them." Another staff member gave the example of Alma Burgess: "I think we might hurt them sometimes by not allowing them to be so independent. For instance, Ms. Burgess, who is in a wheelchair, her legs are swollen, because she no longer walks as much as she supposed to. She can walk, [but] she's scared to walk. She feels as if she might fall. But if we see her waiting by the elevator—she's waiting for someone to push her upstairs—it would be valuable for us to let her realize that she needs to take herself upstairs, but a lot of times we'll say, 'Aw, Ms. Burgess, we'll take you upstairs.' Of course the next day, she's waiting by the elevator again. So I think in that sense, we might be hurting them."

According to Eva, encouraging residents to do more requires taking extra time and developing a personal relationship—both techniques she employs: "I go to their room and I get comfortable. I get me a chair and I sit there and we'll talk and I'll say, 'Don't you know how to do this, that, and the other? You know you can do that, can't you?' You have to do it on a confidential thing; you have to do it on a one-on-one thing." The director at Oak Manor sanctions the additional time it takes to support self-care: "The ones that I know may need more specialized assistance, I'll staff accordingly to them, meaning that I'll make sure they have a resident assistant responsible for them that I know is going to take the extra time to say, 'Ms. X, do you need this or do you need that?'" For Alma Burgess, who often resists asking for help, this strategy is not a reality: "I feel sometimes they bend over forwards in making you do for yourself, and there are certain times when I think they ought to recognize the limitations that some people have. They should be familiar enough with the people themselves to know what they can and cannot do and that they will not just walk out and leave you struggling, which very often happens." The case of Ms. Burgess illustrates the complexity of the independence-dependence conundrum. She both strives for independence and wants help, and at different times the staff give her both more and less help than she feels she needs.

As Eva suggests, an integral part of supporting self-care is getting to know residents as individuals. Knowing them depends on understanding who they are as human beings and also on learning what they can and cannot do. In the small homes, this information is obtained informally, through Eva's "one-on-one thing," observation, and experience in giving care. Only by knowing Bobby's limitations can Esther Adams promote his self-care: "He uses everything excessively. If it's powder, it's coming through the clothes. A bar of soap will last him—I'm talking about a big bar that we would bathe with for a month—about four baths and the bar of soap is gone because he rubs it, so I just buy him the bubble bath. I don't give him the whole bag of Depends [incontinence pads]. I give him like maybe a week's supply at a time."

At Oak Manor, a more formal quarterly assessment procedure also is used to determine care, or self-care, needs. The director considers these tools and "the care staff being knowledgeable of what [residents] can do" essential to supporting independence. The goal of assessment is "to provide care when needed," not "just give everybody a shower."

Although most provider support for self-care pertains to ADL tasks, staff also help residents stay independent in other ways. Providers in two homes support residents' ability to shop for themselves. Cora Greene enlists her brother to take Boss Cook shopping and gives Miss Fannie spending money. Oak Manor provides transportation twice weekly to the nearby shopping center. Ms. Adams has taught Bobby how to take the trash out and roll the big container to the street. At the other small homes, both owners and care staff allow, encourage, and sometimes require residents to help with housekeeping chores. Rosie lets Carole wash dishes, even though "sometimes she dries 'em and put[s] 'em in the cabinets and they're all speckled with food." Workers at Greene's and Blue Skies allow residents with dementia to help fold laundry and insist that certain more able residents have regular chores. Although Oak Manor residents are allowed to perform housekeeping tasks in their own apartments, such tasks are the facility's responsibility, according to the director: "As a part of our promoting independence, we would, of course, allow that, but we do have our regular routine of responsibilities that the caregivers are responsible for doing, certain things in the room every day."

In addition to learning what residents are able to do, a key ingredient in supporting self-care is knowing what they want to do. This knowledge seems particularly important with respect to IADL activities. Lorraine Stokes, the food service director at Oak Manor, tried to involve residents in meal preparation, but her strategy backfired because she had not learned their preferences: "When we first opened, I thought, 'Wow, I am going to buy fresh beans and the residents are going to help me snap them.' I snapped beans for days. They didn't want to be bothered."

Providers in each of these communities facilitate resident self-care through strategies aimed at promoting and maintaining residents' health. Most strategies have to do with encouraging and monitoring compliance with treatment regimens and trying to educate residents about their conditions and how to manage them. Some efforts are more rigorous than others. Esther Adams prepares well-balanced meals at Peach Blossom, complete with meat, fruits, and vegetables, and a big glass of water. Desserts are a rare treat. She closely monitors the dietary intake of all residents, even confiscating Ivera Haygood's contraband peanuts. She also knows her residents' likes and dislikes and tries to prepare healthy foods they will eat. In the other small homes, although special dietary needs usually are attended to, compliance is not so strictly scrutinized or enforced. Rosie, for one, argues for greater leniency for Harold Stamps: "My daughter says, 'Oh, Mama, he don't need no salt, he don't need no sugar.' I said, 'Look, leave Mr. Stamps alone. Give him what he wants. He's 97 years old. If he die, it is time for him to die.'" However, Rosie herself sometimes has to be strict just to get Mr. Stamps to eat: "He don't even really care about eating anymore. I just have to make him come and eat, and I have to talk, like, real strict with him, like, 'Mr. Stamps, get up and come eat breakfast right now,' and he'll get up and come on. But, if I say, 'Mr. Stamps, you want to come eat?' he'll sit right there and miss the meal." Dietary supervision by staff is sporadic at Greene's, and most of the time residents are expected to monitor themselves.

Health promotion is a principal facility goal at Oak Manor, explained Lucy Small, the resident services director: "Well, personal care to me is preventive care, and just seeing someone able to stay healthy as long as possible. That's one thing that we do here. Our activities director spends a lot of time ensuring that everyone is active and not just sitting around with nothing [to do] all day every day, and just trying to promote wellness, you know." Oak Manor also sometimes holds formal educational programs to teach residents about healthy living and how to manage their chronic conditions. One program on urinary incontinence, conducted by a physician, resulted in two residents' adopting new behavioral strategies to combat this problem. Much effort is directed at ensuring the nutritional compliance of the large number of diabetics. Although staff members cannot supervise residents while in their apartments, they carefully monitor their intake at meals and activities where food is served.

Only Oak Manor has a regular exercise program, but providers in the smaller homes urge residents to move around as best they can. Inez Sawyer, a manager at Blue Skies, implores Mamie Hoover to walk more, and Mamie, who is fearful of losing functional ground, appreciates this extra shove: "You make me walk, and I like that." Cora Greene walks with Martha Kominsky, a resident with dementia, when Martha refuses to go on her own.

Valuing Resident Self-Care

Providers promote resident self-care in part for the benefits they believe it bestows on residents. Cora Greene recognizes the boost to self-esteem: "They all have the capability of doing certain tasks, and when they volunteer to do it, you allow them to do that to make them feel good about themselves." Rosie lets Carole wash dishes, despite the extra work it causes her, because engaging in this favorite pastime makes her happy: "She act like she loves to wash dishes. She don't *like* it, she *love* it. I have to wash the dishes over when she wash 'em, but that's the only thing she loves to do." The marketing director at Oak Manor recognizes the value of self-care in keeping residents healthy and promoting aging in place: "[Promoting self-care] is a value, because that resident will be with you longer, actually, if they're doing things for themselves for a longer period of time. It keeps their health up. Their cardiovascular cells are going if they dress themselves; if they can dress themselves [but get used to letting other people do it for them] everyday, then that person might deteriorate quicker than somebody that's working for themselves." Rosie continues to take the extra time to assist Harold Stamps in dressing himself because "the only exercise he get during the day is pulling his socks on, pulling his pants up, and pulling his shirt down. That's it. That's all he does."

Knowing How

Understanding the effect of particular traits and disabilities on residents' self-care abilities and motivations and knowing how to care for residents with these varying conditions are important ingredients in promoting self-care. As noted in chapter 5, owners and staff in these homes vary widely in their education, training, and experience in long-term care. All Oak Manor staff are at least high school graduates, and it is the only facility in our study with registered nurses or licensed practical nurses on staff. The facility has ready access to a nutritional consultant and geriatricians at a local university hospital, and certain caregivers are specially trained in diabetes management. Although as a whole providers in the smaller homes have less formal education, some have gained valuable knowledge during their years of caregiving that aids them in supporting resident self-care. Rosie's training in dementia care has given her the tools she needs to maximize the self-care roles of her three cognitively impaired residents, relieving her own frustration with the task. Because she is diabetic herself and knowledgeable about the disease, Rosie is better able to check Ms. Eubanks's blood sugar and advise her about diet. Rosie's know-how contrasts starkly with that of the usual weekend staff at Greene's, some of whom are illiterate. No providers, however, have had any specific training in the importance of self-care to residents or in how best to promote it.

Staffing

A facility's resources to care for residents affect residents' own roles in care. In the small homes, the care that residents provide for themselves and others can be an essential cog in the care wheel. Cora Greene's very survival depends on resident self-care. The help Rosie gets from Carole and Tracey relieves her painful feet and conserves her energy. Bobby's self-care spares Esther Adams's arthritic knees from daily descents to his quarters downstairs at Peach Blossom. The housecleaning roles of Terry and Marlena at Blue Skies reduce Inez's heavy workload. Such resident "care value" creates extra motivation for providers to promote, and even require, self-care. It spurs Ms. Greene's edict that all able residents make their beds, change their sheets, and clear their plates from the table.

For residents who are less functional, inadequate staffing can create barriers to their self-care. Hassie Hicks's daughter noticed a decline in her mother's self-care capacity when she moved to Peach Blossom. Although she admitted that she did not have a good understanding of the effects of Alzheimer disease, she correctly identified inadequate staff time as one barrier to her mother's continued self-care: "The only thing about moving her to the personal care, Mama lost a lot of her independence, because there were things that they don't have time to wait on them to do. They do everything for them. They was rolling her hair, and Mom know how to roll her hair. She was a beautician. She rolled her hair every night when she was home, and now she don't even care about combing it. She could get her clothes on correctly, and, when she got over there, she was bathing herself. You know, that's the first thing that she said, 'Oh I love there. I don't even have to bathe myself.' But maybe she would have slipped into that anyway. I don't really know the history of Alzheimer people." Although Peach Blossom's owner, Esther Adams, does understand "Alzheimer people," four of her six residents have significant dementia, and it *is* more efficient for her to provide the care herself.

Continuity of staff also is a factor in promoting self-care, since getting to know residents and building resident-staff relationships can be crucial. In all of the small homes, either the owner or manager was present throughout the study year, and, except at Blue Skies, which had been open less than a year, they had been there for years. Clearly, Cora Greene's close relationship with Boss Cook, cultivated over the 10 years he has been living in the home, gives her both greater incentive and greater knowledge to support him. The contrasting high turnover of Oak Manor caregivers clearly affects staff relationships with residents. Elizabeth Bell expressed an often-heard observation: "By the time you get used to somebody and they know what you want and you understand them, you look up and you have a new person."

Physical Environment

A facility's physical environment can either facilitate self-care or create barriers to it. Even a particular aspect of the environment can have both effects. Some features affect self-care directly; others affect it more indirectly, through influence on the social milieu.

Oak Manor, the only home built expressly for assisted living, was designed with residents' independence in mind. It has wide halls with handrails, an elevator, good lighting, shower chairs in all bathrooms, and washers and dryers for resident use. Residents have private bedrooms, and most have private baths, which provides more space for supports such as microwave ovens, ironing boards, hospital beds, rolling desk chairs, computers, and hanging valets. The paved path encircling the building makes a pleasant and safe place to walk. Certain aspects of the environment, though, impede self-care: only a few baths have roll-in showers; closet rods are out of reach for residents in wheelchairs; the chairs in the lobby area are low and soft; the upstairs halls are long; the door to the laundry room is heavy; and the nearby shopping center is up a hill on a busy street with no sidewalks.

Accessibility is decidedly worse in the small homes. Only Greene's and Blue Skies are somewhat wheelchair accessible, meaning they have ramps for entry and exit, but doorways are narrow, and maneuvering space is generally cramped. Although these two small homes are the only ones with walk-in showers, the shower at Greene's has no chair. The number of bathrooms for resident use is limited—more so at Greene's, which has only one full bath for 13 residents—reducing the amount of time residents have to bathe themselves. Greene's is the only home with sidewalks to facilitate walking, but stray dogs in the neighborhood are a hazard.

Some environmental features in the small homes aid self-care. Both Greene's and Sunshine House have convenience stores within a short walk and easy access to public transportation for the more mobile residents. The central location of the kitchen at Rosie's makes it easy for residents to help out. Lack of privacy, room sharing, and generally close quarters also encourage some resident relationships and mutual support.

Provider's Way

Finally, what we call a "provider's way" has bearing on residents' care roles. The term refers to how a provider operates in the overall management of the home and caring for residents. A provider's way is molded to a large extent by personality and care ethic. It wields greater influence on resident self-care in the small homes, where individual care providers have greater power.

A comparison of resident self-care at Peach Blossom and Rosie's Loving Care illustrates the impact of a provider's way. Peach Blossom's owner, Esther Adams, runs a tight ship. Her system for getting things done depends on efficiency and a meticulous schedule, and she believes a resident's appearance must reflect the high standards of care on which her reputation stands. Ms. Adams's system and standards discourage resident self-care, especially for residents who are cognitively impaired. When Hassie Hicks leaves for the senior center each morning at eight o'clock, she is well put together, with no hair out of place, and she is always ready on time. A greater self-care role by Ms. Hicks would most likely have yielded a different outcome. In stark contrast to Ms. Adams's way is Rosie's laid-back modus operandi. Although her residents are almost always neat and clean, Cleo Kellog may leave for the center in the unmatched clothes she donned herself, and Madonna McDowell often rolls her own hair while sitting up late at night, watching TV with Rosie. In this less regimented atmosphere, not only are residents allowed to do more for themselves, they also may do so imperfectly, or even badly.

An individual provider's way at Oak Manor is moderated by the corporate way. Oak Manor subscribes to the philosophy of the new assisted living model, which encourages resident independence and fosters wellness as company policy. Although corporate support for self-care policies and practices is certainly ideal, the individual provider's way may be more vital.

Risk

The phenomenon of risk is a common barrier to resident self-care. Residents sometimes reduce their own roles because of perceived possible risk. Alma Burgess's fear of falling (exacerbated by earlier falls while living at home) dampens her interest in walking. Half-Pint chooses the sink for bathing over the shower, which has no mat, to avoid the fate of a former Greene's resident who fell and broke her hip. Providers routinely restrict residents' self-care activities to prevent risk. Bathing, medication management, and leaving the facility independently are activities frequently targeted. Family members often encourage providers' regulatory role.

Facility owners and administrators also worry about risk to facilities, which includes typical liability concerns regarding residents' behavior as well as risk to their reputations as providers of quality care. A resident who bathes herself runs both types of risk. The marketing director at Oak Manor expressed this dilemma: "People . . . say 'we're independent,' and then they've fallen getting out of the shower because they truly need assistance getting out of the shower. Or they say, 'I can take my own baths,' and then after a week, you're like, 'What's that odor?' Oh well, they haven't taken a bath in two or three weeks because they said they can do it. Looks like we're gonna have to start giving them baths."

The Soul of Self-Care

We have seen that what residents do for themselves—self-care—is a key element of life in these six care communities. Resident self-care encompasses ADLs, IADLs, and health care and promotion activities and has important meaning for residents, providers, and the care community as a whole.

For residents, an important function of self-care is its contribution to preserving their former identities in their new homes. Preservation of identity is engendered by acting on long-held values and enacting customary roles. Self-care empowers residents in relation to their caregivers and gives them greater control over their care. By doing tasks themselves, residents have a better chance of having them done when, where, and how they like. They can, as Julia Shields said, be their "own boss." Self-care boosts self-esteem and overall well-being and provides residents a meaningful way to spend time, or just pass time. Self-care also helps residents maintain mental and physical function and, in Oak Manor, save money—outcomes that promote aging in place. Residents' roles in the support of one another's self-care foster emotional ties. Similar self-care meanings have been found for AL residents in predominantly white communities (Ball et al., 2004a, 2004b).

Resident self-care also has meaning for facilities. Residents managing their own ADLs and helping with facility chores have economic and social value. In small homes, residents' contributions to the care of the home and of other residents help foster a sense of community as well as relieving overburdened owners and managers.

Residents use a variety of strategies to perform self-care. Many of these fit the categories of adaptation (selection, optimization, compensation, and receiving help) identified as important for persons with disabilities who live at home (Baltes & Baltes, 1990; Gignac, Cott, & Bradley, 2000) and in AL facilities (Ball et al., 2004b). An additional, and often critical, strategy for many residents is redefining independence as their abilities decline. In so doing, they are able to perceive themselves as independent by carrying out basic ADLs or, as in the case of Eugene Ellis, by managing care performed by others. The strategy of redefining independence has been reported in other studies of AL residents (Ball et al., 2004b; Carder & Hernandez, 2004; Frank, 2002) and of elders living at home (Ball & Whittington, 1995; Groger, 1994; Johnson & Barer, 1997; Matthews, 1979). Redefining independence is a form of "impression management" (Goffman, 1959, 208), whereby individuals "manage" their identities to give the impression of greater independence, enabling them to repair identities damaged by the stigma of disability and dependency. For some residents, redefining reality reflects a "stretching" of values (Rodman, 1971, 6) in order to give old values new meaning more appropriate to present circumstances. Kaufman (1986, 7) has found such reformulation of values to be highly adaptive and to promote a sense of continuity of self, or an "ageless self."

The desire to retain control of care leads some residents to resist care from others. This strategy, which for some residents leads to unmet needs, also has been reported in other AL research (Ball et al., 2004b) and among elders living at home (Ball & Whittington, 1995). In our study of African American home care clients (Ball & Whittington, 1995), we discovered that clients developed self-care management strategies that, in some cases, resembled those of formal care managers. Those elders able to incorporate elements of care management (for example, assessment, care planning, and taking action to correct problems) into their self-care roles were more successful at both receiving quality care and preserving independence. In the current study, AL residents' self-care roles also include management of their care (from families and facility providers), and we have found that those adept at management are better able to sustain their self-care roles and have their needs met. Eugene Ellis, for example, is more proficient at both determining his needs and communicating them to his helpers than is Alma Burgess, who feels herself misunderstood and neglected.

Dowd (1975) relates dependency in older persons—and the accompanying loss of power—to a decline in resources. Both self-care and self-care management in the six communities of our study hinges on residents' personal resources, including physical, intellectual, social, psychological, and material. Mr. Ellis's mental acuity, health knowledge, family support, assertiveness, money, and value for self-reliance all contribute to his successful self-care role. His relative independence contrasts plainly with that of Miss Fannie, who lacks many of these same resources.

Successful self-care often hinges on support from others. For many residents, family support is a key element in their self-care. For most, facility support is essential. Each of the providers we talked to recognizes their residents' wish to remain independent, and most make an effort to support self-care and maintenance of function. Small's (1993) self-care deficit model of caregiving is premised on a caregiver's provision of needed support to enable self-care. Small argues that it is incumbent upon facilities to assist residents in gaining the necessary knowledge, skills, motivation, and resources to meet their self-care requirements. Although motivation is a strategy used by most providers to promote resident self-care, provision of knowledge, skills, and other resources is less common. Our findings show that most residents do not need further encouragement, but many could benefit from additional knowledge, skills, and physical support. Some providers lack the necessary resources to offer this kind of support, a deficiency more evident in the small homes. Providers also vary in their commitment to supporting resident self-care when it crosses purposes with efficient home management.

This research, as well as other AL studies (Ball et al., 2004b; Fonda, Clipp, & Maddox, 2000; Taylor et al., 2003), indicates that facilities could boost residents' self-care roles through greater attention to promotion of physical exercise. Research in nursing homes has demonstrated the effectiveness of weight training in increasing the strength of frail elders (Evans, 1995).

A key element in supporting self-care is knowing residents' unique needs, wants, and personal histories. In an earlier AL study (Ball et al., 2004b), we indicated that additional training in conducting formal assessments and use of an assessment tool that captures partial task performance, such as the Barthel index (Mahoney & Barthel, 1965), could enhance self-care support. Findings from the more in-depth research reported on here suggest that, although these more formal techniques are useful, getting to know residents informally and over time is probably a more productive strategy. Initial findings from another qualitative study set in small ALFs also has found such informal assessment to be more effective (Carder et al., 2003).

Real or perceived risk inherent in resident self-care influences strategies of both residents and providers. The two types of risk we found in this study—risks to residents' health and safety and risks to operating the ALF—have been described by Carder (2002). The influence of provider risk was more evident at Oak Manor, where the threat of legal repercussions was a more likely reality. Although some newer-model ALFs use negotiated risk agreements (documents that identify risk and propose a strategy agreed upon by residents and providers to reduce the possibility of injury), these vehicles are not legally binding, and little consensus exists on how they should be used (Kapp & Wilson, 1995). No providers in the six facilities we studied had considered using this tool. Negotiated service agreements specify what services will be provided, when, how often, and by whom (that is, by resident, staff, or family member) (Carder, 2002). This strategy, which is based on resident assessment, may be a more practical means of supporting self-care.

Assisted living, as developed in the mid-1980s, is a consumer-based approach to long-term care defined by a shared philosophy (Utz, 2003). This philosophy, which emphasizes a social, rather than medical, model of care, embraces 10 specific points, the second being "fostering" resident independence. Utz's study exploring how well AL practice in Ohio matched its philosophical underpinnings finds that, although providers embraced the philosophy, they struggled to balance its tenets with the reality of running a care facility. Carder (2002), based on her in-depth study of AL in Oregon (one of the first states to embrace and legislate assisted living), suggests that adopting the AL model requires a coordinated effort by residents, families, and facility staff, as well as social service and health care providers, and that all players must be socialized to this end. Our own findings reveal an approach to fostering resident independence that is more scattershot than comprehensive. Although in each facility effort is made to promote resident self-care, barriers remain. Some barriers, of course, are inevitable, but many could be overcome with a true philosophical commitment to the soul of self-care.

CHAPTER 7

Kin-Work

"The most important thing to me right now is my surviving family. They all have just made my life a joy. I can't say anything less," said Ethyl Burns, of Oak Manor. Her sentiment echoes the feelings of most residents of these six communities. Families are important, everywhere. For most of us, family is the first—and most lasting—organizing principle of our lives. The families of many of these residents struggled valiantly to care for them at home and forestall their moves to assisted living. Harold Stamps's daughter Lola spent every weekend at his apartment and, along with other family members, provided round-the-clock care. Michael Waldman's daughter Bernadette drove to Huntsville every weekend to oversee his care. The sons of Hamilton Brewton and Mose Rogers brought their fathers into their own homes to care for them. These families embody the well-documented African American family tradition of caring for its elders (Ball & Whittington, 1995; Gibson & Jackson, 1987; Hatch, 1991; Taylor, Chatters, & Jackson, 1997). In this chapter, we endeavor to establish and understand the uncharted courses of action and meaning involved in African Americans' caring for family members in assisted living. In so doing, we employ the framework of "kin-work."

Kin-work is one of three domains in the "kinscripts" paradigm developed by Stack and Burton (1993). The concept is based on the life course perspective, and it describes ethnic family interaction and support. *Kin-work* is the labor families need and expect from their members to survive over time; *kin-time* is the shared understanding of how and when kin-work should occur; and *kinscription* is the process of assigning kin-work to specific family members. Although the kinscripts framework was developed from ethnographic studies of low-income, multigenerational African American extended families in household settings, it can be used to explore the life course of families across racial, ethnic, and socioeconomic groups. Here, we also extend the application to families separated by the boundaries of assisted living facilities.

The circumstances of the decision to move to AL set off the kin-time alarm clock for many families. The realization that elder relatives need more care than the family can provide signals the need for adjustments to the family's kin-work pattern. In this chapter, we explore the transition of kin-work to the AL setting. For no families do kin ties or care roles remain quite the same, although, as a rule, family members who were supportive of their relatives while living at home continue to provide care in some form following AL placement. In some families, other members are "kinscripted," or enlisted, to share the care burden. In the absence of family members, some friends or neighbors have assumed kin-work roles.

Multiple factors affect the relationships between family members and residents of these six communities and the continuing support that families provide. The homes themselves are key factors in the continuity of the families' kin-work, in providing a culturally compatible care setting—based in a home-like environment and located in an African American community—and an extended network of kin-workers in the person of the providers. Most family caregivers mold their roles to support those of the AL providers to whom they have entrusted their relatives' care. Like residents, they have to adapt to and perform their kin-work in unfamiliar surroundings, but their adjustment can be eased by a home's culture.

We found considerable variation in the amount of kin-work carried out in each of these six care communities and in the level of family involvement in an individual's care. Almost half of all residents receive some type of family support at least weekly; close to one-third receive none. Although having children does not guarantee support, family members providing the most care are children, usually daughters. More than one-third of residents have no living children.

Behind the numbers lies a more complex reality. A fuller understanding of kin ties and kin-work in these homes requires a deeper look at the nature of both phenomena, the multiple factors that influence them, and their impact on these six care communities. The following profiles encompass the range of experiences we found.

Profiles

Hattie Houseworth of Oak Manor

To Phoebe, her mother, Hattie Houseworth, is the "central force" in a family whose members traditionally have not been "a real close-knit group": "It is small, and we are kind of scattered geographically, so I don't know if I would say we were a particularly close family. But, however, there are close units within. My son and my mother are extremely close. We have been very close, all of us, since my mother has moved here. My mother and I got closer when I got sick. It has varied a lot of the time. I don't think we are the kind of family that gathered a lot as a group, but we are a small family, my sister and me. Of course, we all loved each other, but it was not a physical closeness." Phoebe has only one sister, Harriet, who lives in Philadelphia, and they both have two grown children.

Eighteen years ago, Phoebe developed chronic fatigue syndrome. The disability was a determining factor in her mother's move to Atlanta and a turning point in their relationship: "I thought, because I don't have a lot of energy but I have a lot of time, that this might be a better place for her to come. Also it is warmer, and my sister and her family are very, very busy people. I would have more time, even if it is just sitting still. And also my daughter is here, and she was anxious for her grandmother to come. My daughter's wedding last year would give my mother something to look forward to, coming here. It is much more convenient, especially after we found Oak Manor, this being so close to where we live. That was the easiest thing to do by a long shot."

Before Ms. Houseworth's move, Phoebe's illness had prevented her from even visiting her mother, who had retired to her hometown in Louisiana. With Ms. Houseworth now in Atlanta, Phoebe's kin-work has increased exponentially. She described her extensive care role:

> I would say I try to get here at least six out of seven days a week, unless I am sick or something on that order. I usually stay, it varies a lot, it could be just a couple of hours, it could be four or five hours. It depends on how my mother is doing, what is going on around here [at Oak Manor]. Sometimes she participates [in facility activities] more if I stay, so I just stay and participate with her. Often it is just a matter of keeping her company and encouraging her to keep moving and get dressed and get out and come down and see what is going on. Sometimes we just sit downstairs and talk to people, or sometimes the two of us just sit upstairs and talk a little bit. She tends to misplace things, and I spend a lot of time looking for things. Really most of what I do is just to be here, just kind of support. If she is trying to do something, I will try to help her do it. It varies with how I feel. If I can't get here, I call and check, because sometimes she can make it down to meals and sometimes she can't.

In addition to these mostly daily visits, Phoebe does her mother's shopping and assists her with check writing, banking, and laundry. Ms. Houseworth has Parkinson disease, congestive heart failure, diabetes, kidney failure, and narcolepsy, and Phoebe has found a variety of specialists to treat these conditions. Most weeks she takes her mother to at least one medical appointment; toward the end of the study, Ms. Houseworth needed kidney dialysis three times weekly. Being knowledgeable about her mother's health conditions and attending closely to her health care needs have helped Phoebe cope with some of the psychological effects of her mother's illnesses: "She gets angry with me about the fact that people are stealing from her. Geriatric Parkinson's involves lots of problems, including paranoia. I am an expert on that now. As a rule, I try not to say anything because I cannot argue her out of a medical symptom."

Phoebe also incorporates her mother in "all the family events, whatever we do." These include church on Wednesday nights and Sundays and celebrations for Thanksgiving, Christmas, Easter, and family birthdays. If her mother feels up to it, they sometimes go shopping together or to movies, and they talk on the telephone several times a day.

Although Phoebe clearly provides the bulk of family kin-work, her sister and son have vital roles: "My sister takes care of all the financial stuff, most of the bills go to her. And she takes care of renting my mother's house in Louisiana, all that sort of thing. My son says that my sister is in charge of the finances, he is in charge of overall seeing that things go smoothly, and I am in charge of the company and emotional element." Since Ms. Houseworth's move to Oak Manor, Phoebe's sister visits about every three months. Phoebe's son, who lives in New York, calls his grandmother and visits when he can: "If he doesn't call once a week, my mother will track him down. She will leave messages. He is very concerned that everything is going well with her, so he keeps in touch, especially if something is going on or if he is concerned about her health or anything else. He called me the other night because mother had misplaced her dentures. They have always been very close since he was small. He comes down for holidays, and he has come down a couple of other times also, not as often as mother would like him [to]. She is always very happy when he comes."

Despite their ongoing and extensive kin-work, Ms. Houseworth's family entrusts essential elements of Ms. Houseworth's care to Oak Manor. On the whole, Phoebe, who carefully monitors this care, is well satisfied. Oak Manor administrators, in turn, consider Phoebe a model family member because of her active support of her mother as well as her appreciation of the facility's integral role in her mother's care and of her understanding of its care constraints.

Ethyl Burns of Oak Manor

Ethyl Burns's life at Oak Manor revolves around her family, as it always has. "What makes me happy," she said, "is exactly what I have. I've got a loving family. We've always been one." Ms. Burns moved to Oak Manor primarily to satisfy her nephew Everett, who was worried about her living alone. She remembers her childhood as filled with family: "I had a very happy childhood with my grandparents, my mother's family, which was very large. In fact, her mother gave birth to 16 children. Not all of them lived, but those that did live, I think there were about 12 of them, were very close together. We had a lot of family company. My mother's sister lived about three blocks from the family home, and she had six children. They would spend a lot of time at my grandfather's house, which meant I always had someone to be with. My grandfather's mother . . . lived to be 103, I believe it was, Mama Ralston we called her, and, as she got older and senile, she wouldn't do anything but sit on the porch with her cats and this white dog with brown ears at her feet."

Although Ms. Burns has no children of her own, her large family has remained the center of her life. After her husband died, she moved her own mother into her home and cared for her until her death, all the while working as a high school Latin teacher. Her brother, her only sibling, has six children, all of whom have children of their own. Her nephew Everett, her favorite, lived with her most of his younger life, as did a niece, Katherine, whom she sent to law school. Katherine is married to a lawyer and has two daughters, one "about to come out of medical school." Another niece, Melanie, is a teacher and has three children, "one of [whom] graduated out of Georgia Tech last year." Ms. Burns's family "makes a big thing out of this education there," and she has done what she can to support that value.

Now, at Oak Manor, Ms. Burns's family is still the center of her life. She likes to spend her days in her room going through family pictures or talking on the phone to various family members: "I have family here, you see, so I try to check on most of them every day, or they call me. Then I have two family members from out of town to whom I'm quite close. One has had five bypass surgeries, and the other one has had two severe heart attacks, so I try to keep in touch with them. They're my mother's brother's children, and we're just like brothers and sisters really. I spend a lot of time talking to family members."

Ms. Burns does not see Everett, who has a new job out of town, as often as she would like, but he manages her finances and arranges for her medical appointments. Her nieces also stay busy with their families and work, and her brother "doesn't come as much" because "he's 70-something years old," which is "all right" with her since "he gets kind of cranky." When Ms. Burns goes out, it is mainly to family activities and church. Sometimes a niece will take her to visit a cousin who is in a nursing home, and she always spends holidays with family.

Ms. Burns has "never been a person who had to be somewhere else other than home to be satisfied," and she now has made a home for herself at Oak Manor. As was true for her mother, home is her "niche," and her family remains the heart of her home and the key to her happiness.

Mose Rogers of Blue Skies

Before Mose Rogers moved to Blue Skies, he lived with Horace, one of his two sons, in Atlanta. Mose chose Horace, who is divorced and living alone, because the other son, George, has a wife and children, and he did not want to "get in their way." Of Mose's 11 children, four daughters and five sons are still living. Mose moved to Atlanta from his home in Opelika, Alabama, after the death of his wife of more than 50 years. Mose stayed with Horace for about two years, but Horace's work kept him away until late at night; when Mose eventually tired of the long periods of aloneness, he and his sons decided it was best to move him to Blue Skies. Since the move, Mose's sons visit frequently. Sometimes he spends the weekend with Horace, while George provides transportation to doctor's appointments. Lucius, his son in New York, travels to Opelika to keep an eye on the home place and to Atlanta to visit Mose. A fourth son, Daniel, drives several hours from south Georgia for weekly visits, and a niece in the Atlanta area, who is a nurse, also checks on him from time to time.

In addition to providing direct care themselves, Mose's sons oversee the care Blue Skies provides, and sometimes their close scrutiny irritates Clarice Hull, the home's owner. On one occasion, Horace got angry because he found a pair of pants in Mose's closet that belonged to Gary, the other male resident, and George regularly criticizes Mose's lack of daily activity. Their ongoing complaints led Clarice to call a "family meeting" to address care issues and family responsibilities, and the failure of Mose's sons to attend increased Clarice's ire. In the meeting, Clarice's own grievances included the failure of Mose's sons to even greet care staff when they visit their father: "These are the people taking care of your family members. You should show them some respect."

These conflicts with Clarice temper neither Mose's appreciation of his sons' instrumental and emotional support nor their commitment to him. The family's positive relationships, large numbers, nearby residence, willingness to share care responsibilities, and flexible schedules all enable their care roles, and their kin-work enhances Mose's comfort and care quality and allows him to hold on to his role as family patriarch.

Estelle Washington of Peach Blossom

Before Estelle Washington had a "slight nervous breakdown" and moved to Peach Blossom, she lived in her own home with her daughter Elaine, one of her three children. Her other daughter and her son also live in the Atlanta area, and she has 10 grandchildren and "about 18 great-grands." Ms. Washington is "close to everybody" but has a special bond with Elaine's son John because she cared for him from the age of two months, when Elaine returned to her job as a high school teacher. She is also close to a niece, whom she "raised" as one of her own children.

Elaine hopes to retire next year and bring Ms. Washington back to live in her home, and she continually pleads with her mother, who is chronically depressed, not to "give up" before that time comes. In the meantime, Elaine, her siblings, and her cousin, Ms. Washington's niece, cooperate in their kin-work to provide significant and regular care because they do not want her to feel that they were "giving her away." Elaine described the arrangement, which allows Ms. Washington to spend four weekends each month in her own home:

> Since it's four of us, my cousin took the first Sunday. My sister has the second weekend; I take the third weekend; and my brother takes the fourth weekend. We pick her up on a Friday, we bring her home, and, whoever [has responsibility for her that] weekend, they decide whether they want to stay [at the house with her]. My sister leaves her [own] home and comes here on the second weekend, and she stays the whole weekend. Now when my brother comes, he doesn't spend the night. He just comes and picks her up and prepares food and do whatever needs to be done, and then he leaves and goes but come back in the mornings. Most of

the time, my cousin was taking Mama to her house because it was convenient for her to keep her there, but now that her husband is ill, she stays here. Now, when it's five Sundays in the month, I have to take the responsibility of bringing her home. I don't have to, but I do. Now, if it's any time that we got something that we really need to take care of, we call Ms. Adams and tell her that we won't be picking her up.

Because Ms. Washington's son is retired, he accompanies her to medical appointments and orders her medications. Elaine takes care of "everything else: picking up the medication, handling what bills she has, taking care of personal needs, clothing, whatever." Although Elaine has the bulk of the responsibility, she feels supported by the other caregivers: "Whenever we need each other, it's no problem. Everybody does what they needs to do."

Having Ms. Washington at home, however, is often taxing to Elaine, who has regular household chores as well as school papers to grade: "I can be here on the weekends with her, and she wants me to sit up in the room with her. I said, 'Mama, I have things I have to do. I'm still working. I can't come upstairs and just babysit you.'" Her mother's persistent depressive symptoms also are a constant source of worry and frustration for Elaine.[1]

Slick of Greene's Personal Care

Before Slick, at the age of 79, moved to Greene's, he lived alone on farmland in rural south Georgia. The move was precipitated by a heart attack, which landed him in County Hospital, where he was diagnosed with dementia. Slick's twin sister, Iola, was instrumental in his move to Greene's, mainly because of her assessment that "his mind wasn't hittin' on nothing."

Except for Iola, Slick is not close to any of his other family members. According to Iola, Slick, who has always loved "chasing the womenfolks," has children by two different women but cannot remember how many he has and seldom sees any of them. Although Slick contributed to the financial support of at least some of his children while he was in the Army, Iola believes that her brother's early absence in his children's lives led to their present neglect of him: "I don't think n'er one of 'em called since he ended up here, and they ain't studyin' 'bout him. It's different when children are raised up with somebody. These children wasn't raised up with him. They wasn't around that

---

[1] In the end, Ms. Washington had a stroke and spent her final year in a nursing home, not at home.

much, so they don't consider they're compelled to do things like that." Slick and Iola have older siblings but are not close to any of them, either. Iola recounted that when she and her brother were born, their "daddy didn't approve," claiming they "weren't none of his [not his children]." " 'Cause some men go kill [their] children," their "mama got kinda scared that he might hurt them" and left Alabama and moved to Georgia with her twin babies.

Iola and Slick have remained close throughout their lives, and after his retirement from his job as a sanitation worker in Florida, Slick moved back to Georgia to be near his sister. Since his move to Greene's they see each other often and talk regularly by telephone. Because Slick is physically mobile, he is able to ride the bus to Iola's apartment, a trip he makes several times a week. Iola travels less frequently to Greene's because of her own health problems and her part-time work as a sitter and housekeeper. Her life is further burdened by her son, who recently was released from jail and lives with her, in violation of her rental agreement with public housing. Slick sometimes stays with Iola, but she does not tolerate the occasional women he brings to her home. Nor does Iola understand why Slick "can't consider hisself old" and realize the women are only after his money: "They know he got some money, and that's all they worrying 'bout. They get that, and then they through with him till the next time."

Slick controls his income, derived from Veterans Administration benefits, Social Security, and a pension, which is the highest of Greene's residents. After paying his monthly fee of $1,000, he spends much of the remaining $600 on women, and recently, when Ms. Greene took him to the bank to withdraw her monthly fee, Slick had no money in his account. As a result, Iola had to pay his fees from her skimpy savings, and she now is trying to convince Ms. Greene to assume control of Slick's bank account. Although Iola does not feel competent to take on this task herself, because of her lack of education, she sometimes helps Ms. Greene control her brother's often unruly behavior and believes she has a way with him: "Sometime he want to do his way, but me, I think I can handle him very well. I can talk to him, and I tells him things he should do and he should not do." She even can convince Slick to bathe.

Iola worries about what will happen to Slick if Ms. Greene discharges him. She cannot take him into her home but remains committed to this twin brother, who sustained her when she was in need, and counts on their lifelong bond: "Yeah, we still close together. If I don't go see him, he gonna come see me if he can, and that's one thing I can say about him now. I don't care which away the wind blows. I had a pretty tough time after my mama died, and he helped me out. He sent me money for 12 months. He can come anytime he get ready, 'cause I don't scold him too much unless he do something he got no business. But I'm gonna always welcome him over here, because, you know what? There ain't nobody but me and him now and one sister in Alabama, and she blind. Ain't nobody but me and him."

Kin-Work Patterns

These profiles represent a variety of kin-work patterns. The type and level of support these family members provide range from the daily and substantial emotional and instrumental care Phoebe gives to her mother, Hattie Houseworth, to the less frequent and primarily psychological support Iola provides to her twin brother, Slick. In addition, these profiles demonstrate both continuity and change. Each set of relationships is entrenched in long-standing kin ties, yet the nature and degree of contact and support has evolved. Kin-work patterns vary also in the configuration of support delivery. Iola works alone, in contrast to the ordered collaboration of Estelle Washington's family. What these profiles do not reflect are the almost one-third of residents who benefit little, or not at all, from kin-work.

Family Care Roles: Level and Type of Support

The profile of Hattie Houseworth at Oak Manor portrays the range of instrumental and socioemotional care roles that families of residents in these six communities assume. Ms. Houseworth's daughter Phoebe provides ADL, IADL, and health care and enriches her mother's social and spiritual life. She monitors Oak Manor's care and supports her mother's self-care and health promotion. Her daily visits and phone calls offer unfailing emotional comfort. Phoebe embodies the gold standard of family support.

For most of the 43% of residents who have at least some type of weekly family support, kin-work is much less extensive, typically consisting of weekly contact in the form of visits in the home or outings to church, a beauty shop, or a restaurant. Elva, the daughter of Peach Blossom resident Irene Garrett, described her customary pattern: "Usually, I try to stop by in the evening, but most of the time it's on the weekend, because when I get home usually I'm running to pick up my daughter or it's just always something." In addition,

Elva takes her mother to all medical appointments and occasionally shopping, handles her finances, buys her medications, clothes, incontinence supplies, and other necessities, brings her home for holidays, and monitors her Peach Blossom care. Most residents in this support category, and even some with less frequent contact, have at least one family member who takes on similar instrumental and socioemotional roles.

As table 7.1 shows, the proportion of residents in each care community who receive such support varies, but, as noted, these figures do not tell the whole story. Although only three of the eight residents at Peach Blossom have at least weekly support, just one, Bobby Bailey, has none. Each of the other seven has one or more family members (or, in the case of two residents, kin-scripted friends) who undertake key IADL and health care roles, provide at least occasional recreational activities, and involve residents in special holiday and family events. At Rosie's, only four of the nine residents have kin who take on all such tasks. Of the remaining five, three have sketchy family aid, and two have almost none. Rosie described the support Joseph Render, who has no children, receives from a sister, the only family member involved in his care: "His sister sends [by mail] his haircut money, and she sends fifty cent for each bottle of his medicine." This financial aid, totaling $12.50 and deducted from Mr. Render's own Supplemental Security Income check, is her sole contribution. Rosie's daughter Marilyn told us that for residents like Mr. Render, whose families are "not up to par," Rosie "finds herself going to the store, buying them clothes, buying them shoes, and a lot of other things that I told her she cannot afford to buy, whether she wants to or not."

Although each of the small homes has at least one resident with virtually no family support, such marginal kin-work is more prevalent at Sunshine House and Greene's. Less than a third of the 15 residents at Sunshine House have at least weekly support, and almost half have little or none. More than half (56%) of Greene's residents have no children, and some of these residents, like Boss Cook, have no kin support at all. Oak Manor also has residents who rarely see family members and receive little aid, but more than half have regular support, more than three-fourths have children, and all have someone who provides clothes and other necessary personal items and oversees their care.

Continuity and Change

Kin-work patterns represent both continuity and change. For the majority of residents, continuity lies in the enduring ties elders have with their family

Table 7.1. Level of Family Support

Home	No. of residents	Percentage with weekly support	Percentage with no support	Percentage with no children
Rosie's	9	33	22	22
Peach Blossom	8	38	13	50
Blue Skies	8	62	38	38
Greene's	18	39	39	56
Sunshine House	15	27	47	40
Oak Manor	37[a]	53	27	22
Total	95	43	32	35

[a]Family support information was available on only 37 of the 46 residents.

members. Connections are long-standing, and many family members have played prior caregiving roles. Continuity also is found in situations where family members' lack of support mirrors past behaviors.

Change in kin-work patterns most often is typified by a reduction in support with the move to assisted living. Chapter 4 describes the round-the-clock effort Harold Stamps's family put forth to keep him in his own home. Once he moved to Rosie's, his daughter Lola, who previously had spent every weekend at his home, reduced her care role to managing her father's finances, buying his clothes, and taking him to church once or twice a month. Similarly, Lily Porter, before moving to Blue Skies, had lived with her daughter Sharon. Now Sharon visits once or twice a week and takes her mother to medical appointments and occasionally out to eat. A common scenario is a gradual reduction as family caregivers come to terms with the loss of their own role and begin to trust AL providers. Hassie Hicks's daughter Ernestine described the evolution of her role: "When she first got [to Peach Blossom], I visited her every day. It was hard for me to let go of her, 'cause, see, I was used to having to take care of her. I took care of her for two years straight. So it took awhile for me to come off of making sure she was all right. I worried that she was not gonna be all right. I started going three times a week, and now I make sure I go once or twice, but I always go once a week."

In some cases, like that of Hattie Houseworth's daughter Phoebe, family care roles dramatically increased with the move to AL. In all cases in which Oak Manor residents moved, or were moved, from out of town to be near their children, these kin-work patterns reflect the increased mobility of these middle-class families, compared with the relative immobility of the mostly lower-class families in the small homes. Before the move to Oak Manor, these children had little direct involvement in the care of their parents. For some families, the increased kin-work has led to stronger emotional attachment. Phoebe and her mother have become closer since Ms. Houseworth moved to Atlanta. Hamilton Brewton's son Mark also feels a tighter bond with his father, who moved from St. Louis: "I think we're closer now than we've been since I was maybe 14, 15. Adulthood brings, you might say, solidarity and independence, and I think that brings a detachment from family. And then, in later years, we've grown closer now than we ever have been. I'm crazy 'bout him."

Sometimes residents who move to their family member's locale are able to forge new relationships with grandchildren that up to that time had not been possible. Leiva Yarborough's daughter Yvette recounted the experience of her children, who are regularly involved in their grandmother's life: "Well, interestingly, they say that this is the first time they really have gotten the chance to know her, because we have been in Atlanta since '89, and then we were in New York before that. We have not lived in Cincinnati since they were pretty young. So visiting her was not the same as having her here and being able to visit on a regular basis and take her places." In other situations, kin-work has been redistributed among family members. When Eugene Ellis moved to Atlanta to be near his grandsons, they were kinscripted to assume some of the duties formerly carried out by his daughter in Cleveland.

Change in kin-work patterns also is represented by the altered roles of most older persons with regard to their children or other family members. Whereas in the past, they have been more giver than taker, or at least largely independent, these elders are now in a position of dependence, with few resources to exchange for the care they receive, and some chafe at the transfer of power that comes with this altered status. Although Leiva Yarborough's daughter Yvette professes to be mindful of her mother's position, her words belie a biased reality: "She kinda jokingly says now that I'm the mama and I'm making decisions for her, which is not really true. I definitely have a sensitivity about my mother. I don't try to be bossy with her or anything. I try to direct her on some things that I think she needs to do for herself, but I do try to definitely let her know she's still my mother. Even when it comes to her life, you know, I'm not trying to manage her life."

Cooperation, Conflict, and Going Solo

Kin-work patterns vary in composition, structure, and degree of cooperation among kin group members. When multiple family members are available
to provide care, they tend to share the responsibilities, and kin-work often is
distributed among men, women, and children. Some cooperative arrangements, such as that of Estelle Washington's family, are highly structured and
are designed to balance responsibilities and maximize resources. The family
of Sarah Eubanks, a resident of Rosie's, reflects a similar cooperative pattern.
Ms. Eubanks has nine children, some in town and some not, who share duties. Her daughter Judith, who has assumed a primary role, explained how the
local children kinscripted their out-of-town siblings to share the burden of
caring for their mother, who is mentally ill and has multiple physical health
problems: "It wasn't enough of us, 'cause my mother, she's just so demanding.
It's that time, energy, and attention she needs. So what we ended up doing
was drafting a family letter, and we assigned blocks of time for people to make
their phone calls. One of us had to call between the 1st and the 6th, and then
the next person had to call between the 7th and the 15th. When we did that,
it worked out over 30 days—six blocks of time for all of us—and it worked
pretty good." The son who lives in town often takes his mother to church or,
if not, at least stops by Rosie's on Sundays to visit. Judith depends on one sister to help take their mother to her psychiatric appointments: "My sister's
been helping. I'm so glad, 'cause I would have to take off work, and I had to
get her the night before. My sister can go and get her that morning, do the
treatment, feed her, and then take her back the same day. I couldn't do that."

Such arrangements, which capitalize on caregivers' resources while mini-
mizing their burden, also are most advantageous for residents, as well as their
AL care providers. Sarah Eubanks and Estelle Washington are assured contact
with all of their children. Rosie is relieved of having to help Judith get her
mother to psychiatric appointments, and Esther Adams has more time to
devote to other Peach Blossom residents when Estelle Washington is home
for the weekend. Even with less structured cooperation, contributions from
multiple family members greatly increase overall support. When Leiva Yarborough's granddaughters' visits are added to those of her daughter, she often has
company three or four times a week.

Not all kin collaboration is as seamless as these cases, and even these family groups have their moments of dissension. Sometimes, though, discordant

family relations are more entrenched, and such situations are troublesome for all involved and negatively impact residents' care. One example is the family of Oak Manor resident Ida Mooney, who is depressed and in the early stages of Alzheimer's. Three of Ms. Mooney's four children live in Atlanta, but according to her only daughter, Aimee, "there is a lot of family dysfunction." A major problem has been one son's wife, referred to by Aimee as "manipulative" and "evil." When Ms. Mooney first moved to Atlanta from her home in Maryland, she stayed in this son's home where, according to Aimee, his wife isolated her from the rest of her family. When Ms. Mooney moved to Oak Manor, the sister-in-law ceased her kin-work, and Aimee became primary caregiver, but lack of communication among family members, as well as conflict, has impeded her role. One issue has been getting information about her mother's finances: "Right now, to be very honest, that is what we are trying to get a grip on. Because of the situation with my brother's wife, I actually have no idea. I just found two weeks ago what [Oak Manor] costs. I have no idea what my mother has, what has been going on with her money, and it is not a good feeling." In addition, because mail from Oak Manor was going to her brother's house, Aimee missed a number of facility events, which, in her view, "looks like the family doesn't care, because nobody comes."

For most residents with family support, kin-work, as is typical in the United States (Cantor, 1983; Stone, Cafferata, & Sangl, 1987), is carried out principally by one person, who almost always is a child and usually a daughter. In many cases, the older person has only one child, or only one in the vicinity, such as Hassie Hicks's daughter Ernestine, whose sister is deceased, or Hattie Houseworth's daughter Phoebe, whose sister lives in Philadelphia. Even when other family members are nearby, one typically assumes the bulk of the burden. The words of Sybil, daughter of Rosie's resident Madonna McDowell, reflect a common refrain: "My mother has four children. She has a son and three daughters. There is the oldest daughter, who is living here in Atlanta. Myself, I'm the youngest, and I have a sister in Minnesota. My brother lives in Florida, and, so at this time, it's my older sister and I. I have a son, and she has two sons, and my sister in Minnesota has a nephew here, so in total there are five of us. I'm the youngest, I'm the most involved with her, always have been."

The themes of conflict and cooperation can be extended to the relationships residents' families have with the AL providers they have kinscripted to perform care roles. As unofficial members of the families' extended caregiving network, providers are outside the bounds and control of some families' kin-work ethic. In situations where family-provider relationships are mutually supportive, such as the one Lily Porter's daughter Sharon has with Clarice Hull at Blue Skies, all parties benefit. In contrast, relationships fraught with conflict over care ethics and expectations, like Mose's sons' mostly contentious interactions in this same home, have more negative consequences.

Kin-Work Influences

In the kinscripts paradigm, kin-work is viewed as "the consequence of culturally constructed family obligations defined by economic, social, physical, and psychological family needs" (Stack & Burton, 1993, 161). We found such multiple factors to influence the kin-work patterns of residents in all six homes. Obviously, the absence of children or other kin in the vicinity, or at all, is a principal determinant, but other factors have considerable bearing on the level and type of kin-work, as well as its impact. Some factors relate to residents themselves, others to their family members, and still others pertain to their AL communities. Many of these factors interact to determine relationships between caregivers and care receivers and the ultimate meaning of kin-work in these care communities.

Resident Influences

Residents' chronic diseases may be the most important resident influence on kin-work. The disease-related disabilities and symptoms, of course, engender the need for augmented kin care, and they also affect the ebb and flow of that care. Dementia, for example, a major catalyst in AL placement, continues to influence family roles. The disease's psychological impact on caregivers can be a significant deterrent to interaction (Chappell & Reid, 2002; Grafstrom & Winbald, 1995). Hassie Hicks's daughter Ernestine described the emotional strain related to caring for her mother, who has Alzheimer disease: "Mom used to love to dress up, and, when I see her now, I can see the loss in her eyes, and it breaks my heart. It's like this is my mother's body and face, but it's not her. Nobody can really understand that. One day I was looking at a movie, and this man's mother had Alzheimer's. He carried her to a place and he left her, and he said only 'Call me in her death,' and I said, 'How cruel'; but one or two times, that has entertained my mind that, you know, I just wish I didn't have to go back. It's like it's not her. It's like that's her body and that's her voice, and it's not her. She's here but gone. My mother that I knew is gone. See, that breaks my heart. I don't worry now about her being okay. I just want her back."

Ernestine's pain not only diminishes her satisfaction but also has contributed to a gradual reduction in visits from weekly to once or twice a month. Although common among family members of residents with dementia, such feelings do not always deter their care roles. Clarence Morton, the son of Blue Skies resident Marlena, expressed similar distress over his mother's condition—"Sometime your heart just hurt for 'em, because you be so helpless for 'em"—but he never fails to take her to church on Sunday.

Other mental health problems also influence kin roles and their meaning. Estelle Washington's intractable depression frustrates her family's efforts to please her; Sarah Eubanks's chronic anxiety and unrelenting demands tax her extensive kin-work; and Ida Mooney's daughter Aimee finds that no matter what she does, she can "never do enough" to satisfy her mother. The chronic schizophrenia of several residents, such as Heyward North at Sunshine House, has led to the virtual dissolution of family ties. Other disease symptoms, especially limited mobility and incontinence, act as additional deterrents to family support. Sometimes residents with multiple health problems simply "don't feel like going," which is Elsie Joiner's usual reply when her children invite her out to dinner.

Residents' own investment in kin-work, both past and present, affects their chances of receiving family care. The principle of generalized reciprocity, whereby younger family members attempt to repay care provided to them in the past (Wentowsky, 1981), has widespread influence on families' care roles. In other cases, elders still have resources to exchange for care received. A few (all at Oak Manor) provide instrumental aid, such as Leiva Yarborough, who gives regular financial assistance to her daughter, and Rozena Banks, who similarly helps her son. More often, elders assume the traditional African American kin function of mentor (Hatch, 1991; Taylor, 1988). Eugene Ellis moved to Atlanta and Oak Manor to take on this role: "I made the choice of coming here, I would say to you, primarily because of my family. Family I identify first as my great-grands. My great-grandparents didn't live long enough for me to know them, and I made a calculated decision that one of the contributions that I could make in my lifetime is to have my great-grands know what a great-grandpa is like. I thought I could make a greater contribution to those young people, who are yet to develop."

Hamilton Brewton, who has mild dementia, provides ongoing advice to his granddaughter and grandson, a role both they and their parents highly value. Mr. Brewton's son Mark, who has difficulty himself communicating with these teenagers, affirmed his father's role: "My daughter uses him as her, what would you say, not counselor or mentor, her adviser. They discuss things, and she has great conversations with him about what sexual behavior should be, about morals and morality. Same thing with my son—they confide. Well, it's a traditional concept of the village. He's the elder, and he's passing on the wisdom, and so far, knock on wood, it's good wisdom. You know, he may forget from time to time that he already told somebody this, that, or the other, but otherwise it's good wisdom." Conversely, Slick's past absence in his children's lives contributes to their neglect of him. Similar parental behaviors impede support for other residents, such as fellow Greene's resident Boss Cook.

A variety of other resident traits can either boost or curtail kin-work. One is personality. Some individuals are more assertive than others in seeking family aid, a strategy that often is successful but, when overdone, can backfire. Upbeat natures, like that of Rosie's resident Madonna McDowell, whose daughter Sybil enjoys taking her out to dance clubs and watching her "shimmy on the dance floor," promote contact. Some persons, like Greene's resident Beatrice Dove, are just difficult or have physical traits that make them hard to help. Ms. Dove's niece Kate described the difficulty she has helping her aunt: "It's hard to find clothes with her being so big. Most of the time, she prefers to wear the old clothes with the holes in them. I take her new stuff and she won't wear it. Last time I took her some dresses, she told me not to bring her anything else."

Family Influences

Most family members who embrace their caregiving roles do so because they believe it is what families ought to do. Although their values form the bedrock of their caregiving, kin-work values compete with other values, and kin-work rivals other demands. The demands of kin-work also "criss-cross" (conflict with one another) (Stack & Burton, 1993, 164). As a result, many family members experience the role conflict and role strain widely reported in the caregiving literature (Brody, 1981; Cantor, 1983; Stone, Cafferata, & Sangl, 1987).

Leiva Yarborough's daughter Yvette struggles to reconcile her values clash. First, she cannot accept her mother's placement at Oak Manor: "It's difficult for me, I think, being an only child and not having any sisters or brothers to share some of the responsibilities with, and that just puts an emotional burden on me, particularly because I don't feel comfortable with her being there. It's getting more and more bothersome to me. Well, I'm just saying that, as a whole, it is not something that the African American people do. It's usually, families stay with family." Yvette is further conflicted by her desire both to help her mother and, at this point in her life, to find personal fulfillment: "I guess the question you were asking me was, 'Do I spend enough time with her?' No, I would like to even be able to spend more time with her, but I'm almost, well, 50. At the same time, there's things in my life that are just opening up, and, since my children, I was a housewife and mother, the whole time that my children were growing up, and, now that they are on their own—they completed college and all of that—I just feel like my life is opening."

Although Yvette's struggle is quite real and personally difficult, she has a choice that many families of residents in these six homes do not have. She is one of only a handful of family members, all relatives of Oak Manor residents, who are not employed. For all others, kin-work competes with one, and sometimes two, jobs. The situation of Beatrice Dove's niece Kate is common: "I try to see [my aunt] every two to three weeks. It's hard because of my work schedule. I work every day, including Sundays. Most of my days are 12-hour days. I have this business and the daycare." For many families of residents of the small homes, employment is a means of paying the rent and putting food on the table. Others, like most Oak Manor families, are struggling to move up in the world. As Sharon, the daughter of Blue Skies resident Lily Porter, explained, "More African Americans are upwardly mobile, and two household incomes are required."

Additional family caregiving responsibilities compound work demands. Sarah Eubanks's daughter Judith, who has three school-age children and a full-time job, reflects the common predicament of children, usually women, in the "sandwich" generation (Brody, 1981). Others have teenagers, children in college, grandchildren, and even other aging relatives. Eugene Ellis's daughter Caroline also cares for her mother and an aunt in Cleveland, and when she comes to Atlanta to see her father, her children and grandchildren compete for her time.

Some kin caregivers have health problems, common among older caregivers, that influence their roles. Slightly more than a fourth are siblings, and many are old and sick themselves. Slick's sister Iola has diabetes, arthritis, and high blood pressure. Miss Fannie's sister, her only caregiver, is also in her 90s. Others are unable to help because of addiction to alcohol and other drugs. Marlena's faithful son Clarence cannot trust his brother to share his caregiving burden because "he could get on one of his sprees and he'd be gone, and there she is there by herself or something."

Geographic location and access to transportation also affect kin-work. Iola has no car, and unless she can get a ride from her son or daughter, she must travel by bus, train, and bus again to visit Slick at Greene's. Hamilton Brewton's son Mark rarely brings his father to his home because he lives 35 miles from Oak Manor, so "to pick him up, take him to the house, and bring him back, it's roughly two hours of travel time."

Many of the barriers that impede kin-work are exacerbated by poverty. Family members who are poor have been so throughout their lives, and caring for residents who also are poor brings additional burdens. When Harold Stamps's daughter Lola buys clothes for her father and saves for his "opening and closing at Cedarlawn cemetery," the money comes from the income she receives as a nanny. Low-income family members often are in worse health than those with higher incomes, and they typically work longer hours in jobs that are more physically taxing.

No family member is without kin-work roadblocks, but some are distinguished by the superhuman efforts they make, despite barriers. In contrast are the minority of family members who seem to shirk, or outright reject, their kin duties. For these few, the explanation must come down to values. As Vivian, the activity director at Oak Manor, said, "Some, you know, they put the parents up and that is it. Then they live their lives."

Facility Influences

The owners and administrators in each of these homes highly value family support and believe strongly that families have a critical role in residents' care and should be willing to make sacrifices for their well-being. Rosie's viewpoint is the most strident: "It should be made mandatory that they participate with they family members, just like the schools are gonna make sure that you go to PTA meetings and things like that. Like the Office of Regulatory Service make us do what we do, they can make their family member do their part. They should be required to come and take their family member out at least once a month."

Rosie's view is based on her intense personal value for kin-work, including in assisted living: "Children owe their parents a certain amount of time. You don't have any right to take your family member and put them somewhere and, just because you're paying, don't have anything else to do with them, because they taken the time to raise you up and they didn't discard you. They put you in the nursery, and they came and got you and seen about you and fed you and spent time with you, and you still owe that to your parents. I really feel you owe them time, if it's nothing but come and get them and take 'em out and buy 'em a ice cream cone, or take 'em up there to the park and sit with 'em at the table and talk with them and bring them back, at least once a month." Rosie's expectations for families emphasize emotional over instrumental care, because she knows this is a role she cannot fulfill, even though she certainly tries. It hurts her pocketbook when she has to buy clothes for Joseph Render, but it hurts her heart when no family member takes him home for Christmas.

The other owners and operators in these care communities share Rosie's viewpoint, and, like her, all endeavor to promote family involvement. They all understand that for them to be effective extensions of kin-work, they need the support of family members. A primary strategy is to specify family responsibilities and make clear facility expectations. These policies are written in admission agreements and communicated verbally upon admission and later as the need arises. Lucy Small, the resident services director at Oak Manor, affirmed the need to make such policies explicit, a tactic not used when the facility first opened: "Part of the problem that we had in the beginning, because we didn't spend that time explaining it to people, is that the drop-off here was like a nursing home—don't call me for anything; you're expected to handle everything. No, we don't do that. So, I try to let them know what the expectation is while they're at home, for the families, so that when they get here, they don't expect us to do everything, because they will if you don't explain it." According to Lucy, Oak Manor's expectations are "for them to be extremely involved. I always tell families. My question is, 'Who's responsible when Mama needs to go to the doctor, or making sure she has appointments?' They looked at me like, 'You are?' 'No, you need to assign somebody to be responsible for your mom.' I even tell them, 'If you need a case manager, I can refer you to some senior sources,' but for them to know that that's not part of our responsibility. A lot of problems that I think happen, not just here, but in assisted living in general, is that people end up deteriorating because families don't take the initiative of keeping up with their family's care, and that's so important."

Calling family members to request an item or service or discuss care issues as the need arises is a common strategy in all homes. Sometimes more formal approaches are employed. Clarice invited Blue Skies family members to a meeting to explain her expectations for their care roles and to respond to their complaints. During the time of the study, Oak Manor had two family meetings, where facility directors were available to clarify issues related to their particular services and convey the responsibilities they expected family members to assume.

Providers in these homes have learned that their effectiveness as kin-work partners is enhanced by learning about family members and their circumstances. Eva, a care staff member at Oak Manor, who uses this same strategy with residents, expressed this view: "You want to get to know the families as much as you possibly can, and then you can understand what is going on. You want to get a full picture of the family members, as well as the residents, and, when you can do that, you can pretty much establish what is needed." By using this strategy, Rosie is more accepting of, and less frustrated by, some family inadequacies, such as those of Harold Stamps's daughter Lola: "She works like 10 hours a day out in Buckhead somewhere, and so I understand why she can't [come more often], but she does buy him sufficient clothing and shoes." Getting to know family members, of course, is easier in small homes than in large, and in any home it is dependent on some degree of family involvement.

Some providers also encourage family participation by including families in the home's social activities. Esther Adams always invites family members to dinner for residents' birthdays, and Cora Greene encourages family attendance at Greene's annual Christmas Eve dinner. Oak Manor had a family Pokeno night and routinely invites families to special events, such as the Fourth of July picnic and holiday dinners. The facility also sends out a monthly newsletter and calendar of activities.

Although special activities provide an incentive for families to visit in these communities, the "feel" of a home and the degree to which families are free to visit also have an influence. Jordan Taylor, the corporate representative assigned to Oak Manor, expressed this viewpoint: "I think it's creating that feeling. Then your families want to come in and see what's going on, and we encourage families coming in by having 24-hour visitation. If they want to get here in the middle of the night, they can come in, and [we don't limit] their access to their resident." Small homes, of course, cannot have 24-hour visitation, because the owners and operators need to sleep, but certain of these homes are more welcoming—both in policy and atmosphere. Although Rosie's official visiting hours end at 7:30 p.m., she welcomes family members whenever they want to come. The relaxed atmosphere in her home makes them feel comfortable, and she often joins in their family visits. One night she sipped wine until eleven at night with Madonna McDowell and her daughter. Esther Adams, however, who likes to get to bed early, rarely bends her seven o'clock curfew.

A home's physical environment also can affect the extent and type of family support. The private rooms at Blue Skies and Oak Manor facilitate both visiting and care. Hattie Houseworth's daughter Phoebe found her long periods of visiting quite pleasant in her mother's private space, and Leiva Yarborough's two-room suite allowed her daughter to move in for several days and care for her when she was ill. A facility's public space, both indoors and out, and the safety of the surrounding locale also impact kin-work. Sunday visits to Oak Manor by Alma Burgess's niece are encouraged by the attractive outdoor seating area with walkways where her son rides his bike. Homes like Sunshine House and Greene's, which have limited common space for their residents, offer few enticements to guests. Some Greene's family members are fearful of visiting because of its high-crime neighborhood.

Facilities strive to support families in their kin-work. Oak Manor holds educational programs, usually related to health care issues, and individual staff members provide information and emotional support. Esther Adams gives family members advice on how to care for their relatives in their own homes and recently began an Alzheimer's support group for Peach Blossom families. Rosie always has a willing ear to listen to family problems, and she provided information on a source for low-cost protective pads to families of incontinent residents. Lily's daughter Sharon appreciates how Clarice Hull "works with" her: "She found out about a situation where my mother could get some more assistance, and she called me and said, 'Why don't you check this out?' and I think that's great." Sharon also likes the way Clarice calls to ask her opinion about Lily's care. Kay Hughes, the manager at Sunshine House, has developed close relationships with several family members and provides regular counsel. Such support from facility caregivers bolsters families' own care roles.

The Meaning of Kin-Work

Over the life course, kin-work serves to regenerate families, maintain lifetime continuities, sustain intergenerational responsibilities, and reinforce shared values (Stack & Burton, 1993). In this chapter, we have seen that kin-work not only continues once individuals move to assisted living but also maintains many of its time-honored meanings—both for residents and for their family members. When residents, family members, and AL providers share kin-work, or become kin "partners," kin-work takes on additional meanings for the entire care community and adds value to the lives of all.

For most residents, a significant value of kin-work lies in the instrumental support their family members provide. Family assistance with basic ADLs, IADLs, and health care helps residents maintain their health and function and enhances the overall quality of their care. Instrumental support also allows residents to continue valued activities and hold on to former identities. When Lola buys the clothes and "nice shiny, black shoes" that her father, Harold Stamps, "loves," she helps him, at age 96, "be as sharp as he has always been." By taking him to his "home church" once a month, she keeps him socially and spiritually connected to his past. Eugene Ellis's outings with his grandsons hold similar multifaceted value: "When I was home, I was taken out a lot to eat. So, when I'm here, for an example, within this week, Sunday, I ate breakfast at the International Pancake House with one part of my family. Last night I went to a fabulous restaurant—over in some shopping area, casual-living, buffet style. I enjoyed that. Then my grandson went to Home Depot to pick up some windows, and then we went to the barbershop and talked about music and all the old artists. There is an older man there, and he knew about Sinatra and Billy Eckstine and Johnny Hartman, and a lot of the old singers. So we had a good time."

Kin-work helps AL residents maintain valued ties with family members and remain integrated in their family network. For Eugene Ellis and others, who for the first time live near grandchildren and great-grandchildren, kin-work rekindles and deepens family bonds. The value of these new connections is compounded by the mentoring roles they make possible. Residents like Mr. Ellis and Leiva Yarborough, who are able to continue traditional African American elder roles as givers of instrumental and emotional support, derive additional meaning (Hatch, 1991; Stack, 1974; Taylor, 1988). The ability to reciprocate, even in small ways, for the care they receive also helps alleviate feelings of dependency and burden (Ball & Whittington, 1995; Dowd, 1975).

Family involvement sometimes has less positive meaning for AL residents. In most cases, the negative aspects of kin-work relate to restrictions families impose on residents' autonomy, such as limits on telephone access or activities. Even in these family situations, though, the meaning of kin-work is overwhelmingly positive. In sum, kin-work adds considerable value to the lives of AL residents. As Ethyl Burns said, "They all have just made my life a joy."

In an earlier study in AL facilities where the majority of residents were white, we also found that families assumed substantial roles in the care of residents and that this family support was a significant component of residents' quality of life (Ball et al., 2000). More than half of the residents in that study had at least weekly visits from family members, and most received some type of instrumental care. Research in nursing homes demonstrates that families also continue to minister to residents of these more institutional long-term care settings (Bitzan & Kruzich, 1990; Port et al., 2001; Ross, Carswell, & Dalziel, 2002).

In the chapters that follow, we continue to show the impact of kin-work on residents' lives. In chapter 8, we see how families help residents stay connected to the wider community and to their spiritual selves; in chapter 9, we give further evidence of the effect of kin-work, both positive and negative, on residents' autonomy; and in chapters 10 and 11, we further illustrate the role of families in residents' ability to age in place and find meaning in their lives.

Kin-work also has considerable meaning for AL providers and their communities of care. Family support adds to the overall care value of each community. Each task that a family member takes on is one less that a busy owner or staff member has to perform, and the reduction of care burden helps providers conserve their resources or redistribute them to more needy residents. The care that families give their residents also reaffirms providers' own value for family care and increases their well-being along with that of residents.

In addition, the presence of family members adds value to the social environment of the entire facility, particularly in the small homes. A visit to Rosie's from Harold Stamps's daughter Lola makes a brighter day for all residents: "I feel like I brighten up their day when I come in, 'cause I'm so talkative. And by the time I hug everybody, you know, it's like they're always glad to see me. Sometimes I'll take ice cream, sometimes I'll take bananas—and I bet they might need some ice cream on a day like today." Some family members include other residents in the activities they offer their own relatives—for example, Marlena's son Clarence, who takes other Blue Skies residents to church along with his mother. In some cases, providers are able to maintain personal bonds with family members, such as Rosie's friendships with the daughters of Harold Stamps and Pearl Bowman. Others develop new relationships, like that of Kay Hughes, the manager of Sunshine House, with Mayetta Stewart's extended family.

Kin-work holds many of the same meanings for family members as it does for residents and AL providers. Families' continuation of their care roles following residents' moves to assisted living is consistent with their cultural ideal of family support and helps ease their guilt and anxiety about their elders' well-being. Kin-work helps families maintain valued ties to residents and, in cases of cooperative kin-work, keeps extended family members connected to one another. Kin-work provides some family members with useful roles, while others benefit from elders' own kin contributions. The rewards of kin-work for the families of these AL residents are similar to those reported for caregivers of elders living in home care settings (Doka, 2004; Noonan & Tennstedt, 1997).

Yet despite the substantial reward that caregiving brings family members, their kin-work is not without considerable cost. An extensive body of literature confirms the emotional and physical strain associated with informal caregiving in both African American (Cox & Monk, 1996; Dilworth-Anderson, Williams, & Cooper, 1999; Fox, Hinton, & Levkoff, 1999; Mui, 1992) and white (Burton et al., 2003; Cantor, 1983; Stone, Cafferata, & Sangl, 1987) families, and the experiences of the families of these AL residents are no different. Many had reached the limits of their caregiving resources while residents still lived in their own homes, and with the move to assisted living, their caregiving efforts continue to stretch the bounds of their physical, financial, and psychological capabilities. We have seen the pain of losing a parent to Alzheimer's or mental illness, the guilt over not doing enough, the strain of competing roles, the tensions associated with sharing care tasks with AL providers and other family members, the stress of dealing with difficult behaviors related to dementia and mental illness, and the sacrifices of money and health.

Countless studies document similar sources of stress associated with caregiving, including the care recipient's health, especially the presence of dementia (Chappell & Reid, 2002; Tornatore & Grant, 2002), the level of ADL dependence (Newens, Foster, & Kay, 1995), and behavioral problems (Chappell & Reid, 2002); caregiver role strain (Brody, 1981; Stone, Cafferata, & Sangl, 1987); and conflicts between family and formal caregivers (Gaugler et al., 2000). Like many of those in our study, African American families often face additional challenges because of poverty (Dilworth-Anderson, 1992).

Although the struggles and personal costs associated with kin-work deter some families and cause others to reject kin-work outright, most have not, as

Rosie suggests, "dumped their peoples and never come back." They may not uphold the African American ideal of "families staying with families," but they keep giving and caring despite what for some may seem like insurmountable barriers. These families exemplify the well-known complexity of the caregiving situation and the multiple factors that mediate the impact of burden (Chappell & Reid, 2002; Yates, Tennstedt, & Chang, 1999). Among the most important mediators are the meanings attached to caregiving (Noonan & Tennstedt, 1997) and the caregiver's relationship with the care recipient (Yates, Tennstedt, & Chang, 1999). For Marlena Morton's son Clarence, "that love instinct" nourishes his value for kin-work, and that "smile on her face" is the reward of his labors. In the face of burden, the rewards of caregiving, however few, sustain many of these families as they continue the kin-work tradition of African American families.

CHAPTER 8

Bridges to Care

In their monograph on frail elders living alone in their own homes, Rubinstein and colleagues note the increased importance of vectors to the world outside the home for those whose life space, energy, and possibility are reduced (Rubinstein, Kilbride, & Nagy, 1992). Although the primary reason residents move to assisted living is to receive support not available to them at home, the care they want and need often cannot be found completely within their new AL homes, and members of the wider community continue to minister to their social, emotional, physical, and health care needs and enrich the overall quality of their lives. In this chapter, we explore the many-faceted contributions of the wider community to residents and their AL providers in each of these six communities. We speak of "bridges" to the outside world, referring both to community agents who provide support in and out of the AL setting and to individuals who enable residents to "bridge" the gap between facility and community.

Community bridges include a variety of individuals and groups who perform a range of functions. The AL providers who own and work in these six homes are principal players, as are residents' family members. Bridges in the small homes differ in many respects from those in the one large home. Our exploration of community bridges includes community day programs, churches, AL providers, and social service and health care providers. We begin with community day programs, a vital bridge for residents of small ALFs.

Community Day Programs

For almost half the 58 residents of the small homes, community day programs offer the most consistent bridge to the world outside the AL community. In four of the five small homes (all except Sunshine House), a total of 27 residents attend one or more of 13 different community day programs at least some of the time. These programs are of four basic types: senior, adult day health (ADH), mental health, and vocational rehabilitation. All of these programs are operated by private nonprofit agencies financed either through a combination of public and private funding or through private funds alone, and they represent a range in quality of services and facilities.

The senior centers provide a midday meal and a variety of recreational and educational activities for older adults. Three of these centers are operated by the county and partially financed by county and federal dollars (through the Older Americans Act). The Lincoln Center is a newly opened multipurpose center with 30,000 square feet of floor space. A fourth is financed by the Episcopal Church and individual donations. The ADH programs are mandated to provide health-related and therapeutic services and medical supervision for impaired adults of all ages and are funded primarily by federal and state dollars through the Medicaid waiver program (the Community Care Services Program) but also receive money from the county and participants' fees. The mental health day centers have long-range goals for participants to become productive citizens and learn how to manage their illnesses. Two are state funded, and the third is financed by an Episcopal church. The one vocational rehabilitation center is state funded. The following description of residents' experiences in these day programs portrays their role in the lives of residents and owners of the four participating homes.

The Experience of Small Homes

At the beginning of our study, all six Peach Blossom residents participated in four day programs, each quite different from the others. Three residents—Hassie Hicks, Estelle Washington, and Mayetta Stewart (before she moved to Sunshine House)—attended Dawnview Senior Center, housed in a recently renovated city library. All of the approximately 43 participants, other than the Peach Blossom residents, live in their own homes. Activities include daily devotionals, Bingo, exercise, a variety of crafts, and regular monthly outings. Lunches are prepared off-site by a nonprofit organization that provides meals for all the county senior centers. The center has all new furnishings and is well equipped, including even a pottery kiln. Ms. Hicks attended Dawnview before she moved to Peach Blossom, and although she now has some dementia, she still enjoys Bingo and the devotional. Ms. Washington, who is depressed, is more often observer than participant and even brings her own lunch, usually a peanut butter and jelly sandwich. Neither resident goes on center outings, because of Ms. Washington's lack of interest and Ms. Hicks's tendency to wander. Ms. Stewart, who was more engaged in center life than the other two women, was no longer able to attend when she moved to Sunshine House.

Ivera Haygood participated in an adult day care program located in the resource-rich Lincoln Center, which has a full-service kitchen and a swimming pool. Ms. Haygood began attending the program several months after she moved to Peach Blossom and stayed until her death, five months later. Although hearing impaired and unable to communicate verbally, she engaged in all activities, even swimming, and made new friends.

Bobby Bailey, who is mentally retarded and hearing impaired, and Leona Scott, who has dementia, attend two different ADH centers. Bobby's is located in the basement of a former church and has only six participants and few amenities. Bobby's "place" at one of the center's round tables is marked by his coloring book. Ms. Scott's program, housed in a former residence on a large wooded lot, has approximately 30 participants and is known for its "good reputation." Activities are geared for participants with cognitive impairment, like Ms. Scott, and those without.

Getting residents ready to go to these four different programs launches each day at Peach Blossom, and their participation circumscribes the home's and Esther Adams's daily routines: "Usually I'm up about 6:30 in the morning, and I will start by getting the person probably that would go out first. We have four different services coming to pick up, because the residents go separate ways, because we have tried to put each resident in a center, or they were already there when they came to me, that they can get the most out of what that center is offering. In the morning, now, we don't all eat together because of the van service. Some come sooner than the other, so we allow [residents], as they get ready, to come to the table and have their breakfast so that they'll be ready when the transportation comes. And once they're all off to the center, then, of course, we do some [work] here—housework, laundry, and et cetera and run errands and be always back by two o'clock in order to receive them."

Ms. Adams believes strongly that leaving the home each day is "good for" residents. Over the years she has tried to admit residents who share her view and even considered discharging Ms. Washington when she threatened to stop going to Dawnview. It is also, of course, good for Ms. Adams. While they are gone, she has time to take care of housekeeping chores, attend training sessions, and occasionally have lunch with her good friend, a fellow provider; and she has one less meal to provide. But these benefits require effort on her part, and she plays a key role in residents' access and attendance. She helped secure Ivera Haygood's coveted spot at the Lincoln Center and located a program that would take Bobby for $100 per month, paying the fee herself. Because Bobby's center does not offer transportation services, she arranged for his caseworker to pay for Sally, her part-time staff person, to take him back and forth. In addition to making sure residents are ready for pick-up each day, she communicates with center personnel about activities and care issues, makes Ms. Washington's lunch, and sometimes provides transportation when vans do not show up or come too early. She occasionally prepares coffee and a sweet roll for the driver of Ms. Scott's van, in appreciation of his kind attention, but once reprimanded him for giving Ms. Scott cookies. She is mindful of staffing limitations at Dawnview Senior Center and keeps Ms. Hicks and Ms. Washington home on field trip days.

Peach Blossom family members, some of whom play a pivotal role, also extol the benefits of day programs. Hassie Hicks's daughter Ernestine believes the center fills an important gap in Ms. Adams's services and provides continuity with her mother's former life: "Since Ms. Adams doesn't have a lot of activities there, I'm glad that Mom goes to the center. See, they do exercise every morning in the center, and she plays Bingo, which she loves. She walks in, and she signs the book, and she knows that center. I wanted to get her in a place that she could continue going to the same center. I would be unhappy if she had to stay [at Peach Blossom] all day with nothing [to do]." Because senior centers typically bar access to AL residents, Ernestine had to lobby for her mother's entry: "My husband and I had to really work on that, you know, and I had a councilwoman to help me, too. Without one of the council people's help, I don't think I would have been able to pull it off, 'cause they don't want to pick up at personal cares. I don't understand that, and that's what I was trying to tell the lady. My mother is a taxpayer and been going to this same center and, just because she has to go out of her home, doesn't mean she doesn't need the center. She still needs the center."

Other Peach Blossom family members include day program involvement in their kin-work. Ms. Adams expects family members, in addition to helping with access, to handle any resident care or behavior issues, such as when Ms. Scott began coming home with items belonging to other participants or having wet herself.

With the exception of Ms. Washington, who, according to Ms. Adams, "might would just stay at home" if it were left up to her, Peach Blossom residents enjoy, even love, their day programs. A friend of Ms. Haygood's reported after a visit to her center, "She loved it, she loved it. I went there one day, and I didn't know her. She was playing table tennis, and, you know, she doesn't meet strangers. All the people there, the staff as well as those who were there just like she was, they all loved her. And quite a few of them came to the funeral, staff and all."

But AL residents' participation in day programs is tenuous. When Bobby's center closed for financial reasons, Ms. Adams could not find another one to accept him for the amount of money she could pay, and Bobby returned to spending his days at Peach Blossom. By the end of the study, only two of these six residents (Ms. Hicks and Ms. Scott) still attended day programs. Ms. Stewart had moved to Sunshine House, Ms. Haygood had died, and Ms. Washington had entered a nursing home, and no centers had been found for the two residents who replaced them.

Like Peach Blossom residents, Rosie's residents at one time participated in four different programs: two senior centers, one ADH program, and one mental health program. Six attend the Jerusalem Senior Center, a county-operated center affiliated with the Methodist Church. For most of the study period, Rosie drove the residents herself (10 miles round trip) and frequently stayed at the center to help the three who are cognitively impaired. Sometimes, she goes along on field trips to pick apples or pecans, and she pays $40 a week for the "voluntary" meal contribution. Rosie attributes her residents' continued participation, as well as the center's ultimate agreement to provide transportation, to her own role: "They want everybody to be able to do the things they need to do for theirselves. They was taking them because I was volunteering over there and I would be there with them. Mostly all of the centers are like that. They don't want the people like Ms. Burns and Ms. McElhaney and, plus wearing a diaper, they'll tell you right quick, don't bring them. That's the way Jerusalem is, too, because they never take them to the bathroom. If I wasn't there, they would hold their water all day long until they got back here. But I never complain, because, you start complaining, you get your people discharged."

Cleo Kellog for a while went to St. John's Senior Center on Tuesdays and Thursdays and an ADH program on alternate days. She had attended both centers before moving to Rosie's from another small ALF. Ms. Kellog much preferred St. John's, located in the basement of a church, where she developed a close relationship with the young male director, whom she referred to as her "boyfriend"; but because St. John's has no transportation services, Rosie had to take Ms. Kellog to the center herself, a chore that ultimately became too much for her. Ms. Kellog's ADH center is in a new, two-story building, and Madonna McDowell, who moved to Rosie's toward the end of the study, also is a long-time participant. Ms. Kellog's and Ms. McDowell's fees are paid through a grant from the county. Rosie would have liked all of her residents to attend this ADH center, but no additional "scholarship" funds were available. Although Tracey Williams, Rosie's one young resident with mental health problems, at different times attended both Jerusalem and St. John's, about halfway through the study period she began participating in a state-funded mental health day treatment program, much more appropriate to her age and disability. Rosie's daughter, whose son has mental health problems, knew about the program and was instrumental in Tracey's access.

Like Esther Adams, Rosie believes her residents should not stay at home to just "eat and sleep" all day. Even those with dementia "know a little something" and "like getting out." Harold Stamps sings along with the hymns during the daily devotionals, and Dora McElhaney dances when they play music. Tracey benefits from group therapy sessions and medication management at her center and once was given the opportunity to earn $20, which she used to buy cigarettes. Although Sarah Eubanks and Cleo Kellog sometimes say they get "tired of going everyday," they enjoy getting out and love winning Bingo prizes, which they save for gifts to relatives. Ms. Eubanks often leads the devotion at Jerusalem and won the Black History Month contest with her rendition of "The Battle Hymn of the Republic."

Sometimes Rosie has to handle problems related to her residents' mental impairments: Ms. Kellog once "beat up" another lady and pulled her hair, and Dora McElhaney, having refused to put on her seat belt, was ousted from the bus and sent home in a cab (at Rosie's expense). Unlike Esther Adams, Rosie does not involve residents' families in center issues, nor is she quite as careful preparing residents to leave. Occasionally, Ms. Kellog has to take a peanut butter and jelly sandwich or sausage biscuit "to go" because she has not had breakfast when the van comes, or Mr. Stamps may not have had his morning shave.

Five residents of Greene's, all white males with chronic mental health problems, go to a day program at Our Savior's, a neighborhood Episcopal church. The program was created in 1982 expressly to minister to residents of small ALFs, and Cora Greene's residents have always been involved. It is directed by Father Paul, the church's rector, and staffed mostly by volunteers. Father Paul strives to "create an environment of recovery for people with se-

vere and persistent mental illness" by providing "a haven" and "as many opportunities as we can for people." Our Savior's operates on Tuesdays and Thursdays, and services include breakfast and lunch, a foot care clinic, free clothing, facilities for bathing and washing clothes, counseling, an art program, a
poetry class taught by a local college professor, field trips, and parties. Many
of the participants also attend worship services on Sundays and Wednesday
nights. Although the program provides transportation, the five Greene's participants choose to walk the quarter-mile distance. Each of these men, ranging in age from 40 to 67, benefits from the activities and socialization. Edward
Fitzsimmons has principal responsibility for the breakfast service and calls it
his "work"; Burt Hatfield arrives early to shower and do his laundry; and Joe
Kelly has written numerous poems, which he mails to his sister in South Carolina. Mr. Fitzsimmons also attends a county-funded day treatment program
for chronic schizophrenics based at County Hospital. Here, he also assists with
food preparation and often brings leftovers, such as pastries, home with him
to share with other residents and staff at Greene's.

Another group of five Greene's residents attends the Emmanuel Senior
Center, which, like Our Savior's, is partially funded by the Episcopal Church.
One of the researchers, a long-time volunteer at the center, helped them access the program in response to Ms. Greene's appeal for assistance. The center
is open Mondays, Wednesdays, and Fridays from 10 until 2 and provides a hot
lunch and a variety of activities, including devotionals, exercise, crafts, and
monthly restaurant outings and grocery shopping. Because the center does
not provide transportation for Greene's residents, Ms. Greene drives them in
her seven-passenger van. Transporting Boss is a particular challenge, owing to
the combination of his girth and limited mobility and Ms. Greene's bad back.
Ms. Greene also pays the five dollars per resident monthly "dues."

Blue Skies residents' participation in day programs was quite limited, mainly
because the owner, Clarice Hull, had difficulty finding a center, despite her
ongoing efforts. The senior centers closest to the home were full, others do
not furnish transportation, and Clarice has no van. Finally, six weeks before
the end of the study, Clarice found an ADH center, which could both transport residents and furnish "scholarships" to cover fees, but the residents' tenure
was cut short by the center's closing, owing to the death of the director. Even
so, after only one month some of the residents were beginning to tire of the
required daily attendance. Although the center advertised a variety of activities, they consisted mostly of Bingo and board games.

For several months at the beginning of our study, Gary, the 23-year old resident with mental retardation, attended a vocational rehabilitation program for adults with disabilities, where he received a small stipend. His participation ended when, according to his mother, he "got stubborn" and "didn't want to cooperate," but while it lasted, Blue Skies manager Inez Sawyer had some relief from his disruptive presence.

Rewards and Costs of Participation

The rewards of day program participation for residents are numerous (Combs, 2002). Father Paul (the director of Our Savior's), in speaking of his program's goals, stated, "The critical thing here is we've learned we are not just giving people a safe place in which they can come and sit and have dignity but [we are also broadening] the horizons of people." Horizons are broadened, he believes, by exposing participants to activities they otherwise would not have, and may never have experienced, such as field trips to the zoo or a museum and writing poetry and painting. Because most of the residents of the small ALFs are poor and have spent much of their lives working, they have had little experience with creative or leisure activities. Residents who have an opportunity to engage in activities beyond the tired and predictable find them most rewarding; consistent with Rosie's viewpoint, even those who are unable to fully participate derive some benefit.

Special events also are meaningful. Boss, hospitalized in December, was intent on being discharged in time to attend the Emmanuel Center Christmas party, described by Miss Fannie as having "so much food and dancing." This was the only holiday party that these two Greene's residents attended that year. Joe Kelly, who is white, looks forward to the Valentine's dance at Our Savior's because they have "clean dancing with both black and white women."

For some residents of these small homes, particularly those with no family support, day programs may offer the only prospect of leaving the home, save for medical appointments. This was true for Boss, whose description of an ordinary day depicts his confinement: "I might go out on the porch and stand, but I usually get out and go to the center, then come back home, and that's just about it."

As Edward Fitzsimmons's enthusiastic comment—"Yeah, I got friends at the church"—suggests, day programs expand residents' opportunities to make new friends and stay in contact with old. This meaning is important for all residents but especially so for those who are cognitively intact and live among those who are not, such as Rosie's resident Carole Seymour, who looks forward to "getting out among people." Boss met Mandy, his "girlfriend," at the Emmanuel Center, and when he was in the hospital, one of the older ladies called to check on him, which made him "feel special and cared for." Miss Fannie proudly displays the friendship ring given to her by her 95-year-old new friend. Some residents who have moved from their own homes or from other ALFs are able to maintain ties with old friends only through center participation.

Day programs also promote residents' physical and mental health. Volunteer roles and creative accomplishments enhance self-esteem; engaging in recreational activities and interacting with others increase overall well-being and, in the words of Carole Seymour, "help keep your mind together." For some residents, these centers increase opportunities for healthy eating. Meals at the Emmanuel Center and Our Savior's frequently include fresh vegetables, and those at ADH and county senior centers are required to meet one-third of the minimum recommended daily allowance of nutrients. Day programs also expand physical activity. Just walking to and from the house and getting in and out of the van provides some exercise, and three of the centers have exercise classes. In addition, the mental health day centers provide medication management. Tracey has became much more alert since center staff began monitoring her psychotropic medications.

Most residents of these homes are highly religious, and these programs provide some residents their only opportunity to engage in religious worship. Devotional services are a favorite activity of most participants and often the only one that holds meaning for residents with dementia. Miss Fannie described the devotion time at the Emmanuel Center as "the best prayer meeting over there you want to see." Burt attested to the importance of the religious activities at Our Savior's: "I believe you gotta have church to get the food down in your belly or you won't feel good. Your head won't shape right if you don't get the real God in you." The manager of Dawnview Center also affirmed the value of religion to participants: "It's their life. They are very seasoned Christians, I should say, churchgoing folk, and that's very important. And if I am not out there at ten o'clock, they will start themselves."

Day programs also provide goods and services that are critical to the residents living in the lowest-resource homes, mostly those at Greene's. Participants at Our Savior's receive clothes, foot care, eye exams, haircuts, and shaves, and they can wash their clothes and shower in facilities far superior to Greene's. Fellow members at the Emmanuel Center donated clothes to Beatrice Dove and Miss Fannie, and one lady even made a dress for Ms. Dove, who, because of obesity, is hard to fit. Rosie's residents bring home food items, such as bread and yogurt, from the Jerusalem Center.

Although the rewards to residents far outweigh those to providers, home owners and staff derive substantial benefit from residents' attendance at day programs. A principal gain is fulfillment of their goal to enhance the quality of residents' everyday life. Each of these small-home owners feels ill equipped to provide meaningful activities to their residents, yet they aspire to a life for them beyond sitting, sleeping, and watching TV. A second major bonus comes from the resource conservation associated with having some or all residents gone during the day. Providers are relieved of certain tasks, have more time, money, and energy to take care of others, and may even sneak in a restorative nap or recreational activity.

The costs to residents and providers of residents' participation in day programs are few compared with the benefits derived. For residents, costs concern mainly the lack of choice some have about attendance. With the exception of Estelle Washington at Peach Blossom, those who express complaints about going object not to overall participation but to its extent and regularity. For some, attending day after day becomes boring; for others, getting fed, dressed, and out the door is physically taxing. Other costs relate to program inadequacies or to lack of fit between a resident and a particular program. Because senior center programs are not geared to residents with mental impairment, some AL residents are not able to obtain full benefit and risk being misunderstood and neglected by center staff. Even ADH centers, which are intended to serve persons with disabilities, often fall short in their mission because of limited resources.

For providers, costs relate to the effort they expend obtaining access to centers, getting residents ready to go each day, providing transportation, dealing with behavior issues, and paying fees. Rosie probably is burdened most by these tasks, particularly during the period when she was transporting her residents to and from the Jerusalem Center and helping out with their care. For a month during the summer, she kept her residents at home, saying, "I need a rest."

Keys to Access

In each of the homes, the owner's involvement in residents' access to programs and ongoing maintenance efforts are a critical factor in residents' participation. Central to their efforts are knowledge, perseverance, and experience, as well as supporting values. Over the years, the owner of Sunshine House, the one small home with no residents attending day programs, had succumbed to the difficulties of access. Although Louis Ashley's AL home is only two miles from Rosie's, he believes such programs no longer exist and does not seek them out, despite his belief in their value: "There are some things, you know, that I think obviously would make our quality better if we could get that, but it seems as though politics and the way budgeting is going now, obviously we don't have that. Initially when I got into the [AL] business, we had community health centers that were located in the community, day care centers that were located around the community, and so, therefore, it provided health checks, it provided respite for staff, it provided an opportunity for residents to get out, meet other people, move around, and have an exchange. But at the present time, those resources evidently dried up, and, you know, if a person's in a personal care home, then that's the beginning and end of it, and it should not be."

A vehicle to transport residents is another indispensable resource. The owners of Peach Blossom, Rosie's, and Greene's all have seven-passenger vans, whereas Clarice, the owner of Blue Skies, has only a five-passenger car. In some cases, family members hold the key to participation by negotiating access and transportation, paying fees, and handling center care issues.

Program availability and flexibility are, of course, critical factors. No one denies the scarcity of resources for persons who are old and disabled. Programs serving this population have a mandate to serve those most in need, and eligibility guidelines follow this principal. So it is no wonder that those responsible for resource allocation tend to favor elders living alone at home over those in a more sheltered AL environment. One county administrator expressed this dilemma: "With assisted living, we kinda are in a quandary with them. Most assisted living homes have a program coordinator who plans meals and other services. This could be looked at as a duplication of services. We have had assisted living residents in senior centers, but if their home is providing programming and meals, we like to encourage them to take advantage of those services at the assisted living home. The main thrust of our program is to keep people in their homes and as independent as possible, and I'm sure you follow the logic that if a person is in an assisted living home, then they are already out of their home." We found that it takes an assertive and influential family member or a die-hard AL provider to overcome such barriers.

It is the luck of the draw that Our Savior's, the one program developed expressly for AL residents, is located in the Greene's neighborhood. Although Cora Greene has a role in her residents' participation, the program sought them out, relieving her of the toughest obstacle. The flexibility and willingness of the Emmanuel Center to accept a range of persons in need also is a boon to her. The lack of dependence of either of these programs on public dollars, coupled with the skill and commitment of their leaders to make a difference in their participants' lives, increases both their availability and effectiveness.

Churches

For almost all residents of these six homes, religion and organized church activities embody the heart and soul of their past and present lives. Sunshine House resident Mayetta Stewart, who has served as deacon and member of the usher and mother boards of her longtime church, told us, "I love my church more than anything. I told my daughter it was a shame to love it so much." Many residents are able to hold on to spiritual connections through the combined efforts of their families, church communities, and AL providers.

In chapter 7, we portrayed the essential role of families in the preservation of church ties. In each home except for Greene's, at least one resident, and usually more, has a family member who fulfills this role. Ms. Stewart's daughter, granddaughter, and niece ensure her attendance at church every Sunday, as well as other events, such as revivals and homecomings. Marlena Morton's son Clarence takes Marlena to church and also other Blue Skies residents who wish to go. In all homes, family members try to keep residents connected to their "home" churches, but at Oak Manor, where almost half of residents moved from out of town, some "locals" have integrated displaced residents into their own church communities. Hattie Houseworth, who moved from Louisiana, has joined her daughter's church and goes with her as many Sundays and Wednesday nights as she feels able.

Ministers and members of local churches reach out to their own members, as well as to other residents of these homes, in a variety of ways. Edna Nations, an Oak Manor resident with no family help, may receive the most extensive church support. Church members pick her up twice weekly for church activities and also subsidize her AL fees. Viola Wheeler's minister visits Peach Blossom the first Sunday of every month to serve communion. Elizabeth Bell's and Dorothea Buffington's former minister in Chattanooga always includes a visit to them at Oak Manor on his monthly trips to Atlanta to see his parents. George Kelner's church friends visit him weekly at Greene's and take him to church on Sundays. Rosie's resident Pearl Bowman, who has dementia, sits with the members of her mother board on Sundays while her daughter sings in the choir. Ethyl Burns's church friends visit her at Oak Manor and take her to her church clubs and to services two Sundays a month; they would do more if she were not reluctant to impose. On a recent Sunday, her church recognized her many years of service:

> Never did I expect that I would be chosen as the person who was honored on Women's Day at church, because I'm not that kind of church worker. Now, I will work with the children, I will go to Bible school, and, just like you see me around here [at Oak Manor], it's just habit, I can't help it: if I see somebody that needs a little help, . . . here I go. I'm the same way at church with the older people. I belong to two clubs, so we did a lot of service in the church. So, I went to church last Sunday knowing nothing. I started not to go, but I finally went on, and I thought it was kind of queer, 'cause it was kind of crowded, but I sat down, and somebody handed me a program, and I started fumbling through the program, and I got toward the center of it, and there was my picture. It was a complete, absolute surprise, so much so that I could not say a word when they asked me to respond. Nothing came out. In the first place, I didn't think I had done that much, you know; what I did, I did.

Esther Adams, the owner of Peach Blossom, is unique in her role of incorporating her residents into her own church home. Because religion is important to her, she has been careful to admit residents who share that value and even selected her church, which is small and nearby, because of its accessibility to her home and residents. Over the years, she has taken her residents to services on Sundays and to special events. With her current group of residents and her declining energy, she may not get there every Sunday, but she makes it at least once a month, and she praises her church family for their acceptance of her other family: "At Mount Olive they enjoy having the residents come. They do understand that they might need to get up and go to the restroom or somebody might talk a little bit before you can remind them not to, but it doesn't upset them. It's a very understanding church. It's a church that [my residents] seem to also enjoy, and usually, at the end of the service, they don't have to move. The people just come and shake their hands and tell them they're glad. They make them welcome, and they give me a hand, of course; when I go, and they realize I'm there, somebody comes to my rescue and help[s] me to get them seated. So it's a church that I'm proud of in the service that they provide for seniors." One Sunday a researcher accompanied Ms. Adams and four residents to a special Women's Day program at the church, and the experience bore out Ms. Adams's accolades. The church members were welcoming and helpful, and at the end of the service the pastor thanked Ms. Adams for bringing her residents, and the entire congregation gave her a round of applause. For their part, the residents also did her proud during the two-hour service. Only Ms. Hicks spoke up when the organ played, to say, "That's what I love, the organ." Ms. Adams's pastor also comes to Peach Blossom once a month to serve communion.

Three of the other study homes—Greene's, Sunshine House, and Oak Manor—hold church services and prayer meetings conducted by community volunteers. A street preacher, a longtime friend of Boss's, has been coming to Greene's every Tuesday night for more than 10 years. Usually six or seven residents attend the service. Boss, who has not "missed a Tuesday yet," described his weekly visits: "He don't stay but about a hour, you know, have meeting, say the Lord's Prayer and everything, and he go on back. He's a nice minister, too." Although a few residents object to the preacher's "sanctimonious attitude" and "loud gospel music and shouting," those who attend the service value the opportunity to come together as a group to worship and share their fears and hopes. At Sunshine House, a friend of the owner holds regular services, and two church groups visit the home monthly to conduct prayer meetings and Bible classes. Members of one of these groups help with hair care for female residents.

Oak Manor has two weekly religious activities, a Bible study group on Wednesday morning and a Sunday service, both well attended by residents. Sisters Elizabeth Bell and Dorothea Buffington never miss going and are well satisfied: "We have Bible class on Wednesday that we enjoy," said Ms. Bell. "He is real good. We are reading the book of Acts right now. He stimulates us pretty good. Every Sunday morning we have a preacher who comes and we enjoy him. He even gives us communion." Most residents, including Ethyl Burns, find the Sunday service an acceptable substitute for their own churches, especially since a resident donated her piano and plays it for the service: "I'm satisfied with the service they have downstairs. The young speaker's very good, and now we have a piano, which makes all the difference in the world. It really does." In addition to these two activities, Oak Manor has established a partnership with a large church in the neighborhood. The facility's first activity director, a member of the church, was instrumental in forging the tie. As part of its commitment, the church has invited and transported residents to their annual Good Friday passion play and donated tickets and provided transportation to a local theater production. Future plans include one-on-one relationships between church members and residents.

Some churches provide other services that support small homes. Several church groups visit Greene's over the Christmas holidays and bring gifts to the residents. Two churches sponsor annual Senior Day dinners usually attended by Peach Blossom residents. To one, Ms. Adams and her residents rode in style in a limousine.

The church continues to play an important role in the spiritual and social lives of AL residents, providing a spiritual bridge to their past lives and the community beyond the ALF walls. Through the efforts of church leaders and members, together with those of AL providers and family members, residents are able to perform roles and engage in activities they have found meaningful for most of their lives.

Other Facility Bridges

Although we have specified facility roles as bridges to day programs and residents' spiritual lives, AL facilities generate community connections in other ways. A typical means is through a formal activity program, which, of the homes in this study, is found only at Oak Manor. Oak Manor's program bridges the gap between residents and the wider community both by taking residents out and by bringing the community in. Like the day programs attended by residents of the small homes, Oak Manor's activities expand the horizons of its residents.

Over the study year, Oak Manor took residents to 13 special events outside the facility. These included three live theater productions; a movie; lunches at the Piccadilly cafeteria, the Red Lobster restaurant, and the Lincoln Senior Center; and visits to the CNN show, "Talk Back Live," the Coca-Cola Museum in Underground Atlanta, the Margaret Mitchell House, the Jimmy Carter Presidential Library, the Fernbank Science Museum, and a neighborhood branch of the city library. Residents' assessment of these events was enthusiastically positive. Eugene Ellis and Calvin Soames, who rarely participate in on-site activities, attended all three plays, as did Alma Burgess, who before moving to

Oak Manor had been a season subscriber to a local theater company. The major barriers to such trips are the cost and the difficulty of transporting impaired residents. Some expenses come out of the activity budget, but others must be borne by the residents themselves. The facility paid for tickets to the science museum and for two of the plays, but such cash outlays are seldom possible. The facility's partner church purchased the tickets for one play and assisted with transportation to another. Although Oak Manor has a 13-passenger bus with a wheelchair lift, the bus also is used to take residents to medical appointments. Even with the bus, taking a group of residents out requires much planning and effort, and support from care staff usually is not possible.

The Alzheimer's Association annual fund-raising walk, attended by both able residents and Oak Manor staff, allows these residents to contribute to the community as well as participate in it. Oak Manor's weekly shopping trips have the latent function of linking residents to the world outside. Just seeing what grocers have on the shelves and observing other clientele furnish mental stimulation. Hamilton Brewton especially enjoys watching the women.

Oak Manor administrators also invite and entreat the wider community to come to them. They solicit groups and individuals to provide recreational and educational activities for residents, and they make facility space available to community groups for meetings and events. Such activities included poetry readings by students from one of Atlanta's historically black colleges, an AARP program about Social Security and Medicare, tales of slavery from an African American storyteller, a "heart-healthy" program conducted by a registered nurse, concerts performed by high school and preschool groups, a seminar given by an attorney on living wills, and a lecture by a local urologist on incontinence.

Other volunteers contribute on a regular basis. In addition to those who conduct the biweekly religious activities, members of a local garden club help residents with outdoor gardening every other Tuesday, and a woman comes weekly to teach residents how to make greeting cards. For three months during the study year, a student from a local university assisted with activities to fulfill an internship for her social work program. A local supermarket donates flowers each week, which residents arrange in vases for the dining room tables.

Several groups, including the Neighborhood Planning Unit in which Oak Manor is located, have their meetings at Oak Manor. Alma Burgess entertained both of her club groups in the facility dining room, and the kitchen staff prepared and served the meals. An event to benefit Alzheimer disease allowed residents to dress up, sip champagne, and mingle with community civic leaders.

Small homes occasionally have community groups (other than church re-lated) come into the homes to provide activities. Neighbors in the Sunshine House community bring gifts and food on holidays. A woman's service club sponsored parties at Peach Blossom at Christmas and Easter. Esther Adams also sometimes takes her residents out for meals; she and a fellow small-home owner, for example, took their residents to a restaurant for a special Memorial Day lunch. When she has residents who are not attending day programs, she often takes them with her to run errands or have a quick lunch out. Viola Wheeler enjoys these outings, which allow her to reconnect with familiar neighborhoods. Terry Prospect, the 26-year-old Blue Skies resident, often com-plains that Clarice, the owner, never takes residents out shopping or to a movie or restaurant. Like Mr. Brewton at Oak Manor, she feels "trapped" by the walls of Blue Skies and is desperate for a meaningful community connection.

Health Care and Social Services Providers

Community health care and social service providers make important con-tributions to residents and ALF owners and staff. A city the size of Atlanta has a multitude of hospitals, clinics, physicians, home health and social service care agencies, and other health care personnel. Many of these community or-ganizations and agents are specifically noted in other chapters. Here, we sim-ply highlight some of those individuals and services and their sometimes unique contribution to these homes. As with other types of community sup-port, the AL providers often play a central role in securing it.

County Hospital is the principal health care provider for many residents who live in the small homes and even a few of those at Oak Manor. Most Greene's residents receive all health care at one of the many clinics or the emergency room and obtain medications at the hospital pharmacy. Mr. Fitzsimmons's mental health program is there, County Hospital home health nurses visit the home, and Ms. Greene finds most of her residents through the hospital dis-charge planner. County has neighborhood satellite clinics that serve some residents at Rosie's and Sunshine House. Although the County system often is frustrating and can be difficult for impaired persons to manage, the bulk of the hospital's regular clientele would go no other place, and its status as a teaching facility for two medical schools ensures a certain level of care quality. County also provides low-cost incontinence pads, which Rosie helps some of her residents obtain.

Registered nurses with Georgia's Community Care Services Program assist with resident health monitoring and medication management at the two participating homes—Rosie's and Blue Skies. Program social workers also assist with finding new placement for residents who are discharged or are dissatisfied with their homes. Podiatrists visit Greene's, Peach Blossom, and Oak Manor to provide regular foot care to residents. These visits are financed by Medicare, but the podiatrist who visits Greene's, with whom Ms. Greene has cultivated a relationship, treats even residents without insurance.

Workers from home health agencies visit all homes to provide a variety of skilled care, including wound care, urinary catheter care, physical and occupational therapy, and health monitoring after hospitalization. Nurses from the health department provide Rosie's residents with their annual required tuberculosis tests. Cora Greene has an arrangement with a private medical clinic to provide services, both at the clinic and at Greene's. These services include tuberculosis tests, physicals, consultations, and prescribing and delivering medications. This clinic depends almost exclusively on Medicaid and Medicare payments, but residents without coverage are also served. Oak Manor's relationship with a university geriatric hospital provides a source of referral for residents and consultation and training for staff. The facility also has an arrangement with a nearby physician to conduct physical exams and tuberculosis tests, prescribe medications, and authorize home health visits.

Caseworkers from county agencies provide case management services for some residents with mental health problems at Greene's and Sunshine House and for Bobby Bailey and Georgia Mayhew (who are wards of the state) at Peach Blossom. Bobby's caseworker sometimes takes him to medical appointments and visited him in the hospital when he had surgery. A mental health agency provided Cora Greene with discounted training materials and tickets to community events. A local food bank donates food to Our Savior's and the Jerusalem Center, the Emmanuel Center has furnished low-cost eyeglasses to several Greene's residents, and a local service agency (Friends of Disabled Adults) provides them with low-cost assistive devices, such as walkers.

The Long-Term Care Ombudsman Program and the Alzheimer's Association provide free training for AL providers. For the most part, these training opportunities are used by the small homes, where providers have a particularly difficult time fulfilling training requirements. Because representatives of the ombudsman program make regular visits to ALFs and respond to complaints from residents, some providers view them more as regulators than sources of support, but most value the program's educational role. Oak Manor invited a program representative to speak at a resident council meeting about resident rights.

Partners in Care

It is clear from the range of community supports described in this chapter that, like residents' families, members of the community at large serve as partners in the care of assisted living residents. Together, these organizations and individuals make a significant contribution to the quality of care and life of these AL residents, whether through ministering to them or to their AL providers. All residents need and want to remain connected to the world around them, both in ways they have always done and in ways that may never have crossed their minds. They also need the services of outside professionals to supplement those of their AL caregivers. We found that assisted living providers depend on the backing of the community at large. Although their job is to care for the residents who live in their homes, they cannot do it alone. Community support is essential in all six communities we studied, but it is far more critical in the small homes, where most, or all, residents are poor and owners' resources are stretched to the limit and sometimes beyond. In these homes, community bridges go beyond broadening horizons to fulfilling basic needs.

Day programs are an especially valuable resource for small AL homes. We recognize, of course, the scarcity of community resources for such programs and the need for fair distribution, but we dispute blanket assessments that AL residents are less needy than clients still living in their own homes. We found evidence of residents with substantial physical and emotional needs unmet in their AL homes. For some residents with mental health problems, their AL communities have been their only homes for much of their adult lives. In these cases, their need for aid is clear, and their share of community resources has been largely unclaimed.

Community churches are vital bridges for all six of these AL homes. For hundreds of years historically black churches have served as a source of informal support to African Americans (Taylor, Thornton, & Chatters, 1992), especially to elders (Taylor & Chatters, 1986; Walls & Zarit, 1991), and this study affirms the continuation of the church's sustaining role in the lives of AL residents. Earlier research in ALFs in which the majority of residents were white (Patterson et al., 2003) demonstrates similar evidence of vital spiritual connections. Churches have the capacity to make even greater contributions to assisted living communities.

The community at large now makes valuable contributions to these six care communities, and the potential for even greater support exists. Because the future of public funding for long-term care services, and assisted living in particular, looks bleak, the importance of community support for these homes will only increase. Assisted living providers must be vigilant in ferreting out community partners, but communities also must be proactive in their efforts to support these other "communities of care," especially those that care for some of their most vulnerable members.

CHAPTER 9

Control of Care

Although personal control has been labeled a basic need (Baltes, 1994) and identified as an essential element of quality of life (Clark, 1988; Rodin, 1986; Stewart & King, 1994), no person is free from external influences. People everywhere exist in social, cultural, and historical contexts in which multiple factors influence the capacity to act according to individual autonomous will (Collopy, 1995; Hofland, 1995). One's values and actions are inevitably affected by one's past and one's environment, and all institutional structures interfere to some extent with personal autonomy (Lidz, Fischer, & Arnold, 1992). This context dependence is one of the paradoxes of autonomy (Hofland, 1995).

As Peach Blossom resident Hassie Hicks said, "When you live in someone else's house, you can't do what you like." Ms. Hicks has come to understand that moving to "someone else's house," especially because of disability and dependence, compounds everyday restrictions on free will. Numerous studies have confirmed the restrictions on autonomy that accompany moves to both assisted living facilities (Baldwin et al., 1993; Ball et al., 2000; Frank, 2002; Morgan, Eckert, & Lyon, 1995; Utz, 2003) and nursing homes (Agich, 1993; Capitman & Sciegaj, 1995; Kane, 1995; Lidz, Fischer, & Arnold, 1992); it is the threat of loss of control over one's personal life that prompts many elders to cling to their own homes, even in the face of deprivation (Ball & Whittington, 1995; Groger, 1994; Rubinstein, Kilbride, & Nagy, 1992).

In chapter 6, we define *autonomy* as encompassing two dimensions: the psychological, referring to control over one's environment and choice of options, and the spiritual, relating to continuity in the sense of personal identity over time and decision making consistent with an individual's long-term values and life meaning (Hofland, 1990). We distinguish *autonomy* from *independence*, the physical dimension of autonomy, while noting the interrelatedness of these concepts. Independence often depends on far more than ability, and many of the same factors affecting independence also influence autonomy.

For most residents, the significance of choices involves the spiritual as well as the psychological dimension (Hofland, 1990). For decisions and choices to be experienced as real or authentic, they must be consistent with identities developed in the past. The choice must mean something to the chooser. In her examination of the concept of self in old age, Kaufman (1986) emphasizes that old people express a continuity of identity that transcends the physical and social changes that accompany aging. In our previous home care and AL studies (Ball & Whittington, 1995; Ball et al., 2000; Ball et al., 2004b), our informants, like Kaufman's, interpreted and gave meaning to their experiences in the context of their past lives. We found similar values among residents of these six AL communities. Hassie Hicks, who wore red as a child so that her mother could always find her and wore only dresses except when she was picking blackberries, still prefers dresses and likes to wear red.

The concept of privacy, closely related to that of autonomy, concerns the ability to maintain and control access to oneself—either the physical self or information about the self (Lidz, Fischer, & Arnold, 1992). Privacy involves an individual's core sense of self, and having control over personal information is important to developing a sense of personal identity. As Lidz and colleagues (1992) note, violations of both autonomy and privacy occur when an individual is not respected as an independent moral agent, and a violation of one's privacy is often, but not always, a violation of autonomy. In addressing autonomy as it relates to residents of these six AL communities, we investigate what aspects of autonomy are most meaningful to residents, and why; residents' opportunities for achieving autonomy in their daily lives; and the barriers and supports that affect the attainment of resident autonomy.

Realization of Autonomy

One of the questions we asked residents in the in-depth interviews was, "How much control or choice do you feel you have in your life now?" The range of answers we received reflects both individuals' unique situations and the authenticity of their opportunities. Hamilton Brewton's response— "Don't have any. My son has my car, and I can't drive it"—reflects his difficulty in adapting to his circumscribed life at Oak Manor, which, in turn, is influenced by his former lifestyle involving frequent traveling. In contrast, to the same question Ethyl Burns replied, "Control of my life, I have it." Ms. Burns feels in control of what is now, and always has been, most important to her—

connection to her family. In most cases, control is a variable and personal experience for residents.

The areas of control residents find most relevant include food, personal care, daily routines, social relationships and interactions, environment, person, and possessions. In discussing these areas, two things are apparent. One is the variation that exists within areas as to what individual residents find meaningful. The other is the overlap and interaction that occur between areas. Woven throughout the discussion is evidence of both barriers to and supports for realization of autonomy.

Meals

For many residents, it is in the area of meals that autonomy is most central. The basis of this significance is twofold. First, food and mealtimes are a major focus of most residents' daily life. Eugene Ellis's response to the query about his "favorite time of day"—"I like breakfast"—represents a common interest in meals. Second, the schedule of mealtimes bounds the daily routines in each home. The control issues related to meals include what, how much, when, where, and with whom food is eaten. For most residents, what is eaten is most important. Meals at Oak Manor, the large facility, are quite different from those in the five small homes.

Oak Manor has a food service director who plans all the meals, orders the food, and supervises food preparation and service. Residents eat in a formal dining room and choose food from a menu for each meal. Although the restaurant approach to food service is intended to enhance resident choice, comments from residents indicate that this goal, except at breakfast, is not consistently achieved. A common complaint is the repetitive nature of meals. Hamilton Brewton accused the kitchen staff of "playing games with the food": "They serve one food one day and serve the same thing the next day and call it something else. It's kind of childish. The people here are educated."

Another recurring problem is short supply of the chosen item. Rozena Banks expressed it well: "I enjoy the meals because they plan them and you circle what you want. Sometimes they give you what you want, and sometimes they don't have it, and they give you what they got." This problem is more upsetting for Elsie Joiner because it represents not only lack of choice but lack of respect: "One thing that really gets next to me is the fact that they have all these things on the menus, and when the food comes out, you lift up that tin thing [the cover], and something else is on there, but they don't tell you that. At least if they would come out and say, 'We don't have such-and-such a thing today.'"

Those who cook and serve the food try to meet residents' special dietary needs and promote good health, the choice of most residents. The food service director makes sure a comparable sugar-free alternative dessert is available for meals, and dietetic cake and ice cream are served for the monthly birthday celebrations. When serving plates, kitchen workers adhere strictly to the restricted-foods list supplied by Hattie Houseworth's daughter, and they know never to give Ida Mooney beef or pork. All facility staff are vigilant watchdogs, even at events away from the facility. Despite these efforts, a few residents still complain that the food is not wholesome enough, mostly because of the lack of fresh fruits and vegetables and foods low in sodium and cholesterol.

The primary way that residents advocate for more choice is through requests, demands, and complaints, either individually or in resident council meetings, but, in reality, only a few let their voices be heard. Elsie Joiner believes that most residents are "leery" of complaining, and this role is the domain of a few aggressive men: "Then, of course, you have those like Mr. Hughes and Mr. Ellis who loud-talk 'em and say, 'Well, why don't you have this, or you told me you had thus and so,' you know. Whereas there are those of us, women, who don't say anything, fuss among yourselves, talk in the back room." Although complaints appear to be effective for small issues, such as having an egg poached instead of scrambled, Eugene Ellis accurately perceives the futility of pursuing larger issues, particularly those dependent on money: "Too many people don't really take it to heart. They evaluate the change and listen to your complaint, very cordial, very polite, but I don't think they built in the mechanism to bring change. They built in the mechanism of trying not to be ugly, to be polite and listen to your complaint. The service leaves you with a lot to wish for, but I'm not going to make that a chief complaint. I think that you get what you pay for; I don't think we pay for Super Bowl service."

The food budget at Oak Manor is corporately set, and all food is ordered on a monthly basis from a commercial supplier. Lack of money—for fresh foods, as opposed to processed and canned foods, and for adequate staff to prepare dishes "from scratch" and respond to individual requests—is the biggest barrier to realization of residents' choices.

A few residents increase their control over food by preparing meals themselves in their apartments, but this practice is not widespread. All residents have kitchens with refrigerators, which facilitate storage of favorite foods for between-meal snacks. Some have unique strategies, like Elizabeth Bell, who once ordered a salad and a piece of chicken and created her own chicken salad, a menu item she had repeatedly requested.

Meals at Oak Manor are served in the main dining room at eight in the morning, noon, and five in the evening. Each meal is scheduled for an hour-long period, but most residents choose, and are encouraged, to come at the beginning. Some residents complain about the early hour of breakfast, and a few regularly come as late as nine or ten o'clock, which food workers tolerate if they do not demand the full menu. At other meals, residents may request that a meal be saved or a sandwich be prepared only when they have an un-avoidable conflict, such as a doctor's appointment. Residents sit in assigned seats, four to a table. Facility staff make seating decisions, and although they try to place residents according to compatibility and preferences, success is dependent on availability. A few residents have requested and gotten seat changes, but most believe their seat assignments are immutable. According to the food service director, the rationale for the seating policy is efficiency. Typically, only two servers are assigned to each meal, and knowing where to place drinks and salads ahead of time makes this duty less stressful.

In the five small homes, the owner plans the meals and purchases the food. At Peach Blossom and Rosie's, the owner also prepares all, or most, meals. As a rule, residents are served the same menu at each meal. Procedures for eliciting and responding to food choices have both similarities and differences from those at Oak Manor. Size of the home, money, and personal traits of the individual provider account for most of the differences.

In each home, providers attempt to discover what residents want to eat. At Sunshine House, the owner, Louis Ashley, periodically "screens" residents for their likes and dislikes and tries to incorporate their choices into menus. Once a month a resident at Greene's is allowed to pick the menu. When a new resident moves to Peach Blossom, Esther Adams asks about food preferences in her admission interview, and she encourages residents, once they are living in the home, to tell her their "favorite foods" so that she can be sure of serving them "often enough." Although, as at Oak Manor, only a minority of residents are forthcoming, a few residents do assert themselves. Mayetta Stewart often asked for pancakes for breakfast, and Ms. Adams prepared them for her unless she was "in a rush," when she would say, "I can't do it this morning, but I promise you'll get 'em real soon"—and she was good to her promise. Tracey

Williams, the young resident at Rosie's, frequently "bugs" Rosie to buy her the "fast food" she especially loves, and one night Rosie bought Subway sandwiches for all the residents. For the most part, these providers want to accommodate residents' food preferences.

Ms. Adams's willingness is bolstered both by her belief in the golden rule and her understanding of the importance of food: "I treat people like I'd like to be treated and like I would if I was able to take care of my own mother. Had she been in a home like this, then I certainly would have liked for her to be able to have some say-so in her daily activities of living, and particularly including the food." Neither does Ms. Adams want to waste food or effort or see her residents go unfed, and she often prepares a different meal for a resident who does not like the night's offering.

Yet in each home the desire to please residents often clashes with other values. Ms. Adams has a rule of thumb: "I respect each person's individuality and comply as much as I can." She cannot comply, however, when a resident's choice is unhealthy: "I don't serve junk food. I don't even bring potato chips into the house. It's nothing I can do with Ms. Stewart because she brings it with her." As it turned out, Ms. Adams *could* do something with Ms. Stewart, and did: she discharged her, in part for her dietary noncompliance.

In the small homes, it is generally the person cooking and serving who controls the level of resident autonomy with respect to food. At Blue Skies, Inez Sawyer, the weekday manager during much of the study, is much more authoritarian than Clarice Hull, the owner, or the other weekend workers. Inez cooks the Jamaican dishes that she prefers and insists that residents clean their plates, leading Lily Porter to refer to her as "my little Hitler." Inez believes that sugar is bad for the residents, and even though no one is diabetic, she rarely serves desserts and even hides special treats brought by family members or other visitors. At Sunshine House and Greene's, the transient workers who prepare the food tend to pay less attention to whether and what residents eat, partly because of the greater number and mobility of residents but also owing to their lack of competence and commitment and their attitudes toward certain residents. Greene's resident Martha Kominsky, who has no teeth and makes racist remarks, often is hungry because no one takes the time to prepare food she is able to eat, and only Cora Greene, the owner, tries to limit Boss Cook's intake of fattening food.

Residents at Greene's and Sunshine House have greater freedom to bring in and store food. Although no residents at any of the small homes have microwaves or refrigerators, the residents at these two homes are allowed to keep food in their rooms and in the facility refrigerator, and quite a few are able to get out and buy their own food and drinks. Residents with more money and greater mobility have greater choice, such as Boss, who pays more able residents to buy snacks for him at the corner store. Both homes also have vending machines that contain soft drinks and, at Greene's, snack foods.

Similar to Oak Manor, the small homes have set mealtimes, although they are flexible. At Peach Blossom, Rosie's, and Blue Skies, the breakfast hour is determined by when residents leave for senior centers and day programs. On weekends, or other days when residents stay home, schedules are more relaxed, and, except at Peach Blossom, residents who have nowhere to go may sleep late and either miss breakfast or eat later. Times for the other meals generally depend on the convenience of the person preparing them. Sometimes the kitchen workers at Greene's and Sunshine House serve the evening meal as early as three o'clock, when some residents are not yet hungry.

The strictness as to where residents eat and sit varies in the small homes. Although at Greene's residents are encouraged to eat in the dining area, they are allowed to eat in their rooms. Dexter Ross, whose cancer affects his appetite, often chooses this option. In the other small homes, residents are required to eat in the dining area unless they are sick. Because the dining space at Sunshine House is too small to accommodate all residents, they eat in shifts, and the men may eat at the small table downstairs. Only at Peach Blossom are residents required to sit in specific seats. When Irene Garrett tries to assert herself by saying, "I can sit where I want to," Ms. Adams responds, "You are a guest in this house, and you need to sit where I tell you." In the other homes, rigidity in seating is generated more by residents claiming ownership of a particular seat, and conflicts arise when another resident (usually one with dementia) attempts to usurp this right.

Personal Care

Residents' first choice about personal care is to "do for" themselves whenever they can, and those with the greatest independence have the greatest autonomy. Barring self-care, residents want to control when, where, how, how often, and by whom care is provided.

In all homes, providers ask residents at or before admission what kinds of help they need. They do not always ask when and how they want it provided. These preferences more often are discovered over time, if ever. As with food choices, some residents are better than others at asking and telling. Eugene Ellis has a unique strategy for instructing staff at Oak Manor how to make his bed: "I will point to the directions of how to make my bed. 'Do you see a paper above my bed?' They have different people coming in here; that's why it's necessary to write directions. Other than that, you find yourself everyday trying to tell somebody how to make your bed. So you give them directions and be insistent enough to ask them to read it. If they don't understand it, ask them to ask the person who made it yesterday, so I don't have to get into an oral debate of how I want the bed made, 'cause I don't want it made 10 different ways. The way I want it is the way I've written it out. And I ask them to please do it that way." Mr. Ellis has learned to adapt his overall approach so as not to "dissipate" his energy: "If they're not going to change, I'm not going to jump up on the table and make a lot of noise. There's a cliché, 'If you expect too much, you might set yourself up for disappointment.' The only person I have any control over is myself, so I find some little, simple things are very important. I call people by their name. I don't call women 'honey' or 'what-you-call-'em.' I show respect when they serve me. I say thank you." Despite what he himself views as his good manners, some workers still find Mr. Ellis difficult, though he usually gets the service he requests.

Of course, for such strategies to work, care providers must be willing and able to comply with residents' wishes. A caregiver's unwillingness can be an insurmountable barrier. At Peach Blossom, residents are required each day to bathe and dress before coming to the table for breakfast. Most residents are compliant, but when they are not, care becomes a contest of wills, one Esther Adams almost always wins. When Viola Wheeler, aged 88, lived at home, she ate breakfast first thing, did not bathe daily, especially in cold weather, and rarely got "down in" the tub because of her painful arthritic knees. Like Ms. Adams, she is strong willed, and her indoctrination to the routines at Peach Blossom was painful for both. During one early morning visit, the researcher overheard a prolonged battle, during which Ms. Adams and a staff person put Ms. Wheeler in the tub against her will and bathed her. When Ms. Wheeler pled, "I don't take it in cold weather like this," Ms. Adams replied: "That is the way we do it here. I need to take care of you. . . . Honey, you have to wash your bottom. We don't want to offend other persons." During the 30-minute ordeal, Ms. Wheeler wailed several times in distress, "Lord, have mercy on me. Who's going to help me?" Later, Ms. Adams said, "She's quite independent. She wants to do it her way," which, of course, is the problem. Ms. Adams is well intended, and her residents rarely ask for care they do not receive, but they have few opportunities for either decisional or executional autonomy.

In all homes, providers sometimes exert their will. At Oak Manor, Janie Benton, who has dementia, once was observed being taken by force to the bathroom by three staff persons, despite her efforts to resist, including crying and striking out with her cane. Although as a rule Oak Manor workers employ less forceful tactics and are more willing to conform to residents' ways of doing, in this case they deferred to Ms. Benton's daughter, who insists on strict adherence to her mother's toileting schedule. Cora Greene, who often must cajole Martha Kominsky to take a bath, described her less forceful way: "If they're wanting to do something and you're wanting them to do something else, you gotta meet 'em half way, whether you do it or not. But allow them to at least *think* that you're gonna do it. It's just having that patience. You don't just walk up to 'em and say, 'Come on, you gotta get this shower now, and I mean now.' It never works."

Staffing levels are a barrier to autonomy in all homes but especially at Oak Manor. Lucy Small, the resident services director, explained how care needs affect scheduling: "I look at the resident's daily habits. If someone gets up late, I wouldn't schedule them to get a bath in the morning. I'll schedule that bath for the evening before they go to bed. . . . If they need more assistance, then I have to schedule them at a time when I have better staffing." For this reason, Janie Benton, who requires assistance with bathing, dressing, and toileting, is awakened at five in the morning by night staff for her morning care. At Greene's, where residents often exhibit signs of neglect, too few bathrooms and the need to conserve water also are impediments. The absence of bathtubs at Oak Manor interferes with some residents' preferences. As Elizabeth Bell said, "[My sister and I] just kind of like to get in that tub and soak."

Family members also exert influence over resident care. They can enhance autonomy by supporting self-care, advocating for the resident's preferences, and providing information about what the resident wants and needs. When their definitions of quality clash with residents' own, they also can restrict residents' care choices, especially when providers give greater credence to the wishes of family members.

Daily Routines

Schedules for meals, care, and community day programs structure residents' everyday routines, but facility policies governing when residents should get up and when they should go to bed also wield influence. The rigidity of this structure varies across homes and usually from one resident to another within each home. In some homes, residents may choose to get up in time for breakfast, while in others they must arise at a set time, no matter what. The precise time may depend on whether and how much help they need. Residents at Peach Blossom may sleep in (until eight o'clock) only on weekends, because it is important to Ms. Adams that things operate in a "timely manner." Going to bed has similar influences. Only Blue Skies has a strict curfew of nine o'clock, but Peach Blossom residents who need help (all but one) must be in bed early enough to allow Ms. Adams to retire by her preferred bedtime of nine. Within this structure, residents in all homes have variable amounts of "free" time.

Residents in all homes want to choose how they pass time, and they want their choices to be authentic. Probably the most significant barrier to resident autonomy in this area is disability. Many are no longer able to carry out activities they deem meaningful. What matters most to Hattie Houseworth, after "peace and not having any pain," is playing bridge, which she "really, really loves," but her Parkinson disease hampers her ability to follow this mentally challenging game.

Facility rules exert varying degrees of control. Rosie explained the relative lack of structure at her home: "I don't have enough rules. I let them do things that they like to do. Mr. Stamps, he likes to go in his room and sit in the chair and nod. He don't care about watching TV." Madonna McDowell concurs about life at Rosie's: "Well, I do whatever I want to do. If I want to go out, I go out. If I want to lay in the bed all day, I do. I do whatever I want to do, which makes it nice." Rozena Banks feels similar freedom at Oak Manor: "I know you have to get your meals, but you can do whatever you want to afterwards. I don't feel compelled to do anything." Residents at Greene's and Sunshine House have comparable liberty. More restrictions are in place at Peach Blossom and Blue Skies, where providers are more concerned that residents stay healthy and in their beds at night than that they are able to exercise their rights. As Blue Skies resident Jane Smithers said, "A lot of times I like to lay down, and they make you get up. They want you to get exercise, they don't want you to just lay around." It is most likely when the more authoritarian worker, Inez, is on duty that such freedoms are curtailed.

Residents' freedom to pass time in meaningful ways also is influenced by the facility's recreational activities. In the small homes, watching television is often the only "activity" available, and some residents say they would be "lost" without TV, while others are bored with it or, because of dementia, find it meaningless. Even TV choices are restricted, mainly by the financial resources of residents and facilities and by facility rules. Among all the small-home residents, a total of only seven have their own TVs. Ms. Adams does not allow individual TVs at Peach Blossom—because she wants to "foster togetherness" and does not want to get up at night to turn one off if a resident forgets how or falls asleep—and she chooses the programs she believes residents like and are appropriate for them to watch. Louis Ashley, the owner of Sunshine House, does not allow residents to have TVs or radios for fear they will disturb other residents, and programming on the communal TV in the living room usually is determined by what staff persons want to watch. The nine o'clock curfew at Blue Skies restricts the viewing choices of some residents, such as Hannah Tilly, whose favorite programs come on later at night. Autonomy in TV viewing is impeded also by old equipment and lack of cable access in all homes except Peach Blossom and Rosie's, although cable service at Rosie's varies with her ability to pay the fee.

Oak Manor, in contrast, has a full-time activity director and a half-time assistant, who plan activities for each day of the week, yet barriers to residents' choice are evident here, as well. Although the activity director tries to involve residents in planning, she must limit their choices to what she can reasonably provide: "So what you may do is give them maybe four or five options. 'Pick three of these that you would like to do.' That way they would still have independence and making up their own minds; still, you are not stretching yourself to where they are making unreasonable demands that you can't meet." The diversity of residents at Oak Manor, including some with dementia and others in wheelchairs, adds to the difficulty of planning for all. Again, some residents are reluctant to express preferences. Sarah, a caregiver, explains that residents are more likely to confide in those with less authority: "I told them this: 'During your resident council meetings, you should bring these things up. Just bring them to the table. Let them know how you all feel. You tell us [care staff] how you feel, but when you get around a lot of people you're scared. You hold back, you won't say anything.' It's easy for us to sit around and listen to them because we are the ones more closer to them, so they come and talk to us and tell us how they feel."

In the end, the bulk of activities are geared to the level of most residents, a strategy that is less costly in terms of staff and money but reduces resident choice. Jordan Taylor, the corporate representative assigned to Oak Manor, explained the dilemma: "Well, obviously there are going to be specific things that are important to each resident. What's going to be important to Mr. Ellis is not important to Ms. Banks, in some cases. Some cases they run together. However, I think you have to be as general as possible so that you please the crowd, and you have to be as specific as possible so that you meet those individual wants and needs." Oak Manor offers residents much greater TV choice, because all residents have private rooms with their own TVs. The facility does not charge extra for cable access, and residents vote on the channels included in the cable package.

Many residents value passing time outdoors. The principal barriers to this choice are the facility's physical environment and residents' mental and physical disabilities. Rosie's resident Carole Seymour describes herself as an "outside" person, and she enjoys being in the front yard, just sitting or watching the cars go by or the planes fly over. This choice is not available to Pearl Bowman or Dora McElhaney, residents with dementia, who in the past have wandered off. No residents are allowed outside at Peach Blossom, but all like sitting on the glassed-in front porch, where they can watch the dog in the neighbor's yard and people getting on and off the bus at the corner stop. Blue Skies has a carport area with chairs, and Oak Manor a front porch and large patio with comfortable seating, plants, and fish pond, as well as sidewalks that circle the building. Neither Sunshine House or Greene's has a safe place for residents to experience, or even view, the outside world, which limits spending time out-of-doors to those more mobile residents.

Only a minority of residents are smokers, and smoking is prohibited inside all the homes, a rule that generates complaints only in inclement weather. The primary autonomy issue—access to cigarettes—involves two residents, Tracey, at Rosie's, and Jane, at Blue Skies. Both Tracey and Jane have mental problems, which increase their need to smoke, and neither has sufficient money to buy a satisfactory supply. Rosie, who understands Tracey's dependence on smoking, buys cigarettes for her, often with her own money, and even permits Tracey to smoke in the bathroom with the window open when the weather is cold or rainy. In contrast, Jane must beg visiting family members and neighbors to take her to purchase cigarettes, which Inez then confiscates and doles out as she sees fit, causing heated disputes between the two. Ultimately, Clarice, the owner of Blue Skies, ruled that Jane should be able to smoke when she chooses, partly because she believes Jane's "background" as a "beer-drinking chain-smoker" prevents reform.

Less discord surrounds the issue of alcohol consumption. The rules are clear, and no residents abuse the privilege. Three homes—Blue Skies, Peach Blossom, and Sunshine House—do not allow drinking, period. Although Rosie's written policy states a similar ban, she thinks it is "OK" for residents to drink if they are not "taking medication," and one night she served wine to Madonna McDowell, who is accustomed to drinking when she goes out with her daughter. Cora Greene ensures Miss Fannie's autonomy in this area: "If Fannie gets bored, Fannie gonna ask you to go to the store and get her a little nip. Fannie's around 91 years old. She say, 'That's what has kept me living this long.' So occasionally I go down to the store and get her her gin, and she enjoys that. I mean, she's still living; that's what she would have done if she was at home." The policy at Oak Manor is that residents may drink, with physician's approval and facility oversight. As one staff person said, "If they were socializers with alcohol before they came to the facility, 9 times out of 10, it'll be the same once they got here. It is their right." Each night after dinner, a staff member brings Calvin Soames his customary glass of vodka.

Social Relationships

Most residents who move to these six communities are thrown together with a group of people they do not know and did not choose. Some have more choice than others. Residents with greater resources, both in terms of money and physical and mental ability, have greater choice over their facility and, presumably, over the type of residents they are joining. For individuals like Eugene Ellis, commonality with other residents in terms of race and class was a principal reason he chose Oak Manor. The population is less diverse in this facility than in some others, all residents being older and African American and most middle to upper middle class. Blue Skies has the most heterogeneous resident population, with variations in race, class, age, gender, and disability; when the Jamaican culture of the owner and primary staff person is added, the home's diversity increases. Yet small size may temper the discordant effect of heterogeneity. Lily Porter's daughter Sharon made this observation: "It's more like a family environment, I think. My mother fusses about Terry sometimes, because she's still a young woman and she likes to listen to pop music and she has opinions, and she can be a little loud and boisterous sometimes, but that's what young people do. I don't think it bothers her that much, but it does lend for a more diverse environment." Residents in smaller settings tend to be more tolerant of those with dementia and other mental problems, viewing them, as Sharon suggests, as "family."

Some residents in the small homes develop kinlike ties. Lily has achieved the status of wise family matriarch at Blue Skies, and she worries about other residents, which she believes indicates "family-like" bonds. Carole describes other residents at Rosie's as "like family," and when Sarah Eubanks moved to a nursing home, she mourned the loss of her AL "family." In Rosie's view, small size is critical to kinlike ties: "To keep it, you know, like family settings, for just like six, like, for instance, I had seven kids. It was homely."

Yet small size limits the pool of residents from whom to choose in forming relationships. The lack of opportunity for a little romance is bemoaned by a number of residents, both young and old, who see no prospects among their fellow residents. One is Rosie's resident Madonna McDowell, aged 72, who said, "It would be nice to find a nice man in my life, somebody to go out with and talk to. There's not one in it now." The larger resident pool at Oak Manor increases residents' chances of finding an in-house love interest. The relationship between Elsie Joiner and Eugene Ellis is probably more than just friends, and Eleanor Winfrey is "in love" with Watkins Orr. Mobility increases residents' opportunities for romantic encounters, as does attending day programs. Hewitt Washington, a resident at Sunshine House, has a neighborhood girlfriend, and although Boss is not able to get out and meet "the girls" as he once did, he has developed a relationship with Mandy (whom he met at the senior center) since she came to work at Greene's. He also finds female companionship among the frequent temporary residents, whom, because of his relative wealth, he is able to woo with money and small gifts.

Some facility owners and staff sanction such male-female relationships. Eva, a staff member at Oak Manor, affirms residents' rights in this area, at least for those who are mentally competent: "There do be some intimate relationships, and it might be some sexual relationships, and that depends on mentally where they are at the time. This is their home, you know, if they want to have, even if it's a resident-resident thing, or if it's a resident and outside, if they're alert, what happens behind those doors is their right." Cora Greene does not interfere with Boss's relationships, but he is aware of his limits: "Ms. Greene don't have no girls hanging 'round unless you got your own girl. They can come see you if you want to, but just girls on the street, she don't have that." Although we found no instances of intimate relationships in the other homes, it is unlikely they would be permitted, mainly because of the lack of opportunity for privacy and the potential for disruption to the community.

Autonomy in social relationships also means the opportunity to be alone. When asked about the importance of privacy, invariably residents speak of having some way of controlling contact with other residents. Hamilton Brewton expressed this viewpoint: "Yes, that's very important, and I can go shut myself off from the people when I get tired of them. If I'm not tired of them, I can find people that can't stop talking, and I talk with them." A private room is the principal way residents achieve privacy in AL, and residents who have this option place high value on it. Residents' health problems increase the value of not being "bothered." Elsie Joiner, who has Parkinson's, said, "Nobody bothers you here. I'm sleepy in the morning, because some of the medication that I take makes me sleepy, and I can come on up to my room and nobody bothers me."

Only a few residents in the small homes have private rooms. One is Lily Porter in Blue Skies, whose daughter chose this home principally for this reason: "My mother is social to an extent, but she's still a very private person. That's part of who she is, and I think to take that away from her would begin the steps toward dehumanization." Lily no doubt is less bothered by Terry because of her private room. Jane, who rooms with Marlena, a chronic snorer, is less lucky. Without private rooms, residents must hope for a "good roommate," which is how Cleo Kellog describes hers at Rosie's: "Yeah, she's a good roommate. We tell each other goodnight. I don't bother her, she don't bother me." Although Boss is less "bothered" by the lack of privacy in his everyday life at Greene's, at times he wishes for more: "I try to be in a good mood every time I see people, you know. I love people, [but] when I don't feel like being bothered with somebody, I still be bothered with 'em."

Eugene Ellis's private room at Oak Manor allows him both to contract his social interactions and to expand them—through his computer: "I am an outgoing person; however, this place provides an opportunity to be with people when you want it and also provides the privacy of going to your apartment when you want it. I don't need this facility to furnish all my needs, particularly in light of the fact that I'm an active person on a computer. I'm busy answering e-mail for people all around, locally, my alma mater, so it's a vicarious visit with me when I go to the e-mail."

Other residents who are not computer literate augment their social connections by telephone. Except for Terry at Blue Skies, only Oak Manor residents have private telephone lines, which greatly increase their choices for keeping up with family members and former friends. Almost every evening, Ethyl Burns goes to her room and talks until bedtime to her much-loved relatives and church members. Until her phone was disconnected because she could not pay the bill, Terry also enjoyed the freedom to talk at length. Each of the small homes has only one line, and although residents may use the telephone when they wish, competition can be stiff, conversation time is limited, and in most of the homes, long-distance calls are blocked. In all homes, some residents, because of physical or mental disability, are dependent on busy providers or other residents to exercise this choice. Family members of several Oak Manor residents refused to let their telephones be connected, preventing vital connections to friends and family.

Some residents want the choice to interact and have relationships with providers. Both possibilities for building such ties and residents' value for them are greater in the small homes, where, in most cases, providers' presence is more stable and they are more available. Rosie's habit of watching TV in the living room with residents and Kay's of letting Mayetta visit with her late into the night at Sunshine House are examples of how providers increase residents' opportunities for developing meaningful ties. Sybil McDowell describes her mother and Rosie as "hanging buddies," that is "you know, [they] hang out together." These connections sometimes even serve as substitutes for family relationships that are wanting. At Oak Manor, the prevailing preference of residents is for a more professional relationship with providers, though most still value interactions. More sociable residents often seek out conversation with staff members when they are bored or lonely. Before the furniture in the lobby was rearranged, the two chairs adjacent to the reception desk were always occupied by residents. No doubt Eugene Ellis summons a staff person each night to give him a snack from his refrigerator to fulfill a social, rather than instrumental, need.

Environment

A significant autonomy issue in all homes is control of, and access to, space, both common and personal. Rosie's is the only small home where residents have free access to all parts of the house. In Rosie's book, this freedom helps make her ALF "homely": "Being able to use the whole house, being able to sit down and be comfortable, relax yourself. Nothing is off limits to you." Although she once said she does not allow residents who "wet on themselves" to sit in the living room, this rule is not enforced. Residents are free to watch TV, either on the sunporch or in the living room, use the dining room to play games, go to their own rooms when they wish, enter the kitchen, and even open the refrigerator. Facility access is most restricted at Peach Blossom, where Esther Adams requires residents when at home to spend waking hours either in the living room or on the porch. They may sit at the dining room table only for meals, and her personal quarters and the kitchen are strictly off-limits.

Ms. Adams also denies residents with dementia access to their clothes, if they have the habit of creating disarray. When Hassie Hicks first moved in, Ms. Adams turned her wardrobe toward the wall to block Ms. Hicks's access to it, an upsetting event, her daughter Ernestine recalled: "When she first got there, that was an insult to her. She was very hurt. She was very happy there the first days, and then she told me that they had locked her clothes up. They had turned her clothes [closet] around, but, see, she did [dress herself] at home. She would get up and, like, I would bring her clothes washed and ironed, straighten out all her drawers, and when I come, she had moved things. So I understood that, but I just asked them, since that was her first week, to please try to turn 'em back around. Because you take a person out of their home and all of their things and then you put 'em in a place where they can't get to they little personal things, to me that's cruel, you know."

At Blue Skies, Clarice Hull instituted a rule barring residents from the living room, allegedly to preserve the new furniture but more likely to provide a haven for Inez, the live-in manager. Since this room is where the choice TV is located, this ban restricts residents' TV viewing, as well. Gender influences access at Sunshine House, where women sleep upstairs and the men downstairs. Since no women indicate they wish to enter the male domain, and men seem to like their segregated digs, where they are free to stay up and watch TV as late as they wish, this space allocation is not a problem. On occasion, though, Mr. Ashley banishes Lewis Howell to the downstairs, except for meals, because of inappropriate behavior toward women.

At Oak Manor, although residents have free access to all common areas, one thorny matter, which links access to use, is a policy forbidding sleeping in the lobby. The basis of the policy, as explained by the executive director, is essentially "the bottom line": "From a marketing aspect, corporate, and those internally, say when people [visitors] come in, let's say residents are really comfortable sleeping in the living area, it doesn't look like a healthy environment. The residents say, 'Well, this is our home,' which is rightfully so, but it's just how it appears." Residents are split in their opinion of this policy. Some, like Alma Burgess, agree with management: "I think that is fine. They can find somewhere else to sleep. You may nod off, but to actually sit there and sleep. . . ." Malcolm Harding vehemently disagrees: "Most elders cat nap. They may be up and prowling during the night. They don't just sleep eight hours like everybody else. So if they get to this point, hell, what I usually say is, 'Whenever somebody [is] 80 years old, whatever in the hell they wanna do, as long as they don't kill me, let 'em do it!' So they sleepin' in the living room. Hell, they paying $3,000." In reality, the policy is seldom enforced, mainly because of the difficulty of "teaching" some of the major offenders, most of whom have some dementia.

Control of personal space affects control of person and possessions. Having a private room with a lockable door increases control of both but guarantees control of neither. At Oak Manor, all suites have lockable doors, but residents' control over their space sometimes is thwarted by facility staff. Residents are upset that staff members sometimes enter their rooms when they are out and fail to follow their instructions about locking the door. According to Calvert Hughes, "If I ask to lock, they unlock. If I ask to keep open, they lock." Elizabeth Bell attributes this problem to worker turnover: "They change them so often that by the time you get one person and say, 'Be sure you lock my door when you come out,' some of them will come and do what they have got to do and leave your door open. You don't know who is going to walk down that hall or come in that back door. We just like to keep it locked."

A number of residents at Oak Manor make regular complaints about theft. Although many are unfounded, some are not. The loss of even small items has import for residents, as Hamilton Brewton remarked: "At our age, the few precious things we have. . . . We don't have many possessions. We are very poor people. This is all we've got. To steal from us is unconscionable." Although the facility has not been able to solve the theft problem, the management is responsive to complaints and replaces lost items when possible. Yet it is not just the loss of the items that troubles these residents but also the violation of their personal space. In Rozena Banks's words, "It is not right for them to go through our things." Oak Manor residents also complain about invasions of privacy by staff persons who enter their locked rooms without knocking or waiting for a response. Mr. Harding reported that one walked in on him when he was "buck naked."

The few small-home residents with private rooms have no means of locking them. Only those residents at Greene's who manage their own medications have any personal space they can lock. Theft is an ongoing problem at Greene's, mainly because of the temporary residents and the generally low-income status of the residents and the neighborhood. Residents keep possessions they prize on their person during the day and under their pillows at night. At Blue Skies, theft of small items (nail clippers and a dollar bill) led to a ban on residents' entering one another's rooms. That Cleo Kellog has no secure place to keep her dentures led to their "theft" by a resident with dementia. Residents in the small homes also cannot lay claim to a particular room to call their own. Providers move residents around to enhance compatibility or care; some residents at Greene's have even been shifted to another house.

Sharing bedrooms and bathrooms, of course, impedes privacy, and Rosie's is the only home where any bathroom door has a lock. Rosie understands the importance of privacy, even for residents with dementia, and takes precautions to enhance their safety: "Joseph Render lock the bathroom door because he don't want anybody coming in the bathroom when he in there, but, anything happen, I have a knife outside the door; I just stick it in there and unlock it. Even the ones with Altimer's, they like they privacy, and I have a sign on the door say, 'Before you enter, please knock.' Don't just burst in the door. You knock on the door and treat the people with dignity and respect, which I would like. I wouldn't like anybody busting in my room and I might be dressing. I might be scratching somewhere I ain't supposed to scratch."

Residents in all homes want control of temperature, and their success in achieving it depends on a number of factors, including the design for heating and cooling in each home, the willingness of a provider to grant residents' choices, and AL regulations. Each room at Oak Manor has an individual thermostat, but some residents' choice of temperature is limited by their competence in operating the control mechanism, which differs from the kind most had at home. So many residents have difficulty that Eldon, the maintenance director, proposed taking a replica of the device to a resident council meeting and demonstrating the operation, a strategy he never employed. This solution quite likely would not have worked anyway for confused residents, but even Calvert Hughes, a former electrician, has difficulty with the device and complains that he alternately "freezes" and "burns up."

Two additional ongoing problems are the coldness of the dining room and the water temperature in the bathroom. The executive director, Kathy Wall, who suggests residents simply wear sweaters for meals, alleges the need to consider the servers, who, because of the fast pace of their meal duties, tend to overheat. Eldon claims that state AL regulations are the primary impediment: "To be honest, I think regulations interfere a lot, because if this building is 83 or 85 degrees, we supposed to pass out water and do all that kind of stuff, because the state law requires the building to be cooler than 83 at all times during the summer. Residents, especially in the dining room, they don't understand that. Even when it came to the water, the state requires that the water be 110 degrees. Anything higher than that, we can be in trouble. And the state don't understand that some people blood content, or red or white blood cells, are not enough to circulate to keep them warm, so they are cold all the time. That's the laws we have to live with." Residents' primary way of dealing with these concerns is to adapt to the situation. Many take Kathy's suggestion and wear sweaters. Hamilton Brewton takes his bath at night, when water is hotter, and others summon staff to adjust temperature controls.

In the small homes, control of temperature is in the hands of the owner or staff person in charge. All providers seem to be aware of residents' preferences, and no one considers state regulations when adjusting the thermostat, turning fans on or off, or opening or closing doors. On many visits to these homes, researchers felt the oppression of summer heat while residents continued to wear long sleeves or sweaters. Only at Greene's, where the owner is ever vigilant about energy consumption, and Blue Skies, where Inez exerts her will, do residents sometimes suffer. Inez's practice of keeping doors and windows open, as she did "to catch the breeze" in Jamaica, is not popular with residents, particularly Terry, who said, "It makes me mad that I have to ask Inez if I can close the door. I should be able to close the door if I am cold. We have to ask permission for everything we do around here."

The Whys of Autonomy

Residents experience and perceive autonomy over a wide range. Some feel that they have substantial control both psychologically and spiritually, some only one or the other, and some neither. Some have autonomy in certain aspects of their lives but not in others. The foregoing discussion has touched on the many factors that affect residents' ability to realize this important value. Next we describe some of the principal barriers and supports.

Barriers to Autonomy

Rosalie Kane (1990) identifies four R's in long-term care settings—routine, regulation, restricted capacity, and resource constraints—that interact to impede personal autonomy, and numerous studies confirm her argument (Agich, 1993; Beck & Vogelpohl, 1995; Lidz, Fischer, & Arhnold, 1992; Shield, 1995). We, too, found these four Rs to be determining—though variable—forces in these six AL communities. The organizations and individuals who define each home account for much of the variation.

The effect of routine on resident autonomy is well documented in the nursing home research literature. Agich's (1993) comprehensive discussion of nursing home life offers clear evidence of residents' being controlled by authoritarian staff and a rigid time schedule determined more by the work needs of the staff than the preferences of the residents. Lidz and colleagues' (1992) ethnographic research also found that strong adherence to a medical model of care and a staff emphasis on institutional order greatly restricted resident autonomy. Routine affects autonomy in all six of these AL homes but more so in Peach Blossom and Oak Manor. Esther Adams's "system" based on rigid scheduling is designed for efficiency but gives residents at Peach Blossom little choice about when they get up, go to bed, or bathe and dress. Schedules at Oak Manor are predicated on the most efficient use of staffing resources, and residents' autonomy varies with their level of dependency. The impact of routine on autonomy at Rosie's, Blue Skies, and Greene's depends on the particular staff person in charge and whether residents attend day programs.

Regulations governing care practices and other aspects of residents' daily life, such as temperature of air and water and the timing and content of meals, although designed to protect, also restrict (Kane, 1995). Those regulations expressly mandating protection of residents' rights to make everyday choices lack effectiveness because they compete with standards for resident care, which providers tend to favor out of fear of legal and regulatory repercussions (Agich, 1993). Moreover, as Kane (1995) argues, autonomy-enhancing regulations often are difficult to enforce.

Regulatory barriers to autonomy are most notable at Oak Manor, where they are invoked to justify both the chill of the dining room and the tepid bath water. Although small-home providers struggle to keep required records, they pay little attention to regulations when making decisions regarding care, even with a clear understanding of state law. Esther Adams restrains Viola Wheeler with bed rails, Cora Greene runs an unlicensed home next door to Greene's, and no one adheres to posted menus. This variable adherence can be accounted for in part by the scant likelihood of getting caught. Both the state regulatory agency and the Long-Term Care Ombudsman Program make only annual routine inspections of ALFs. All other visits are complaint driven, and the chances that a complaint will be filed with either program is much higher at Oak Manor, where residents are more numerous and they, and their family members, are both more knowledgeable about regulations and more assertive. Oak Manor resident Gwen Runnels received transportation to a doctor's appointment on an unscheduled day by threatening to call the ombudsman program. In contrast, at Peach Blossom, Viola Wheeler lacks the resources for effective protest of the violation of her rights. Regulations related to reimbursement also affect autonomy through control of funding. In Georgia, only limited public financing is available through the Medicaid waiver program to pay for care in ALFs, which significantly restricts the resources available to these small homes.

Residents' restricted capacity has an obvious and significant effect on autonomy in all homes. Impairment interferes with a resident's ability to make and execute decisions and to articulate and negotiate choices, and it interferes with a provider's capability, and sometimes willingness, to support those decisions and choices. Supporting the autonomy of residents with cognitive impairment presents even greater challenges. Beck and Vogelpohl (1995) note a number of barriers to autonomy for cognitively impaired nursing home residents, which also are present in these six homes: including, on the part of caregivers, assumptions of low self-care functioning, lack of understanding of dementia, and inadequate skills to communicate effectively with cognitively impaired residents, and on the part of impaired persons, their inability to express their needs and wishes and their learned behaviors, which cause them to acquiesce to authority figures. The effect of restricted capacity also is dependent on the authenticity of the type of autonomy it denies. Limited mobility has minimal effect on Eugene Ellis's computer activities, whereas it denies Boss Cook the "street life" he most misses.

Although all providers have difficulty supporting meaningful choices of residents with significant impairment, some are more able and willing than others. Cora Greene explained how she provides a meaningful choice for Frankie Johnson, a resident with dementia: "Some can't make decisions. If they make decisions, it's not for the best, because they're not decision makers. Their decision-making skills are pretty much stopped, you know. So if Ms. Johnson says, 'I want to go to my house,' we know she don't have a house, so we take her for that walk. Sometime the walk is not good enough for her, so we take her for a ride." When confronted with the same dilemma at Peach Blossom, Ms. Adams's strategy is to solicit sedating medication from Viola Wheeler's physician.

Resource constraints restrict residents' autonomy in all homes, but the effect is most critical in the small homes, where both fees and residents' incomes are lower. Most limited are environmental features, such as bathrooms, private space, and accessible outdoor areas, transportation, recreational activities, food choices, and staffing. Of the small homes, Greene's and Sunshine House are most lacking, with deficits in each of these areas. The interaction of barriers is again evident: the realization of autonomy in each of these settings is a function of both resource availability and resident characteristics, that is, values and behaviors regarding resident autonomy tend to reflect the extent to which the facility's resources are adequate to meet the demands for care imposed by residents' dependencies. This finding is consistent with research in nursing homes and home care settings (Hennessy, 1987; Kane, 1991) and with the tenets of resource dependency theory (Hasenfeld, 1983, 265), which views organizational behavior as adaptive responses aimed at acquiring and maintaining the resources necessary to carry out the organization's assigned functions. Providers in this study face significant challenges caring for residents and surviving financially. Although Oak Manor is far richer than the small homes, as Jordan Taylor, the corporate representative, said, "It is a business. It is not a nonprofit, and we have promised investors a specific return on their investment, and we've got to provide that to them."

Because autonomy is such a complex and ethically problematic value—and sometimes produces harmful and risky choices as well as wise, responsible, and prudent ones—caregivers often face their own moral dilemmas when trying both to respect a person's autonomy and promote his or her well-being (Collopy, 1988, 1995). The help that caregivers provide frequently impinges on the very freedom and independence that persons value, creating tensions in the caregiving situation between the self-determination of the dependent person and the decisions and standards of the caregiver. Collopy (1990, 9) suggests that this choice "is nettled with dilemma, since it requires not simply choosing right from wrong, but choosing right from right, choosing one value over another."

Considerable research gives evidence of the conflict between autonomy and beneficence in a variety of long-term care settings, including the home (Ball & Whittington, 1995; Hennessy, 1989), assisted living (Ball et al., 2000; Rutman, Baron, & Tatem, 1987; Schiman & Lordeman, 1989; Utz, 2003), and the nursing home (Kane, 1995). A caregiver's concern for the safety and well-being of a resident inevitably creates barriers to the resident's independence, and we find the same to be true for autonomy. In each of these homes, providers impede residents' choices because they believe the choice is not in the residents' best interests, even when a choice is mandated by law and a resident is cognitively intact. In some homes, the values of one caregiver clash with those of another. Rosie disagrees with her daughter over serving fried as opposed to baked fish, and Inez's austerity regarding desserts at Blue Skies is not endorsed by Clarice. The value of justice also compounds the value of doing good in settings where the fair distribution of resources, including staff, is a significant issue and places inevitable constraints on how much autonomy is possible for any individual.

As in nursing homes (Kane, 1995; Savishinsky, 1991; Shawler, Rowles, & High, 2001), individual autonomy in ALFs also rivals the rights of other residents and the concerns of family members. At Blue Skies, Lily's choice to listen to her radio at night competes with another resident's right to peaceful sleep, and residents vie daily over who gets to watch a favorite soap opera. Janie Benton's daughter's insistent demands about her mother's toileting regimen encourages the forcible actions of her Oak Manor caregivers, and Mary Overton's son prevents her having a telephone and leaving the facility with her friends.

In chapter 6, we describe what we term a provider's way, which influences residents' success in achieving independence. Although a provider's way is molded by a variety of influences, including the four Rs described above, it is firmly rooted in a provider's value for, and definition of, quality care. Rosie believes her residents should be clean and well fed, but her value for these elements of quality does not dominate her value for resident autonomy. Rosie believes that residents love "homely" more than "convalescence" and that her home is "like home" to her residents. "Homely" means care is not "a production line," nothing is "off-limits" to residents, rules are ethereal, and relationships are "like family." In contrast, in Esther Adams's definition of quality, resident autonomy is given lip service, but it is not paramount. Although she too considers residents her "extended family" and Peach Blossom their "home," she defines home differently and organizes her family in a different way. No doubt, Ms. Adams established a similar system when raising her own children and the many foster children who shared their home. Now (and probably then) what she does "best" is provide care in a systematic, and mostly non-autonomy-yielding, way. Few can quarrel with the quality of the care in her home, but residents who move to Peach Blossom must be prepared to toe the line.

It is corporate, rather than individual, values that have the overriding in-fluence on resident care and life at Oak Manor. The facility mission statement, which affirms resident choice and respect for residents' individuality, is sup-portive of resident autonomy. Yet similar to the situation at Peach Blossom, other values often take precedence. When asked to state the corporate view on balancing autonomy and beneficence, Jordan Taylor replied, "There's no formula for that. You've got to create—I mean I'm talking in sales terms, but it's also in care terms—you've got to show the value in what you're doing and why you're doing it. And I think by being keenly aware of the residents' needs and what their concerns are, and the families' needs and what they perceive the needs to be, and you translate that to your staff, you are going to provide a happy medium." Families tend to have more influence at Oak Manor than in the small homes because they are more critical to the home's bottom line.

We would add a fifth R to Kane's list of autonomy impediments: risk. Bar-riers to autonomy often boil down to risk, either to resident or facility. Risk, as Kane and Levin (1998) note, can be incurred to varying degrees. Some choices obviously are more risky than others, and some are so dangerous they should not be allowed. We saw how some Greene's residents without deci-sional capacity sometimes incur risk when they are allowed to skip meals or exit the facility. However, curtailing residents' autonomy unnecessarily can cause harm to both their physical and mental health.

Supports for Autonomy

Collopy (1995) makes the distinction between negative and positive au-tonomy to refer to either noninterference with a person's choice or behavior or the provision of resources that sustain an individual's ability to be free. We prefer the terms *passive* and *active* to denote these two ways of conceiving of autonomy. Active autonomy requires relationships with others who enhance and support autonomy. Chapter 6 describes how care providers support resi-dents' self-care roles, and we know that promoting independence is one of the most effective means of enhancing residents' opportunities for choice and control. Many of the same strategies that enhance independence, such as getting to know residents as individuals, encouraging them to express their needs and preferences, and providing a supportive physical environment, also directly support autonomy. But fully supporting both the psychological and spiritual dimensions of autonomy requires additional tactics.

Many states, including Georgia, have enacted "bill of rights" statutes that detail the rights of residents in ALFs (Hopkins, 1989), similar to those found in nursing home regulations. These statutes state that residents have the right to choose activities and schedules consistent with their interests; be treated with respect; have access to a telephone; fully participate in care planning; be free from physical and chemical restraints; have access to the Long-Term Care Ombudsman Program; and be provided with information that relates to their quality of life and care, such as explanation of rights and care options. Notwithstanding the difficulty with enforcing such autonomy-enhancing regulations, we found they do motivate providers in these communities to support autonomy, at least in small ways and in some areas. For example, when residents at Oak Manor demanded that salt shakers be returned to the tables, the food service director recognized their right to this choice. We believe the effectiveness of these regulations could be improved if greater effort were made to educate residents and their families about the legal rights of residents to make choices in their daily lives. Providers are required to inform residents about their rights upon admission, typically a perfunctory process, but this education should be ongoing. Providers also should educate residents about the Long-Term Care Ombudsman Program and how to contact a representative. Most residents seem oblivious to the required ombudsman poster displayed at each facility.

One significant support for autonomy at Oak Manor is the resident council, which provides a forum for residents to complain about issues important to them and for facility staff to respond to their concerns. Residents elect officers and conduct the meetings, leadership roles residents like Eugene Ellis value. Although some facility administrators find the heavy emphasis on complaints bothersome, they are committed to the council and its purpose of empowering residents and have invited the ombudsman to help educate residents about their rights. Research in nursing homes has found an active resident council to be an effective means of increasing residents' control over activities (Grossman & Weiner, 1988). Although formal resident councils are not practical for small homes, providers could facilitate informal resident meetings to discuss issues of concern.

Hofland (1995) suggests that in addition to rights residents in nursing homes have responsibilities that are complex and involve both other residents and staff. Such responsibilities can include self-care, expressing gratitude and complaining appropriately to caregivers, following facility rules, assisting other residents, articulating needs and preferences, participating in resident councils, and maintaining contact with friends and relatives outside the facility. We found here, as in earlier research among home care clients (Ball & Whittington, 1995), that residents who make such responsibilities a part of their resident roles are more successful in realizing meaningful autonomy. Facility providers can support autonomy by guiding residents in understanding and enacting this aspect of their roles.

Supporting authentic choices for residents demands that providers make special efforts to learn about a resident's past character and persistent values. Although this task is easier in the small homes, a smaller resident population does not guarantee success, especially if residents are cognitively impaired. Oak Manor has a comprehensive tool for gathering such data about residents in the special care dementia unit, but it is not used for AL residents, though the executive director regrets the absence of the practice. Rowles and High (1996) have found family members to be a valuable resource in providing information to nursing home staff about the true preferences and values of persons with cognitive deficits. Families are used in this way in each of these six homes, but not to their full potential. In addition, care must be taken when using this strategy, because family members who have not recently been in close contact with residents may not have accurate knowledge. Studies in nursing homes (Shawler, Rowles, & High, 2001) and assisted living facilities (Reinardy & Kane, 2003) show that residents, family members, and facility caregivers can have different views on the relative importance of day-to-day choices.

The role of the physical environment in relation to autonomy is most often viewed in terms of environmental support and resources for control of ambient conditions (regulating air temperature and noise to personally comfortable levels), control of access to self (visual and acoustical privacy in bathroom, lockable bedroom doors), and individual expression or presentation of self (means to display personally important objects). The physical environment also plays a role in other realms of autonomy in more subtle ways. Personal control in the type or timing of baths depends on adequate bathing facilities, and choice and control in social situations require places for residents to socialize and to be alone. Oak Manor, similar to the typical purpose-built ALF, provides the most supportive physical environment of these six homes. Our findings confirm other research that demonstrates that residents overwhelmingly prefer private rooms, primarily because of the control such space affords over social interactions and daily recreational and self-care activities (Ball et al., 2000; Kane et al., 1998). Easy access to community services—drugstore, community center, church, library, public transportation—facilitates autonomy in instrumental activities, leisure, management of personal affairs, and continuity of lifestyle. Greene's and Sunshine House have the easiest access to the wider community, as well as more residents able to take advantage of it.

Miniaturization of Autonomy

In their book on elders living alone, Rubinstein, Kilbride, and Nagy (1992, 143) describe a process they term the miniaturization of satisfaction, whereby people for whom few possibilities remain lower their expectations and find satisfaction in the realm of small, rather than large, events. Other research gives evidence of what we might call the "miniaturization of autonomy." Among elderly home care clients and residents of ALFs (Ball & Whittington, 1995; Ball et al., 2000), we have found acceptance of restricted options and keen satisfaction from controlling the smallest tasks of everyday living. A number of nursing home studies also demonstrate that even in restrictive environments, individual choice and control can be introduced in ways—some quite small, such as choice of clothing and activities—that residents find meaningful (Barken, 1995; Groger, 1995; Shield, 1995). These studies also indicate that persons who are able both to maximize their resources to achieve autonomy and to adapt to their restricted options are more satisfied with the quality of their lives.

In each of these six communities we found evidence for the miniaturization of autonomy. For most residents, life is carried out within, or very close to, their new homes, and it is the choices related to daily living that loom large—the when, what, where, how, how often, with whom, and by whom of ordinary activities. Viola Wheeler cares very much about when she bathes and what she has for breakfast; how her bed is made (without a wrinkle) is a chief concern of Lula Merriwether; who takes her to the bathroom matters to Pearl Bowman; and where and how often she smokes is central to Tracey Williams's day. The importance of small choices, though, does not mean that the larger choices are not missed or desired. Boss Cook laments the loss of his former persona of "ladies' man," and Hamilton Brewton misses his car and the freedom it gave him to come and go, but residents who use the adaptive process of miniaturization are more satisfied. When Eugene Ellis's eyesight fails him, he can be happy with decisional control over how another executes his computer tasks. He also miniaturizes his strategies for achieving autonomy by focusing on smaller, more manageable requests.

By understanding the process of miniaturization, providers also can be more successful in realizing residents' psychological and spiritual autonomy. Cora Greene uses this strategy by taking Ms. Johnson for a walk or a ride when taking her home is not possible. Viola Wheeler might have been happier with her bath if she could have sat in a shower chair or bathed later in the day.

Advance Planning

Clark (1987) argues that support for autonomy should begin with advance planning for long-term care, and we certainly concur with this argument. Residents and family members, when looking for a facility, should search for a good resident-facility fit, and the findings presented in this chapter confirm the worth of this endeavor. Mayetta Stewart "fits" better and feels freer at Sunshine House than she did at Peach Blossom, and the young men at Greene's and Sunshine House would be sorely constrained at any of the other homes. Eugene Ellis's authentic autonomy is made possible by the physical and social environment at Oak Manor.

So, Whose Home Is It?

The realization of resident autonomy hinges to a degree on how the various stakeholders define ownership of the home. The official version at Oak Manor is that the facility is, in fact, the residents' home. When residents move in they are told it is their new home, and management trains staff to treat it so. Although no residents consider Oak Manor really home, a few do think of it as *like* home, at least within the confines of their private space. When asked if Oak Manor felt like home, Ethyl Burns replied, "Sure, it does. I can't be at somebody's house and do what I want. But here, it's just like me being at home. Here you feel more free." Frankie Johnson experiences a similar freedom at Greene's: "I just like it 'cause I got my own house, you see. I can get up when

I get ready and lay down when I get ready, you see. I don't want no boss." To Hassie Hicks, Peach Blossom is "someone else's" house, and Ms. Adams reinforces this view when she says, "You know what the rules are in my house and follow them."

Although those residents who feel more at home also seem to feel more free, the question of whose house it is, of course, is more complicated. Some people live in these six homes. Others own them. Still others only work there. So, whose home is it? In reality, residents, owners, and staff members all can lay claim to some authority over the fabric of everyday life in these communities. Each has rights to some say-so about the home's operation. Each also has responsibilities. Providers must care for residents and follow regulations. Residents must pay their bills and follow certain rules. Corporations must be watchful of investors' money. We have laid out the many barriers to autonomy, and we know it can be challenging to give residents meaningful choices. But we also know it can be done. Some factors that limit autonomy in these homes are immutable. Attitudes are not. Facility providers and family members who are truly committed to maximizing resident autonomy achieve greater success.

CHAPTER 10

Continuity of Care

When Esther Adams opened the doors of Peach Blossom more than 20 years ago, one of her first residents was Bobby Bailey, then aged 58, mentally retarded, hearing impaired, and unable to communicate verbally. Ms. Adams thinks he "probably never went to school because he doesn't write." Since Bobby had no family to speak of, he became a ward of the state, and Ms. Adams became his "family."

Over the years, Ms. Adams fed and clothed Bobby, saw to his medical care, found day programs to enrich his life, and incorporated him into the life of her home. Bobby experienced no significant decline until December 2000, when he had surgery to relieve a urinary blockage. He came home from the hospital with a urinary catheter and, for a couple of months, needed help bathing, dressing, and toileting. Although Bobby recovered from this episode and regained function, several months later he began to lose his appetite and weaken. He was diagnosed with cancer and, in September 2000 (six months after the end of our study), Ms. Adams and Bobby's caseworker made the decision to place him in a hospice care facility, where he died a week later. Ms. Adams visited Bobby in the hospice, so that he would know that the "same people still loved him even though he was in a different place." "He was a special person," Ms. Adams recalled, "and every time that I might have decided that, well, maybe someone else would meet his needs, it never worked out. So then, I came to the conclusion that I guess it was meant for this to be his home until."

Bobby's 20-year tenure at Peach Blossom represents the ideal of "aging in place" in assisted living. Although the term "aging in place" traditionally has been applied to individuals growing old in their own homes (Pynoos, 1993), recently the concept has been expanded to include assisted living. One of the key philosophical tenets of the newer model of assisted living is the promotion of aging in place by maximizing resident independence and providing services to accommodate residents' changing needs (Citro & Hermanson, 1999); 28 states include such a philosophy in their statutes or regulations (Mollica & Jenkins, 2001). But if the concept means that residents may stay in a facility until death, aging in place thus far has been an illusion for most residents (Chapin & Dobbs-Kepper, 2001; Hawes, Rose, & Phillips, 1999; Phillips et al., 2003). National data show an average length of stay of only 18 months (American Seniors Housing Association, 1999), and most providers view a resident's stay as only a way station to nursing home placement (Frank, 2002).

Elsewhere (Ball et al., 2004a), we describe a conceptual model for aging in place in assisted living that identifies management of resident decline as the cornerstone of residents' ability to remain in this setting over time. Multiple resident, facility, and community factors influence the capacity of residents and facilities to manage decline, and the ability of residents to age in place is principally a function of the "fit" between the resident and facility capacities. Management of decline involves both prevention and response. Prevention entails health promotion and adherence to treatment regimens, and response includes balancing needs with resources, extending (sometimes overextending) resources to meet needs, and acceptance of the fact that some residents' needs will be unmet. Assessment of potential risk to both residents and facilities is a key factor guiding strategies for management of resident decline. This model builds on that of Bernard, Zimmerman, and Eckert (2001), which also explains the role of community-, facility-, and individual-level factors in AL residents' ability to age in place by illuminating how and why various factors operate within and between levels.

Our model for aging in place is based on a study of five facilities, which varied in size, design, geographic location, resources, and resident profiles and included Oak Manor (Study II). With the exception of Oak Manor, the resident populations of these homes were either all or mostly white. In this chapter, we extend our exploration of residents' ability to age in place to the five small homes in the Andrus study (Study I) and compare the experiences of residents in these homes with those of Oak Manor residents. We describe the pathways of residents who leave and of those who stay, and we identify factors that influence the capacities of residents and facilities to manage decline over time. In addition, we examine the impact of staying and leaving on residents and their families and on facilities.

Table 10.1. Changes in Resident Census during Study Period
(number of residents)

Home	At start	Moved in	Discharged	Moved on own	Died	At end
Rosie's	7	2	1	1	0	7
Peach Blossom	6	3	2	0	1	6
Blue Skies	5	3	0	2	1	5
Greene's	14	4	1	2	2	13
Sunshine House	7	8	2	2	0	11
Oak Manor	20	26	9	9	0	28
Total	59	46[a]	15	16	4	70

[a]Includes one resident who moved from Peach Blossom to Sunshine House.

The Experience of Aging in Place

Going, Coming, and Staying

At the beginning of the study, a total of 59 residents were living in these six communities. Eighteen of these residents moved out, four died, and 37 remained until the end. Over the course of the study, 33 new residents moved in, and another 13 moved both in and out, leaving a total of 70 residents at the study's completion.[1] Some, like Bobby Bailey, have lived in these homes for many years. Although Bobby was the most long-term resident, Sarah Eubanks was the first resident at Rosie's when it opened 10 years ago, Arney Stokes has been at Greene's for 15 years, and Lewis Howell at Sunshine House for seven. Both Blue Skies and Oak Manor also have charter residents, but those homes have been open only a short time. Table 10.1 shows the movement of residents in and out of each home.

Residents Leaving

Of those who left, almost half (15) were involuntarily discharged. Two-thirds of these went to nursing homes, four Oak Manor residents were transferred to the home's dementia care unit, and one Peach Blossom resident moved to another ALF.

[1]One resident (of Peach Blossom) moved to another facility (Sunshine House) during the course of this study.

Problem behaviors and increased physical care needs accounted for all discharges. Most problem behaviors were dementia related. Dora McElhaney, who lived at Rosie's for about a year and a half, is typical. Ms. McElhaney had always been challenging—losing Cleo Kellog's dentures, clogging up the bathroom sink with pieces of tissue, and pulling the trim off the curtains and the buttons off her clothes. But Rosie began to think about discharge when increased dementia led to her trying "to fight someone" at the senior center and using the bathtub for the toilet. Rosie issued a 30-day discharge notice in November 1999; but when Ms. McElhaney's daughter Trudy shed tears, Rosie gave her until February 2000 to find another place, because she did not want to see anyone "on the street." In the end, it was Ms. McElhaney's hospitalization after a fall that finally led to her departure. Rosie could not bring herself to put her out but was steadfast in her refusal to take her back, despite Trudy's considerable anger.

Discharging Ms. McElhaney was difficult for Rosie, because her tradition has been to "keep the people until they pass." But Rosie herself has declined physically over the years and is no longer able to maintain her ideal. Ms. McElhaney's challenging behaviors were compounded by her ADL care needs, and three residents needing heavy care became more than Rosie could handle without compromising her care standards.

The bar for dementia-related problem behaviors is lower at Oak Manor, one reason being that its special care dementia unit still is not full. The resident services director explained the criteria for transfer: "Walking the halls up and down, wandering [into] other residents' rooms, you know, that shows me that there's some confusion. You should be able to function without us directing you. You should, once you've got acclimated to the building, be able to go down to the dining room for meals. You can read the calendar and know the activities going on. You know, if you need all that cueing and redirecting, you need to go to a smaller, structured environment." Although one resident, Rose Bowman, was transferred for wandering from the building, the other three residents sent to the dementia unit needed only "redirection."

Not all problem behaviors leading to discharge were related to dementia. One exception was Mayetta Stewart, who was discharged from Peach Blossom because, in Esther Adams's view, her "ways" were "disruptive to the home." Ms. Adams prefers "people who are compatible . . . and don't create a fuss." Instead, Ms. Stewart "would do what she wanted to do and say what she wanted to say." Her unacceptable behaviors included wearing unmatched outfits, bringing junk food into the home, and eating fried chicken in her Sunday clothes. Although Ms. Stewart missed the smaller size of Peach Blossom, she found the less regimented atmosphere at Sunshine House more suited to her taste and personality.

Edgar Allgood, who moved in and out of Greene's during the study, is representative of a resident whose physical care needs increased beyond what a home was able or willing to manage. Mr. Allgood moved to Greene's straight from County Hospital, where he had been taken after suffering a stroke. At that time, he could manage all of his ADLs, albeit with difficulty; but over the next three months, he steadily declined, and his incontinence and other care needs became too taxing on Greene's staff. Cora Greene explained his discharge: "When he gotten to the point where he was wetting on himself every night and he can't even bathe himself, he can't do the everyday things in order to keep himself going, that's when I try to find nursing home placement for them." Yet Ms. Greene expressed regret for this and similar decisions: "It's always painful for me to let them go into the nursing home, because that's not what they wanting to do. And they really be sad about it." Although Ms. Greene hoped that, with therapy, Mr. Allgood would improve, his decline continued in the nursing home, and, when last visited by the researcher, he was comatose.

The four residents who died during the study period, like Bobby, were able to truly age in place, remaining in the home until their deaths. For Ivera Haygood, a resident of Peach Blossom, death was both sudden and unforeseen. One Sunday morning after breakfast, Ms. Haygood got up from the sofa and headed toward the bathroom. Ms. Adams, who was in the dining room, seeing that she had vomited, hurried after her. Ms. Haygood appeared to be in pain, and Ms. Adams made her lie down on the bed and then called 911. When the paramedics arrived, they administered oxygen and rushed Ms. Haygood to County Hospital, where she died that night, the result of a heart attack. Ms. Haygood had no family, but Ms. Adams was able to locate two of her church members to go to the hospital to be with her. Ms. Adams attended the funeral, took three of the residents to the funeral home the night before, and displayed one of the floral sprays at Peach Blossom. Although distressed over Ms. Haygood's death, Ms. Adams believed that the swiftness of her passing was "a beautiful way to go." Ms. Haygood was 78 and had lived at Peach Blossom for only nine months.

Lily Porter's death, a little more than a year after she moved to Blue Skies, was more predictable. She was 92 when she moved in, had suffered a stroke in the past, had a pacemaker, and frequently used oxygen because of chronic shortness of breath. Her first serious crisis, another stroke, came after she had lived in the home for 11 months. Inez, the staff person, heard Lily call out one night and quickly went to her room. Lily "looked strange," and "her teeth [dentures] were falling out of her mouth." Inez administered oxygen and then called 911 and Lily's daughter Sharon, who met Lily at the hospital. After a week-long hospital stay, Lily returned to Blue Skies, but less than a month later she suffered another stroke. This time, she stopped breathing, and Angel (the staff person who replaced Inez) gave her mouth-to-mouth resuscitation until the ambulance arrived. Angel had witnessed her own mother's death and was determined to keep Lily alive. Lily again returned to Blue Skies, but after only three weeks she had yet another stroke. This time she did not recover.

Sixteen residents chose to move out of these homes, or submitted to their family members' choice. Four of these improved in function and no longer needed the assisted living environment: Mr. Kelner, who according to Ms. Greene "didn't need personal care by no means, never needed it," moved from Greene's to his stepson's house; Spike, a young resident with mental illness, left Sunshine House after only five months to try living on his own; Louisa Walden moved back home from Oak Manor after a six-week rehabilitative stay; and Frances Bates left Oak Manor for a senior apartment close to her daughter's home. All of these residents made their own decisions to leave. Ms. Bates explained hers: "I want to live my life. I am too active. I am not ready to just lay down and die. I wanted to try assisted living, and now I have had the experience. This is costing me too much." Cost was the primary impetus for three other residents who moved from Oak Manor to a nearby, independently owned African American ALF with lower monthly fees.

Family members made the decisions to move seven residents. One was Sarah Eubanks, who moved from Rosie's to a nursing home. Although Ms. Eubanks has nine children, it was two of her daughters who decided it would be best to move her to where she had access to skilled care and was closer to their homes and before, as her daughter Judith explained, she got "worse": "She's not gonna get any better than she is now, and we don't want to wait until she's much worse and then we're running around like chickens with our heads cut off trying to find her a place to be." Ms. Eubanks suffered from manic depression, a heart condition, and diabetes and had been hospitalized twice over the past year, once as the result of a sugar imbalance and the other because of a mental "breakdown," but each time she recovered fully. Although Ms. Eubanks was a habitual complainer, Rosie knew she did not want to move from the home where she had lived for 10 years. In Rosie's view, complaining was her "nature" and, if she "was laying in a bed of whipped cream with God on one side and a rose on the other, she still would complain." Rosie worried sometimes about keeping up with Ms. Eubanks's seven medications and monitoring her blood sugar, but neither she nor her daughter thought the move was best for her.

The day before her move, Ms. Eubanks expressed anxiety about the transition. She worried about who was going to help her pack, whether she should wear a dress or pants, put on her wig or "go natural," and how the doctors would know what medications to give her or how many "amps" were needed for her shock treatment. About her stay at Rosie's, she declared, "I enjoyed being here. I know I ain't gonna find better than here. I'm from a big family, and all ya'll make me feel at home." On the day of Ms. Eubanks's departure, fellow resident Carole Seymour reported, "She cried. We all shed tears, too. She really didn't want to go." Three months later, Ms. Eubanks died. According to Rosie, "Her sugar had gone to 600, and she had gone into cardiac arrest."

Two other residents were moved by family members from Oak Manor to nursing homes. One was Corrine Wallace, whose family chose this option over the home's dementia care unit because of the unit's higher fees. The other was Mabel Crosby, who had rheumatoid arthritis and was wheelchair bound. Although Ms. Crosby was happy at Oak Manor, according to the business manager, her children were "stressed out" over the inevitability of further decline and moved her after only a five-week stay.

Three residents with dementia were moved by daughters (one a "play daughter," a common term for fictive kin) to their own homes. Although future discharge was likely for each resident, their family members chose to pre-empt this outcome. In Frankie Johnson's case, her family feared for her safety after she wandered away from Greene's for the second time. Ms. Greene described her departure: "Ms. Johnson wandered out of the home about one o'clock in the morning. Her family member got so angry 'cause we allowed her to get away. She end up at County Hospital that night, and her daughter went to pick her up and she moved her out. They said that if we was taking care of her better, that it wouldn't of never happened. I was apologetic to her walking out, but I tried to explain to them that I felt like we had done all that we could do for her, 'cause not only was staff having to watch out for her all day, all night, everybody in the home was chasing her, 'cause she'll be sitting in one spot this moment and the next moment she on up the street."

Residents Staying

Although 35 residents left these homes during the study, 70 residents remain. For some, particularly those who moved in relatively young or healthy, decline has been minimal. Such was the case for Bobby Bailey for all but the last year of his life at Peach Blossom. Arney Stokes, diagnosed with schizophrenia, at the age of 40 has experienced little change since he moved to Greene's 15 years ago, nor has Curtis Lowell in his four years at Sunshine House. But decline is ongoing and largely unavoidable for most residents in these six homes. The decision to move to assisted living is typically the choice of last resort. Prior decline is the impetus for entry, and once there, though the pace varies, decline tends to continue as residents age. The decline trajectories of residents who stay resemble those of residents who leave. As stated earlier, how decline is managed—by residents, their families, and facility providers—has significant influence on residents' tenure in assisted living. The cases of Eugene Ellis and Boss Cook illustrate typical trajectories.

Mr. Ellis had significant health problems when he entered Oak Manor in September 2000. His congestive heart failure had led to five heart attacks and a pacemaker; he had diabetes and cataracts, took 10 medications, and used a walker for mobility. Mr. Ellis plays an integral role in his health care. He is knowledgeable about his conditions and adheres to prescribed treatment regimens. He is accustomed to good medical care and assertive about getting it. When he moved to Atlanta, he asked his former cardiologist in Philadelphia to recommend a new doctor. He keeps up with appointments and schedules transportation, uses his computer to order medications and record blood sugar levels and clotting times, and seeks information from Oak Manor's consultant dietician about the correct diet for a person taking a blood thinner. When he needs help, he asks for it. He leans on his grandson to take him to get his prescribed orthotic shoes and on Oak Manor's executive director to fill his medication box.

But Mr. Ellis's conditions are serious and intractable, and at this point in his life, preventive measures go only so far. In November 2000 he was hospitalized for three days because of swelling in his lower extremities. The following spring he began to have problems with incontinence. Once, after returning from the doctor, he urinated in front of the building in plain view of several residents, a performance that earned him a discharge threat. In June 2001 he returned to the hospital with swelling in his legs and ankles. While there, the doctors discovered that his kidneys were failing as well as his heart, and he was anemic. When Oak Manor's resident services director assessed him on June 20th, she deemed him not ready to return, and on June 25 he was transferred to a nursing home.

Mr. Ellis's daughter Caroline, who came down from Cincinnati, helped find the best possible facility for his hoped-for rehabilitation and continued to visit him in the nursing home and communicate regularly by e-mail with the facility's director. Caroline said about Mr. Ellis at the time, "I think my father has a strong will to live. He says, whatever I say, he'll do." During his nursing home stay, Mr. Ellis contracted pneumonia but recovered, and with daily therapy and medication adjustments recommended by his cardiologist, after two months he improved enough to return to Oak Manor. Once back, he received physical therapy and nurse visits from a home health agency several times weekly, and the resident services director increased his care level from "independent" to "enhanced," meaning limited bathing and dressing assistance. Although Mr. Ellis is continuing to age in place at Oak Manor, he has lost ground, and his continued stay is tenuous.

Boss Cook moved to Greene's from County Hospital after a stroke at the age of 50. Now 60, Boss has aged in place for some time, but he is declining. At the beginning of the study, Ms. Greene expressed concern about his weight gain and limited mobility. Even then he used a walker and could walk only short distances. He can dress himself but needs help with bathing, mostly supervision to prevent falling. Boss's main health problem is hypertension, aggravated by obesity, which he seems unconcerned about managing. Despite ongoing opposition from Ms. Greene, he persists in sending other residents to nearby fast food restaurants to buy him the unhealthy food he loves. Except for his trips to the senior center, he usually sits and watches TV from early in the morning till late at night, though sometimes he squeezes a rubber ball in hopes of increasing the strength in his hands.

Boss receives medical care at various County Hospital clinics, which means he has no regular doctor and clinic visits are daylong ordeals he rarely elects to brave. During the study year, he experienced increased swelling in his ankles and shortness of breath. Finally, early in the morning on December 17, 2000, Ms. Greene took Boss to County Hospital because he was having difficulty breathing and left him in the emergency room with Jesse, a staff person. When Ms. Greene returned later that day, Jesse reported that the doctors were keeping Boss overnight "for observation." During a hospital visit from the researcher, Boss said he had had a "lot of tests" but no one had given him any information, although he did know that the support hose he was wearing were for his badly swollen legs.

Boss was anxious to get back to Greene's. He was worried about his money, which he had given Jesse for safekeeping, and he wanted to attend the Christmas party at the Emmanuel House senior center. He returned on December 23, with four new "pills," knowing neither their names nor their functions. Ms. Greene, who knew little more, was frustrated that County doctors had sent him home "without any instructions" and with his legs still badly swollen and his breathing labored. The doctors told Boss they did not know the cause, just that "it wasn't his heart." He also was having difficulty "holding his water." Since Ms. Greene "didn't know anything else to do," she put him on a strict salt-free, sugar-free, low-calorie diet and instructed him not to "go against her." She also urged him to use his walker as much as possible, because she knew she could not keep him at Greene's if he became wheelchair dependent.

Boss showed no improvement, and about two weeks later, Ms. Greene took him to a private hospital, where he again was admitted. Laney (a staff member) reported that, before he left Greene's, he had been doing "very poorly" and "wetting on himself and stinking real bad." She praised Ms. Greene for taking him: "She knows her clients, and she knows when things are not right." According to Laney, doctors at this hospital diagnosed Boss with a "bad bladder infection and fluid around his heart" and sent him home with an order for physical therapy visits from a home health agency. At first, Boss was diligent about adhering to his diet and staying out of his wheelchair. Staff served him boiled eggs and toast for breakfast, salads for lunch, and half portions of meat for dinner. But by February, Boss had reverted to supplementing his diet with junk food, and new staff members refused to prepare his special food. By the end of the study, Boss was unable to walk, bathe, or dress on his own. Although Ms. Greene wanted to send him back to the hospital, Boss begged to be left at the home, and she agreed to a reprieve. Over the years, Greene's had become "like home" to Boss—and where he wanted to stay—and both he and Ms. Greene knew that another hospital admission would most likely end in nursing home placement.

The Capacity to Manage Decline

According to our conceptual model (Ball et al., 2004a), assisted living residents' ability age in place hinges on management of decline. Decline management involves both prevention of further decline and response to existing decline. Our descriptions of residents who left and those who stayed illustrate both kinds of strategies. These descriptions also indicate that both strategy choice and effectiveness depend on the decline management capacities of residents and facilities. Also consistent with the model, the capacity to manage decline is influenced by multiple interactive, and sometimes mutable, resident, facility, and community factors. As noted earlier, the research on which the model is based included data from Oak Manor. Data from the five small homes lend substantial support for this model.

Resident Capacity

A resident's health status has obvious influence on his or her capacity to manage decline and age in place. Residents are entering assisted living older and more impaired (Hawes, Rose, & Phillips, 1999), and the residents in these six communities are no exception. Harold Stamps at Rosie's, Eugene Ellis at Oak Manor, Lily Porter at Blue Skies, and Viola Wheeler at Peach Blossom, whose age at entry ranged from 85 to 95, represent this progression. Esther Adams reflected on the change in her clientele over her 20 years in the business: "I might say that the clientele has changed over the years. When I started out, they were people who needed assistance, but basically everyone could get up and go to the bathroom, do their own care in the morning. I'll call my first group of people the "first era"—then we got into what was really more residents who needed more personal care. Really, when I started, Alzheimer's was sort of new. I mean, it wasn't talked about. If it was present, which it might have been then, we didn't get referrals for that. Then all of a sudden, it turned around, and, maybe out of 10 referrals, 8 would be Alzheimer's."

Ms. Adams speculates that her residents' increase in frailty is related to a change in their families' willingness to keep them at home longer: "Well, the only thing I can say is, I think sometimes the residents like we first had, their families might have decided that they wanted to work with them [keep them at home]." The data presented in chapter 4 attest to the efforts of both residents and their family members to delay the move to assisted living as long as possible.

A resident's particular health condition, of course, also affects the nature and effectiveness of decline management. Decline trajectories vary. Those with a primary diagnosis of mental retardation or mental illness have the potential of being long-term residents, assuming they take prescribed medications and enter, like Bobby and Arney, before old age, but little can be done to brake the steady course of Dexter Ross's colon cancer. The pace and direction of Hattie Houseworth's Parkinson disease is less decipherable. Ms. Houseworth's daughter Phoebe expressed hope, but also uncertainty, about her mother's future at Oak Manor: "I hope that she can stay here and be at least as functional as she is now for as long as possible. I hope, never having watched anyone with Parkinson's. She has changed radically over the year. When she first got here, she was very sick. When she got medical treatment, she got better. After about midsummer, there was a little bit of a slide again. I am hoping that she can retain as much of her independence and ability to function as possible. Unless something goes terribly wrong and she is beyond the level of care that they have here, I would see her staying here as long as possible."

This study confirms other research findings of the significance of financial resources in residents' ability to age in place (Ball et al., 2004a; Hawes, Rose, & Phillips, 1999). At Oak Manor, money is necessary to pay both basic fees and add-ons related to increased service needs. According to the executive director, "Denial [of need for additional services] and money," which "go hand in hand," are the biggest barriers to aging in place. Hattie Houseworth has sufficient money from her government retirement and the sale of her house to live out her years at Oak Manor, but not all residents are so fortunate. Some have already moved out for lack of funds, and others worry about what lies ahead. When asked her thoughts on her mother's long-term care future, Ida Mooney's daughter Aimee replied, "I don't know. It is terrifying. When I think about the financial responsibility, I see it mounting as her needs change. I can see that happening. She is healthy, but I can see [her abilities] diminishing. I hope we can pull together as a family, because I know the financial responsibility is going to be tremendous." Although Ms. Mooney has four children, one a physician, the family's combined resources may not be sufficient to keep Ms. Mooney, who is relatively young (aged 77) and has dementia, at Oak Manor for her remaining years.

Julia Shields, a retired nurse, is able to afford Oak Manor fees only because of her long-term care insurance, which pays $1,200 of her $1,945 fee. According to her younger sister Maude (aged 88), her primary caregiver, the insurance is a key factor in her continued stay at Oak Manor: "That's one of the main reasons we tell her she got to stay out there, because she'd been carrying the insurance for a long time, and after they put that rider on there that you could use the assisted living, they would pay for that. See, she's always saying, 'I'd rather be at home.' Well, I said, 'Now if you were at home, they wouldn't be paying,' because she had used up all her home health care insurance from years before."

But the AL benefits also are not forever: "The thing is, though, they would pay for two years, and waive your premium for those two years, but then for the next six months, you have to come off and you pay [the premium], and then they evaluate you again, and, if you able, then they take you back up again. So she went in last June and, the 13th would be a year that she's been out there, so she'll have another year, and I don't know what we are going to do at the end of the two years. She has pretty high medical bills. She has this problem with her bladder, and then that Aricept for her memory." At least one Oak Manor resident moved to a nursing home because the care would be covered by Medicaid payments, and three others moved to lower-cost ALFs.

Money also affects the decline management capacity of residents in the small homes. Hassie Hicks's continued stay at Peach Blossom is dependent on her daughter's willingness to supplement her $600 monthly income from Social Security. Since Ms. Hicks arrived in September 1997, her monthly fees have increased from $750 to $1,000. The ability of Campbell Jenkins and Slick (both with Veterans Administration benefits) to pay higher fees ($1,000) at Greene's induces Ms. Greene to be more tolerant of their increased needs and aggravating behaviors. In contrast, Edgar Allgood's low fee of $600 held no sway with her and could not, in the end, protect him from discharge. Participation in the Medicaid waiver program enhances the payment ability of six of the nine residents who lived at Rosie's over the study year. The majority of residents in the small homes participate in the Medicaid program, which ensures their access to health care (though it is most likely not of the highest quality) and medications. However, the lack of access to quality—or any— health care throughout their lives influences both the health status and treatment regimens of these low-income residents. For several Greene's residents, the lack of money to buy incontinence pads threatens their continued stay.

In chapter 7, we discuss the critical role of families in these communities of care. Suffice it to say here that residents who have families involved in their care have a better chance of remaining in each of these communities. Family members provide care, money, and even the will to keep going. Eugene Ellis's daughter Caroline furnishes both instrumental and emotional support, as do his three grandsons and their wives and children who live in Atlanta. When he was in the nursing home, Caroline stayed in his room at Oak Manor on her visits from Cincinnati, made friends with residents and staff, and lobbied for his return. Hattie Houseworth's daughter's devoted presence in her mother's life, as well as her support of the wider Oak Manor community, no doubt fortify her mother's longevity. Lack of family support, however, quite likely hastened Mr. Allgood along his path out of Greene's and will contribute to the imminent discharge of Miss Fannie from there, too.

Chapter 6 explores the strong value for independence that motivates most residents to practice self-care. This value has clear impact on residents' ability to stay in each of these homes, but even more so in Greene's and Sunshine House, where hands-on care is at a premium. The desire to remain in these homes also prompts residents to hold tight to their remaining independence. Except for the few residents who improve or are dissatisfied, almost no one wants to leave, at least not to enter a nursing home, a psychiatric hospital, or a homeless shelter. The overwhelming preference of most residents and their families is for residents to stay where they are. Lula Merriwether's niece Georgiana, who had cared for her own mother before she died and for Ms. Merriwether before her move to Oak Manor, expressed this aspiration: "I would hope that she could stay at Oak Manor until she dies. And I know that's inevitable, but my hope would be that she would not be in the situation where she would have to leave and go to another facility. I have said, and I firmly believe, that I will not take care of another terminally ill person in my home. She is happy there, and I would hope when her time comes to go, whether it's a year from now or 10 years from now, that she just goes right there, 'cause I think she'll be happy."

A few family members, though, all daughters, held on to the hope of bringing their parent to their own homes. The daughters of Peach Blossom residents Irene Garrett and Estelle Washington and Rosie's resident Pearl Bowman all viewed these homes as stop-gap measures until they could retire and provide the care themselves. Pearl Bowman's daughter Fannie expressed the strongest resolve, particularly in the event that nursing home placement becomes the alternative for her mother, who has Alzheimer's: "I am going to keep her myself. My children will help. She's *not* going in a nursing home. I have sung [with a visiting choir] in too many of them. I know the kind of mother I had. She don't need to suffer. She always been a very sweet person. Everyone who knows her loves her."

Residents' knowledge about their health conditions and medications, access to formal health care and insurance, and health promotion also influence their abilities to manage decline. Eugene Ellis, with his greater education and wider experience in dealing with formal systems, is more able than Boss Cook to obtain quality care and carry out treatment regimens.

In other research (Ball et al., 2004a), we have found that social ties with other residents and providers can enhance and thereby lengthen residents' AL stays, and evidence of similar influences exists in these six communities. These relationships contribute both to providers' willingness to retain residents and residents' desire to stay. Cora Greene tries so hard to keep Boss because she has grown to love him over his 10 years in her home, and her affection for Martha Kominsky mellows the offense of her racist remarks. Esther Adams's love for Bobby has a similar effect. The family-like bonds Sarah Eubanks developed during her long-term stay at Rosie's contributed to her grief over leaving. Rosie is loath to discharge Harold Stamps and Pearl Bowman because their daughters are her old friends.

Friendships between residents also promote mutual support, which in some cases increases tenures. Although such relationships have the best chance of developing and wielding influence in small homes, some evidence of the effect of relationships on aging in place is present at Oak Manor. Executive director Kathy Wall indicated that the impact of family support on a resident's ability to stay in AL is enhanced by understanding based on relationship. Using Hattie Houseworth's daughter Phoebe as an example, she said, "It's a relationship thing. Her daughter knows that Oak Manor is doing the best they can. She understands how long it takes to get her to breakfast in the morning. She wants [the care staff] to get her up, but she understands they don't always have time to accomplish it."

Facility Capacity

Admission and Discharge Policies

Policies governing admission and retention demarcate the boundaries for aging in place in each facility. These policies, as in ALFs nationwide, are circumscribed at the community level by state regulatory requirements for admission and retention, which specify the characteristics of residents who may be served and the types of services that may be provided (Mollica & Jenkins, 2001). Although states vary with regard to these requirements, most states, including Georgia, do not permit residents who are nonambulatory or require a two-person transfer or continuous skilled nursing care. Facilities may request a waiver to keep residents with needs beyond those allowed, but they must demonstrate they have the capacity to meet those needs. None of these six homes is using, or has used, the waiver process. Neither do they keep residents with needs beyond those allowed by law, though Rosie's has in the past.

Specific admission and retention policies in ALFs often are more restrictive than stipulated by state law (Chapin & Dobbs-Kepper, 2001; Hawes, Rose, & Phillips, 1999; U.S. General Accounting Office, 1999), and this is often the case in these six homes. A major policy determinant is the home's capacity to meet residents' needs. As Esther Adams said, "Once I have a resident in the home, I go out of my way to accommodate them to the very end, and that is the end that I can still provide the care that they need. When the point comes that I know that I can't provide or meet their needs, then of course I don't mind letting someone know to make further arrangements." The AL literature describes facilities as following "retention" versus "transfer" (Bernard, Zimmerman, & Eckert, 2001) or "extended care" versus "lite" (Carder, 2002) models, depending on the extent to which their policies support keeping residents as they age and their needs increase. Although evidence indicates that most facilities subscribe to a "lite" or "transfer" model (Hawes, Rose, & Phillips, 1999), one study of 366 ALFs finds that 65% allowed their residents to receive hospice services (National Center for Assisted Living, 2001). Of these six homes, only Rosie's might be described as following a "retention" model.

Similar to our findings in other research (Ball et al., 2004a) and as noted in chapter 5, admission and retention policies and decisions in these homes are influenced by both economic and personal factors. These factors guide both the policies and consistency of adherence. Personal factors such as relationships, personalities, and values exert more pressure in the small homes, particularly in the family model homes. Rosie keeps residents whose care needs exceed her economic and energy potential, and Esther Adams banishes residents who do not "cooperate" and refuses admission to smokers, nonchurchgoers, and people under the age of 60.

Service Capacity and Care Strategies

Admission and retention policies in ALFs typically reflect service availability, and limited service capacity is the cause of most resident departures (Ball et al., 2004a; Mollica & Jenkins, 2001; Phillips et al., 2003). Service capacity is determined largely by staffing. In the small homes, "staff" usually is one person, and the optimum strategy is to balance residents' care needs with care resources. In Greene's and Sunshine House, with lower staff-to-resident ratios, that usually means discharging any resident who requires more than minimal ADL care. Sometimes at Greene's, balance is not achieved, and residents' needs are not fully met. In the smaller, family model homes, owners try to balance residents requiring heavy care with those who are less taxing on their resources. When Estelle Washington had a stroke and went to a nursing home, Esther Adams said she would leave her bed empty rather than take in another resident with heavy care needs, even for "good money" ($1,500 a month). At that time, Bobby was recuperating from surgery, and all five remaining residents needed hands-on care—two more than she considers a manageable number. In each of these homes, at times, providers have to overextend themselves to meet care needs as residents decline. Although all small-home owners try to charge fees commensurate with residents' care needs and admit those who can pay higher fees, this tactic often is not feasible because of the limited resources of their typical clientele.

Staffing at Oak Manor follows the minimum staff-to-resident ratio required by state law—1:15 in the daytime and 1:25 at night. The "à la carte" pricing system is designed to balance resident care needs with staffing resources. Although residents who deny the need for increased services or cannot pay the commensurate charges ultimately are asked to leave, according to Kathy Wall, the executive director, "quite a few" are behind in payments for housing, care, and medications. Kathy indicated that, because the facility is "all African American," they "bend over backwards to be lenient with families who do not pay on time." She cautioned, though, that as the facility reaches capacity, management will probably be less tolerant. Fees at Oak Manor are lower than at comparable homes owned by the same corporation, where most residents are white, a policy Jordan Taylor attributes to the fact that assisted living is "new to the African American community."

Staff quality, as well as quantity, affects a facility's ability to manage resident decline. Assisted living staff in Georgia must receive basic training in first aid and cardiopulmonary resuscitation before beginning work and 16 hours of continuing education annually, but ample leeway is given, and enforcement is fairly lax. Hiring quality staff is a particular challenge for the small homes. The two homes where the owners provide the bulk of care themselves—Rosie's and Peach Blossom—have the most-qualified staff. Although Cora Greene, the owner of Greene's, is quite capable, she is often away from the premises, and other staff members, particularly on the weekends, have limited competence to handle medications, deal with health crises and problem behaviors, monitor health conditions, and even provide protective oversight. Obtaining the required continuing education is extremely difficult for most staff in small homes, and some employees begin work without even the basic training. Only Esther Adams has the money, necessary staff support, and interest to take advantage of a wide variety of community educational opportunities. She believes strongly in the value of training and over the study year attended 18 workshops or lectures provided by a variety of organizations. She also obtained instruction in blood sugar monitoring and other aspects of diabetes care from her personal physician to equip her to care for her diabetic residents.

Staff at Oak Manor, on the whole, are better qualified than those in the small homes. A registered nurse or licensed practical nurse is on duty during weekday shifts, and certain staff persons receive special training to handle medications, monitor blood sugars, and inject insulin, skills necessary to manage the large number of diabetic residents (14 during the study). The facility provides regular training on-site, either from facility or corporate personnel or from an expert from the wider community.

As our descriptions of residents who leave and those who stay show, dealing with health crises is a significant component of a facility's decline management role. Each home had at least one such event during the study, and typically they have more. Rosie summoned emergency personnel to her home four times. Although we have no record of the number of 911 calls made at Oak Manor, from individual data we know they are not uncommon. At least three calls were made on behalf of Alma Burgess, all related to chronic swelling of her legs owing to congestive heart failure. Prompt response to a critical event can make the difference between life and death, and the closer quarters of the small homes may be an advantage. Esther Adams's quick action did not prevent Ivera Haygood's death, but a similar response no doubt saved Estelle Washington when she had her stroke. Possibly, earlier detection would have saved an Oak Manor resident who was found dead behind the closed door of his private room.

Regulations require that providers call 911 in emergency situations before notifying family members, but family support often is an essential element in managing health crises. Providers depend on family members to provide follow-up in the hospital or emergency room and communicate essential information about future medications or care. When Rosie sent Joseph Render to County Hospital after an episode of nausea and difficulty standing, the hospital sent him back at nine o'clock that night, no better off than when he left. After complaining to a social worker about his early dismissal, Rosie returned him to the hospital, where he stayed for two days. Mr. Render, like Boss, has no family support, and because of a speech impediment caused by an earlier stroke, he was unable to communicate with emergency room physicians. Although Mr. Render returned to Rosie's with an order to follow up "with neurology," no appointment had been made, an omission remedied only after Rosie expended much time and frustration navigating the labyrinth of County Hospital's bureaucracy.

Management of residents' problem behaviors, which is an essential component of the provider care role, has significant impact on residents' ability to age in place in AL settings (Ball et al., 2004a; Hawes, Rose, & Phillips, 1999). Some providers in these homes are better able than others to tolerate annoying or dangerous behaviors and devise workable strategies. Much depends on their knowledge, time, energy, and personality. Rosie has learned to let Pearl Bowman (who has dementia and is leery of water) bathe in the shower, rather than sit in a tub, so that she can "step away from the water." Cora Greene promises Frankie Johnson her walk or ride and puts Slick in a private room and threatens to withhold his money. Esther Adams lobbies family members and physicians for psychoactive medications and keeps the front door locked at all times. Most residents at Oak Manor who wander or exhibit other signs of confusion are transferred to the special care dementia unit, which still has vacancies. Both administrative and direct care personnel for the most part demonstrate patience and skill in dealing with resistant or otherwise trying residents.

In previous chapters, we have discussed additional aspects of these facilities' capacities to manage decline. Providers' willingness and ability to promote residents' self-care and healthy behaviors have obvious influence, as does their role in residents' access to health care professionals. The capacity of a home's physical environment to support independence is also a key factor.

Community Supports

Chapter 8 describes the substantial contribution of senior centers and day programs to the lives of both residents and providers in the small homes. These programs not only improve residents' quality of life, they also expand providers' care capacity and help them tolerate challenging residents over time.

Community resources are known to buttress the health care functions of assisted living (Ball et al., 2004a). Although small-home providers experience certain frustrations with the Community Care Services Program, this program nonetheless offers support. At Blue Skies and Rosie's, a registered nurse makes bimonthly visits to review participants' medications, weigh them, and check their blood pressure. Such visits are especially helpful for residents with complicated health problems and multiple medications. When Sarah Eubanks returned to Rosie's after a hospital stay, the nurse communicated medication changes to the pharmacist and helped Rosie institute a new diabetes management regimen.

Home health care agencies, hospitals, and individual health care providers supply critical support for decline management in all homes. A home health nurse visited Blue Skies weekly for a month after Mamie Hoover fell, cutting a four-inch gash in her leg. The nurse cleaned and dressed Mamie's wound and taught Inez (the staff person) how to monitor her leg for infection. Veterans Administration nurses made daily visits to Greene's to treat Martin Self's periostitus (a skin inflammation characterized by open sores), and Boss's physical therapy treatments shored up Ms. Greene's rehabilitative efforts. For a period of time at Oak Manor, one home health agency provided daily management of the home's numerous diabetics. This service relieved facility staff members of this burden, and residents benefited from the close monitoring. Oak Manor's relationship with a university geriatric hospital furnishes additional resources for staff training, consultation for disease and behavior management, and referral of residents for therapy. Podiatrists visit four of the six homes to provide regular foot care. A physician friend of Ms. Greene's also brings medications and provides consultation. Despite numerous complaints about County Hospital, it is a stable resource for residents with limited or no health insurance coverage. In many cases, access to these community health resources depends on facility personnel playing an active role.

Managing Risk

Our model of aging in place (Ball et al., 2004a) specifies the relationship between managing decline and managing risk. That is, when choosing strategies to manage decline, residents and facilities assess the potential risk of a particular strategy and the degree of risk, if any, that is acceptable. Because risk appraisal guides strategy selection, resident and facility risk are both intervening conditions and consequences of the process of managing decline.

Weighing risk takes place on a regular basis in these six homes. Before discharging Dora McElhaney, Rosie compared the risk of Ms. McElhaney's daughter's threats to sue with the stress of her continued care. Frankie Johnson's daughter chose to risk her own well-being by bringing her mother home, rather than jeopardize her mother's safety by leaving her at Greene's. Alma Burgess weighs the risk of caring for herself at Oak Manor against the threat of running out of money. Louis Ashley, the owner of Sunshine House, assesses the relative merits of discharging residents requiring heavy care versus keeping beds occupied; and Cora Greene accepts some resident neglect rather than risk possible financial ruin. Risk management influences all aspects of the provider care role, and it affects residents' abilities to engage in self-care and maintain control over their lives.

Other assisted living studies have found risk management to play a key role in aging in place (Frank, 2002; Kane & Wilson, 2001). Two kinds of risk are possible—risks to residents' health and safety and risks to facility operation (Carder, 2002). Risks to residents result from their own behavior and from that of other residents. Providers risk liability with regard to residents' risky behaviors, and they risk financial loss associated with balancing occupancy and the desired level of resident impairment. In this study, both resident and facility risk influenced the strategies of residents and facilities to manage decline.

Resident-Facility Fit

Our model of aging in place (Ball et al., 2004a) depicts the "fit" between the capacity of residents and facilities to manage decline as central, and additional data presented here support this notion. We have described similar actions of resident, facility, and community factors on decline management and have shown how shifts in these factors affect resident and facility capacity and, in the end, their fit. Like risk, resident-facility fit is both a consequence of decline management and a factor influencing the process. Other research corroborates the importance of person-environment fit in ALF residents' ability to age in place (Bernard, Zimmerman, & Eckert, 2001; Heumann & Boldy, 1993; Lawton, 1980; Moos & Lemke, 1994). These studies, like ours, highlight the need to interpret environment broadly—in terms of both the physical and social aspects and resident, facility, and community factors.

Although a good fit is the ideal outcome, periods of "misfit" related to aging in place do occur, and this is another factor in risk management. The degree of misfit that is tolerated, by either resident or facility, depends largely on the degree of willingness to incur risk. We have seen that the "window" or margin for fit varies in these six homes. It is wider in homes with a greater capacity to manage decline, such as Oak Manor, with its expanded service capacity and supportive physical design, and Rosie's, where flexibility reigns. Conversely, the margin is much narrower at homes like Sunshine House and Greene's, which lack the resources to manage ADL decline.

Resident-facility fit has significant bearing on the meaning of aging in place for both residents and facilities. Clearly, maximizing residents' tenure is a worthy goal when fit is achieved, but the appeal of aging in place is less clear with misfit. Esther Adams understood this maxim when she sent Mayetta Stewart packing to Sunshine House, where she fit better. As the following chapter shows, assisted living residents can find meaning in their lives and even feel "at home." Fit is a principal factor in the success of these endeavors. When advocating for aging in place, we need, as Rowles (1993) argues, to be ever watchful of the role of place in aging.

Part IV / Conclusion

CHAPTER 11

Creating New Meaning in Assisted Living

"I made a calculated decision of what I wanted to do with the rest of my life—either hang on to old memories or be creative and productive and do something that I would enjoy that was different. That was come to Atlanta and be with young people who were still developing, like my great-grandkids and my grandchildren." Eugene Ellis's reflection expresses both his optimism about his move to assisted living and his openness to change—a key theme in residents' transition to assisted living. Achieving a meaningful existence in the assisted living environment involves an interplay between continuity and change. Maintaining a sense of continuity is central for residents, but being open to change has equal merit. Although individual residents experience the transition to assisted living in different ways, most accept and adjust to the change, and a few, like Mr. Ellis, have even welcomed and embraced it as a positive turning point in their lives.

The concepts of continuity and change are important themes in the study of the life course, particularly in studies of adaptation to change in old age (Arbor & Evandrou, 1997; Kaufman, 1986). Our findings provide insights into the differing social, economic, and cultural contexts surrounding elders' transitions into assisted living and contribute new understanding regarding the meaning of such transition in residents' lives.

Defining Meaning in Assisted Living

To understand how individuals interpret and give meaning to their life changes, some contemporary life course researchers draw inspiration from symbolic interactionism (Hatch, 2000; Holstein & Gubrium, 2000). Elder (1985) suggests that an individual's "definition of the situation" (Thomas & Thomas, 1928, 572) can provide important insight into the effect of life course transitions. This classic concept posits that what we define as real is real in its consequences. That is, if an individual assesses a situation negatively, the outcome is likely to be so. The definition of the situation can reflect objective facts or be highly subjective. As individuals participate in social life, they may amend their definition of the situation based on changing circumstances and cues from others.

To explore meaning for residents in assisted living, we asked them how they defined their transitions into this care environment. Eugene Ellis, who made his own decision to move to Oak Manor, viewed his transition as an opportunity to contribute to the lives of his younger family members. Fellow Oak Manor resident Ethyl Burns expressed the sentiments of most: "I don't think anybody would say they are happy to be here, but since I needed to be somewhere, I'm glad I'm here." This definition of the transition as necessary and accepted (but not necessarily welcome) is commonly held regardless of social class or cultural background. Although Greene's resident Beatrice Dove had less choice than Ms. Burns regarding care options, she defined her transition similarly: "It's all right. The social service folks had me to come here. I had to have a place to stay." Several factors highlighted throughout this book influenced residents' transition to assisted living, including achieving a good resident-facility fit, having support from families and the community, and maintaining control in decision making. Most residents learned to adjust over time, and regardless of the length of the adjustment period, an important factor in their ability to adapt was being open to change.

Some residents viewed their transition to AL as an improvement over past conditions. Cleo Kellog, who lives at Rosie's, credits "the Lord" with taking her away from another facility where the provider "picked on" her. To Joe Kelly, Greene's is a step up from his former unlicensed facility, which was closed by the state: "It needed a lot of repairs and the roof leaked and the policeman hangs around every day, two or three police cars. They were fighting and Ida [a female resident] was mean. She did a lot of heavy cursing, and she slammed a chair on my head." Although Joe objects to regularly relinquishing his bed to accommodate temporary residents, living at Greene's is "better than being out in the streets or in a homeless shelter." In some cases, residents' disadvantaged backgrounds have mitigated their difficulty adapting to problematic features of their new environment (for example, the lack of privacy and the high rate of theft at Greene's). The miniaturization of satisfaction (Rubinstein, Kilbride, & Nagy, 1992, 272) is applicable here. According to Boss Cook, who believes he can "live no better," Greene's "ain't what you call bad."

Some residents not disadvantaged by poverty, such as Hamilton Brewton, also viewed the AL transition as an improvement over past conditions. Because of severe depression, Mr. Brewton had left Detroit to live with his son in Atlanta. Although initially happy, he began to feel lonely and isolated while his son and daughter-in-law were at work and their two teenage children at school. Things got worse when his son hired a "babysitter," and Mr. Brewton, who never has been inclined toward religion, found himself subjected to her daily proselytizing: "Because they were all working, I was home by myself, and I had to have a babysitter. She read the Bible to me every day for about a month, and I told [my son] to get me out of there." Now at Oak Manor, Mr. Brewton feels less dependent on his family and more in control of his life. Other residents felt similarly freer living in AL than they would have in a family member's home. Many also found relief in not being a burden.

When examining the meaning of environmental transition, an important theme in recent research is the concept of place (Cutchin, Owen, & Chang, 2003; Rowles, 1993; Rowles & Ravdal, 2002). *Place* may refer to a variety of community settings, including neighborhoods, towns, cities, and houses. A central question is what makes a place home. *Home* is a complex construct that evokes emotional meaning. An individual's recollections of home are tied to personal events and experiences throughout the life course (Gurney & Means, 1997). For most people, the concept of home evokes positive meaning. It is an important symbol of the self, a personal place, the setting of intimate relationships and significant life events.

Rowles and Ravdal (2002) argue that the ability to maintain a sense of place is important for quality of life and may be related to well-being in old age. They define *sense of place* as a level of consciousness gained both through "place-making" (McHugh & Mings, 1996, 540) and maintaining continuity with the past places of our lives. Although these researchers acknowledge that the meaning of place may not be the same for everyone, they maintain that place can be an important source of meaning in old age and posit that elders who relocate can gain substantial benefit from maintaining connections with the past places in their lives.

Recently, researchers have begun to examine the meaning of place in assisted living (Ball et al., 2004a; Cutchin, Owen, & Chang, 2003; Frank, 2002). These studies have focused on whether AL residents are able to feel "at home"

(Cutchin, Owen, & Chang, 2003; Frank, 2002) and the importance for them of aging in place (Ball et al., 2004a; Frank, 2002). Although findings from these studies show that, given the choice, most residents want to remain in the AL setting until they die, the question of "at-homeness," or feeling at home, is less clear-cut. Cutchin, Owen, and Chang (2003) find that residents develop a meaningful attachment to the AL environment, suggesting some level of "at-homeness," but they acknowledge that the specific meaning of this attachment varies among residents. Frank's (2002) findings show that, despite residents' desire to stay in AL, many essential elements that they associate with "home" are missing.

Our research confirms other findings that, although many residents develop meaningful attachments to the AL environment, few define it as "home." Some may describe certain aspects as "like home" or say they feel "at home," but most do not equate living in AL with being in their own homes. The few residents who do consider these settings "home" in the intimate sense of the word live in the small family model homes, and most of them refer to those living there as "family."

Miss Fannie describes Greene's as a "care home," and her use of the word "building" is instructive: "This is a good home right here, especially for an old person like me. It's quiet, you don't have no fussing and fighting and cussing and stuff going on in the building, period." Even Boss Cook, who never settled in any place for long, defines a "home" as something intimate and distinctly different from his present circumstances at Greene's. Referring to Greene's, he said, "This place is like a home," but "home" evokes an earlier time when he was living with a favorite girlfriend and one of his many children: "If I was at home, my little girl would be making a lot of noise, running around the room, tearing up things, and my old lady, she would probably be in the kitchen cooking, getting ready to feed us a meal. That's one thing I miss." We found that, for the residents of these six care facilities, the concept of "community" is more meaningful than that of "home."

Attachment to Community

Historically, African Americans have relied on family and significant others in their communities for support and day-to-day survival. For the African American residents in our study, this tradition of mutual support and collective unity remains active after the transition to assisted living. Other disenfranchised groups, such as persons with mental illness, sometimes develop similar community ties. For most residents in this study, including those who have been homeless or have mental illness, community is an important source of identity and emotional support.

In chapter 3 we define the concept of "community" broadly to include families and significant others who make up residents' social worlds. Many residents include in this definition significant others in the AL environment. Although Hamilton Brewton calls his fellow residents "inmates," like many Oak Manor residents he values living in a "nice," all–African American care environment, and the common bonds of class, culture, and race he shares with residents afford him a sense of belonging he would not have living in a "mixed place." This sense of belonging has helped him overcome his depression and motivated him to involve himself in Oak Manor's social life. Residents at other facilities who, like Mr. Brewton, have achieved a good resident-facility fit have found a similar sense of community within the AL setting. For some residents, community connections that extend beyond the AL walls carry greater meaning than those found inside. Many residents from Atlanta highly value staying active in former churches, social clubs, and civic organizations. Edward Fitzsimmons stays connected to persons from his past by living at Greene's and attending mental health programs. Through common histories and experiences battling mental illness, he and other residents have developed a shared sense of community, both inside Greene's and in the wider community.

Maintaining Meaningful Social Relationships and Activities

Given the choice, most residents prefer spending time with family over anyone else. Quite a few, like Hamilton Brewton, have family members living nearby, or even in the facility, and others maintain meaningful connections with relatives despite geographic separation. In the absence of family, some residents have developed family-like relationships inside their AL homes. As illustrated throughout this book, such relationships are more common in the family model homes. At Peach Blossom, Esther Adams has become Bobby Bailey's family, and Rosie is Cleo Kellog's "Mama."

The development of meaningful social relationships inside ALFs is most common among residents who share similar histories. Numerous residents have been reunited with people they knew in the past and in some cases have found meaning in building on these former relationships. Since moving to Oak Manor, Alma Burgess has become friends with Gwen Runnels through connections in Ms. Runnels's hometown. Other relationships have been fostered by common community affiliations, geographic ties (for example, having grown up in the same neighborhood), and similar career and work backgrounds.

Meaningful relationships also are based on similar abilities and interests. An example is the relationship that has developed between some residents who have dementia. At Peach Blossom, Hassie Hicks and Irene Garrett spend hours together retelling each other the same stories about their past lives. Although annoying to some, this repetitious chatter is meaningful to these residents. Mose Rogers and Gary Cotter, the only male residents at Blue Skies, spend time together because, according to Mose, "Guys have to stick together." At Greene's, Boss Cook and Edgar Allgood have forged a close relationship based on shared interests and mutual need. Soon after moving to Greene's, Mr. Allgood began to rely on the more streetwise Boss to survive in that environment. Boss, in turn, craved conversation with someone knowledgeable about old movies and music, two of his favorite subjects. A number of residents have developed helping relationships, some of which are reciprocal, such as the women at Greene's who help one another bathe. In more unilateral relationships, residents find meaning in their altruism. Hamilton Brewton values "taking care of" Ophelia Cantrell, who in her confused state is drawn to him because he resembles her late husband: "I see that she gets food and goes to bed, that sort of thing. At 98, she's confused at times. For some reason or another, she trusts me, so I hang onto her."

Some residents find meaning in actively distancing themselves from fellow residents. An example is Mr. Brewton, who describes himself as far superior to other Oak Manor residents, though some are as well traveled as he: "I have had a whole lot of experiences and have been everywhere. Who am I going to talk to? [The other residents] have never been anywhere." This strategy, like that of "redefining independence" (discussed in chapter 6), is a form of impression management (Goffman, 1959) whereby residents maintain a more positive self-image by disassociating themselves from the negative status of living in an elder care facility. Although Eugene Ellis has developed close bonds with some residents at Oak Manor, he avoids ties with others: "Naturally, there are some people here that I can talk to without being personal. Some people are at the level that you have to be very careful, because, if you are not interested in developing personal relationships, it could be misunderstood." Loners Half-Pint and Beatrice Dove continue lifelong behavior patterns at Greene's by remaining aloof from other residents. As Ms. Dove said, "I don't have many friends, [but] I do very well."

In a few cases, residents have developed friendships with staff. Typically, these relationships occur in the smaller homes, where residents and staff tend to share similar backgrounds. An example is the friendship that blossomed between Greene's resident Edgar Allgood and staff person Laney, who both had lived in the Old Fourth Ward neighborhood and knew many of the same people.

As we note in chapter 8, a variety of bridges to the wider community furnish residents with a pool of potential new friends and help them stay connected to old ones. For residents in the small homes, day programs also provide meaningful activities. Ms. Dove, who rarely speaks or shows any form of emotion, often displays visible signs that these activities are meaningful for her.

Most residents attach greatest meaning to activities that are consistent with long-held values and interests. Religion has played a prominent role in most residents' lives. Some residents, especially those without family support, deem religion and participation in spiritual activities as "what matters most in life." For many, religion provides a source of strength as they age and confront life changes, including the transition to AL. Churches, families, and volunteers from the community enrich residents' lives by providing spiritual activities both inside and outside these homes. Some Oak Manor residents have remained actively engaged in various academic clubs, alumni groups, social clubs, and professional associations. Membership in these groups, which symbolizes success and professional standing in the African American community, continues to be a source of racial pride and identity, as well as a means of preserving lifelong friendships.

Although most residents have access to at least some meaningful activities, many struggle to find meaning in daily routines. Planned activities at Oak Manor are geared to the lowest common denominator in residents' physical and mental function, and so many residents' authentic interests or abilities are not met with appropriate activities. Ethyl Burns expressed the feeling of some: "Whoever is planning them just cannot conceive what it's like to be in a wheelchair, or a walker, or disabled. They think in order to make old people happy, what they need to do is have some kind of teenage activity." Although a loyal contingent of residents truly enjoy Bingo, others long for greater intellectual challenge. As we have illustrated throughout this book, residents in the smaller homes have no access to recreational activities in their facilities, even Bingo. Unlike residents at Oak Manor, many of the small-home residents also do not have adequate personal resources, such as a television or a radio in their rooms, to help fill this void. Residents in all homes achieve meaning through maintaining their health and independence.

Maintaining Meaningful Roles and Identity

Many age-related life changes, including a move to AL, involve role transitions (Holstein & Gubrium, 2000; Settersten, 1999). Some roles are valued more than others, and roles that carry the greatest personal meaning are those most integral to an individual's self-concept (Holstein & Gubrium, 2000; Zurcher, 1983). The move into assisted living constitutes what Rowles and Ravdal (2002, 98) refer to as a "dependency move." This type of move, usually perceived as "a final move," often is involuntary and traumatic and typically is precipitated by increased functional decline. As the final move, it prompts a reconceptualization of social identity as one transitions into the role of AL resident.

The ability to maintain meaningful roles has been a crucial factor in residents' capacity to adapt to the AL environment. Some residents find meaning in adopting new roles: Hamilton Brewton and Eugene Ellis have both assumed the role of "wise elder," mentoring their younger family members. For most residents, retaining former roles is key. By maintaining meaningful roles, either by creating new ones or holding on to those from the past, residents are able to preserve a viable sense of self. As noted, some residents also use the strategy of impression management to disengage from the role of AL resident in order to preserve their self-image.

A central value of most residents is maintaining some sense of independence. In addition to valuing self-reliance, most avoid burdening others. Such values increase the meanings residents attach to their self-care roles, as well as to their roles helping others. Many residents living in the smaller homes, who have experienced little leisure time during their lives, find special meaning in carrying out facility chores. Even those with significant cognitive impairment, such as Bobby Bailey at Peach Blossom and Frankie Johnson at Greene's, value such helping roles.

At Oak Manor, participation in the resident council gives residents an opportunity to meet as a group and voice their opinions and concerns regarding facility services. Their collective efforts, which are an important factor in community formation (Keith, 1977), reflect a long-standing tradition in the African American community of working together as a group to overcome problems and promote change. This forum also allows Mr. Brewton and Mr. Ellis, both of whom have served as resident council president, to maintain the leadership roles that have always been an important part of their identities.

Facility roles are shaped to some degree by participants' backgrounds and each facility's culture. At Greene's, Boss Cook's leadership role, though equally satisfying, stands in stark contrast to those of Mr. Brewton and Mr. Ellis, which match their former careers as professionals in the affluent African American community. In addition to showing new residents the ropes and supervising residents' behavior, Boss's position as the "houseman" gives him control over the television and other Greene's operations. Boss's personal operations include brokering staff services for residents with less power and making interest-bearing loans to those who need money to tide them over till their next check. This godfather-type role mirrors the leadership role Boss held "on the street."

Creating New Meaning in the Assisted Living Environment

Traditionally, culture has been defined as the shared values, beliefs, customs, and practices of a group, community, or society. Recently, researchers have begun to view culture as a dynamic process rather than a static condition (Lopez & Guarnaccia, 2000). This new definition of culture recognizes the active role individuals play in establishing their own cultural worlds. Culture thus emerges out of group norms, values, and experiences and is shaped by individuals' values, behaviors, and life histories.

The meanings providers attach to their roles and the strategies they use to negotiate risks form the bedrock of culture in each care home. Eugene Ellis defines Oak Manor as possessing "a common thread of culture." This cultural commonality reflects corporate investors' target group of middle- and upper-middle-class African Americans. Similarly, the culture of the smaller homes represents their low- to moderate-income populations. Providers' admission and discharge policies also affect clientele and culture. Other factors that shape the culture in these six care communities include the geographic location, the staff, and people in the wider community.

Rosie's and Peach Blossom symbolize "home" to the owners and to many of their residents, and their owners' lifelong commitment to caring and family has influenced the culture within. Although these homes are similar in many ways, their differences lie in each owner's unique personality and management style. Ms. Adams partiality to residents who "sit quietly watching TV" contributes to Peach Blossom's tranquil, if constrained, milieu. In contrast, the atmosphere at Rosie's is looser and livelier, sometimes downright loud.

At Blue Skies, Greene's, and Sunshine House, similar forces shape the social environment. Blue Skies manager Inez Sawyer is competent but controlling. This facility's diverse population, including Jamaican providers and residents of varying ages, races, and functional abilities, also shapes its culture. Confinement to the home encourages residents' dependence on one another for companionship and diversion in an otherwise humdrum world. At Greene's, as at Blue Skies, residents are a mix of old and young, black and white. Residents here, though, include a group who remain active in the culture of the neighboring streets, which sometimes spills over inside. Staff members and residents at Greene's are more like peers because of their similar societal positions. The culture at Sunshine House is influenced by the two factions that rarely interact: the mostly elderly female residents who live upstairs and watch TV in the living room during the day and the younger male residents who inhabit the downstairs and spend their daytime hours on nearby street corners. Neither Greene's nor Sunshine House is characterized by family-like relationships, yet Greene's possesses a sense of community.

Holding On to Meaning

Examples of life with little meaning can be found throughout this book, but in the end, we believe that most residents have adapted and achieved a measure of meaning as residents of these care communities. An important factor in residents' ability to adapt has been their willingness to accept change. As these individuals have done throughout their lives, many continue to build community within their AL environments, and the unique culture of each home reflects these community-building efforts. Although many residents do not define these communities of care as "home," most have developed a sense of belonging and a sense of place.

The transition into AL is an ongoing process marked by change. Over the course of this study, we witnessed many changes. We watched staff come and go and observed changes in the cultures in these homes and in the health of both residents and providers. Inez has left Blue Skies, and Angel has taken over, leading to a more relaxed environment. Staff changes and reduced care resources at Greene's have led to stricter discharge policies, which have resulted in residents turning to one another for help and becoming closer as a consequence of their reciprocity. Boss's diminished function has decreased his power as the houseman, and Rosie's declining health has weakened her resolve to keep residents "till they pass." Many changes saddened us, including the deaths of residents we had grown to love. Residents of these communities must continually adjust to change, often including change in their own functional abilities, but most draw on their communities of care in their ongoing struggle to confront life's challenges. Miss Fannie, who has lived in poverty all her life and recently experienced significant decline, expressed a view held by many: "I'll just live a happy life till I leave it. If the Lord come get me, he can carry me on home."

Strengthening Communities of Care

"I think [assisted living] is a good solution for African Americans." said Sharon Avant, the daughter of Blue Skies resident Lily Porter. "It helps relieve you of that burden of guilt because you're putting your loved one outside of your home. But it also allows you to have some comfort level 'cause you know they're being cared for, if it's the proper facility." Sharon expresses both her relief and her lingering doubts about moving her mother to assisted living. She appears to share the feeling of most African Americans: that it is a violation not to take care of your own parent. Yet she is reassured that the place she has chosen is "the proper facility." Her mother will be all right. Sharon herself will be all right. We have to believe that what we must do is the right thing to do. Usually, it is.

The concluding chapter of *Surviving Dependence*, our earlier book about what it is like to be a poor, black, disabled home care client of the Community Care Services Program, began with the sentence, "Sometimes nothing helps." We did not mean to say that all such clients are hopeless or that their caregivers should just give up. We only wished to issue our main caveat before drawing conclusions from our data: it is well to remember that old and sick people may not respond to efforts to help them, either because their problems are so overwhelming as to be beyond help, because helpers' approaches to care are flawed, or because clients simply reject help in order to maintain their treasured sense of control.

We also noted in that book that some of the low-income African Americans we had met during that study, despite their physical, mental, and social challenges, retained a keen value for independence and autonomy and effective skills for survival; they worked so successfully to adapt to their losses that we developed a deep admiration for them. Some, though not all, were so committed to the idea of self-care and making their own decisions that they managed to incorporate the physical and mental deficits age had brought, taking advantage of whatever care was available and holding fiercely to the ideal of being whole persons in charge of their own lives. In short, sometimes, when the desire and commitment to help dovetail with the client's wishes and supports the client's own efforts, success—as defined by the care recipients and by their family members—can be achieved.

In the present book we have explored similar themes in a different care setting. Some residents, often with the dedicated help of providers and family members, have been able to hold on to past patterns of life, while others have not. Social class (as it affects both past and current resources) plays a role in this process. We have tried also to confront the often contradictory implications of our findings for residents, for providers, and for family members. African American elders and their families are dealing with the increasingly public dilemma of a traditionally private responsibility—caring for themselves and their loved ones. In this final chapter we discuss the public policy implications of our findings and conclude with recommendations based on them.

Policy Implications

Regardless of neighborhood or class, the black community in Atlanta, like ethnic communities everywhere, prides itself on "taking care of its own." Some families go to great lengths to keep their elders at home. Others are less able or less determined to avoid institutional placement, indicating perhaps that for some African Americans resistance to care by strangers has begun to weaken as the pressures of two-career family life and dependence on two paychecks render at-home elder care more and more difficult for black families. Until recently, most African Americans seeking professional care short of skilled nursing homes have turned to small AL homes, many of which still are scattered through the African American community. These facilities have been the black community's primary source of "disability care" for many decades. In just the past five years, however, developers, some black, some white, have begun to venture into the middle- and upper-middle-class market for high-end assisted living targeted to African Americans. In 1999 two such facilities were opened near each other in one of the several commercial nodes serving a sprawling, largely black suburban Atlanta area. These competitors claim to have been—and possibly were—the first of their type in the country. Certainly, they represent the leading edge of the commodification of care in the black community, a trend that can only intensify.

In our earlier book (Ball & Whittington, 1995) we framed the crucial dilemma of African American elders in declining health as that of "surviving dependence." Here we have extended that argument from the home setting to what is typically the first formal level of care—the assisted living, or personal care, facility. Most of the African American–owned homes we studied are small, older, modest facilities with mostly low- to moderate-income African American residents. During the two studies we report on in this book, we could find only one African American facility in all of Atlanta that was large, new, and owned by a corporation, though, as noted, another was to open shortly. These two types of homes—small and modest, large and affluent—are quite different care environments with very different populations.

Our findings suggest that African American AL residents, families, and providers have many similarities to their white age-mates. In most ways the experience of aging, disability, and decline is the same regardless of race, and the cultural imperative of family responsibility and care is similar for all ethnic groups. Certainly, the effort and the pressures of running a small business, especially one that requires so much personal and interpersonal investment, are no greater for blacks than for whites.

Yet the experiences of African Americans in assisted living, both as residents and as providers, are distinctive in one way: their lives have been circumscribed by race. Although it was not our purpose to explore their views of the racial divide or how it may have affected their old age, we can hardly ignore the limited resources of many of these residents and their families, the continuing limitations of the communities in which they live, the type of care they can afford to purchase or provide, or the level of expectation they bring to their late lives. Among both residents and providers of the small homes, discontents are common, but overt complaints are rare. This a group that is not used to seeking or receiving special favors from the authorities. The more affluent residents of Oak Manor, of course, were more comfortable voicing their needs and dissatisfactions, even to those in charge. Because their history had been more privileged, they were able to pay for better environment and better service, and their expectations were decidedly higher.

Yet we now know (Gornick et al., 1996; U.S. Department of Health and Human Services, 2001) that, independent of socioeconomic status, the race of all these African American residents created in them a higher lifetime risk for chronic disease and disability, especially diabetes, heart disease, and hypertension. Whether the mechanism was intentional discrimination, cultural patterns, or both, the power of race to influence life chances is still apparent. We hardly need to extrapolate from this fact to social policy. It is sufficient to point out that racial disparities in health and health care persist and that, while the goal of reducing them is now policy, public action in that direction remains limited and inadequate.

In addition, the small homes in our Andrus study (Study I), and even the large facility in the National Institute on Aging study (Study II), have been established and run against a backdrop of racial discrimination and its resulting limits. Moreover, the professional history of each of these providers is relatively brief; none inherited from parents either the business or the stake to establish it. Theirs is a first-generation industry still in its infancy, and consequently these African American entrepreneurs (at least the small-home owners) appear to have few professional resources to draw on for advice or support. For the most part, they do not belong to or participate in the largely white—and expensive—trade associations, even to obtain the mandated training for themselves and their staffs. A relatively small association of black providers exists, but that, too, appears to have limited appeal. It is hard to find time for professional training, networking, or political action when the job at hand is all-consuming. The situation is much different for the corporate owner and the administrator of the large facility, but even they are new at the AL business and found it necessary to begin their enterprise with a managing partner, a white-owned firm with years of experience in the assisted living industry. The future will doubtless bring many more black entrepreneurs into the field, and a critical mass of expertise and a network of experienced professionals will develop. For now, however, the lack of such a network is a significant disadvantage, especially to the small providers.

In addition to the cumulative effects of racism across the life course, many of the small-home residents are also poor, or nearly so, and have been all their lives. Although we recognize the strengths and skills available in these residents, in their families, and in their AL communities, we also note the difficulties produced by limited income and financial assets. The physical environments are not as nice, privacy is in short supply, activities are severely limited, transportation is a struggle, medical care is less available, and neighborhoods are resource poor and sometimes dangerous. Perhaps the most significant impact of such shortages is the limitations they place on personal choice and control. The socially and emotionally rich environment evident in Oak Manor is possible because of the residents' greater financial resources. The universal truism applies: money confers choice.

Perhaps the most important policy implication of our findings flows from the stark differences between the small homes we studied and the one larger facility. Despite their common racial heritage, the two types of AL facilities appear to be headed in opposite directions. The large home represents the future of assisted living: modern, managerially complex, service rich, and profit oriented. The small homes are our past and a significant part of our present: they embody a simple, if powerful, idea—caring for the old and weak—but they are struggling to meet obligations and barely holding on to what they have, with their very survival in doubt.

Their dilemma is most apparent in their dealings with the public regulatory agency. In our studies we learned how the public's impulse to insure quality of care for elders and to prevent abuse, expressed through regulation, can contradict the real needs of lower-income assisted living residents and render the job of managing these homes with limited financial resources difficult at best. In fact, we believe an inherent contradiction exists between an economic system that has traditionally discriminated against and penalized African Americans, affording many of them in old age only poverty-level accommodations and care, and the dominant cultural system that mandates that such care be first class. While the intent of the regulations is certainly the safety and well-being of residents, their impact is often a heavy financial and time burden on the small-home entrepreneur. Several of these small-home owners complained about the regulatory burden, especially the difficulty of record keeping and adhering to such requirements as the posting of daily menus and preparation of a written disaster preparedness plan. While none disputed the necessity of regulations, all expressed a need for support in both interpretation and compliance. We suggest more attention be paid to the context of care and the economic realities of these facilities, and we argue for regulatory equity rather than equality between single-provider, shoestring operations and those run by modern corporations.

Small African American–owned AL homes are an important part of the long-term care system. By providing a significant portion of the care needed and preferred by black elders, they perform a crucial support function for both

African American families and their employers. They (and their white-owned counterparts) are the third, more affordable, alternative to nursing homes and expensive AL facilities. This combination of functional importance and the mounting strain noted earlier creates real dangers for these facilities and the individuals, families, and communities that depend on them. In Georgia, support for assisted living from the Medicaid waiver program is quite limited, and State Supplemental Payments (SSP) support is nonexistent. Yet assisted living facilities already divert some consumers from nursing homes, where they clearly do not want to go anyway but where the bill is likely to be picked up by Medicaid. Given Medicaid's continuing fiscal crisis in every state, and especially in Georgia, inattention to the needs of small, less expensive AL homes seems wrongheaded.

For the past 10 years, legislation has been introduced in Georgia's General Assembly to establish a second level of assisted living, between personal care and skilled care, that could provide limited health-related care; we are chagrined to note that each year that proposal has been rejected. Of course, a powerful and effective nursing home lobby is responsible. The industry fears competition for residents (probably with good reason) and for the Medicaid dollar. Although Medicaid funding for such mid-range care has not been part of the proposal, nursing home owners clearly think they see the camel's nose through the tent flap. It is their inalienable right to oppose policies that could harm their interests, just as it is the public's interest to secure a wider range of health care choices that could be obtained at a lower cost to both families and states. The care clock is ticking, however, and at the end of the day we may find that our long-term care choices have dwindled to two: publicly financed care in nursing homes, where we would rather not be, and privately financed care in large, congregate facilities that we cannot afford.

Recommendations

The findings of these studies form the basis for a number of practical and policy recommendations for improving the quality of care in African American–owned assisted living homes; strengthening those homes—in fact, all assisted living facilities—as an important element of the long-term care system; and, most important, improving the quality of life for the residents of assisted living homes. We direct these recommendations at five groups that make up these communities of care: residents, family members, providers, communities, and policy makers. We are acutely aware of the irony (and possibly the futility) of publishing these recommendations in a scholarly book unlikely to be read by many consumers of care or even many providers and policy makers. Our hope is that those of our ideas that resonate with other scholars or industry professionals may be disseminated further and eventually find their appropriate audience. In some sense, too, these are not so much recommendations to the actual participants in these communities as recommendations on their behalf.

For Residents

One of the core themes of this book has been the importance of independence (largely related to self-care) and autonomy (choice and control) to residents' quality of life. Despite residents' clarity about the importance they attach to these values, most residents move to assisted living because of self-care deficits; once there, they experience significant limitations in their choices and personal control. Obviously, some limitations of personal freedom are necessary, but we observed many occasions in these facilities when residents were unnecessarily deprived of choices in when, how, and by whom they would receive care, when and what they would eat, and how they would spend their time; some were not even accorded a say in whether they would move in or move out. Often these usurpations of rights were inadvertent, resulting from caring and concerned family members anxious to make a "good" and quick decision about care for their elder or simply underestimating the elder's wish and ability to be involved. Other times, they occurred because providers were "in charge": the facility did, after all, belong to them, and their decisions about how the home should be run, even how residents should live, became the rule. Sometimes elders appeared to acknowledge their lack of social power to influence their own situation and simply withdrew from the process, registering little or no objection to the decisions of others.

We recommend that all potential residents (that is, everyone) be educated and advised of their right to self-determination and encouraged to exercise it, from the decision to move to assisted living, through all the little choices of daily life, to the final important choice of whether to stay "in place" or transfer to another living arrangement. Of course, the resident's role partners must cooperate in this, but a collaborative process will not be possible unless the resident is prepared to express her or his wishes, expect they will be respected—and, wherever possible, met—and object clearly when they are not. African

American elders, in particular those who have little experience getting what they want out of life, may not be prepared to assert their wishes, even with other African Americans. Ways must be found to encourage them to do so, because our evidence shows it makes a huge difference in how happy they are with their care.

Independence and autonomy are the results of behavior that is part of a process of taking charge, what some of our colleagues call self-directed care. Residents must be permitted and encouraged to take charge of their own care, and many will have to be taught to understand how important it is, especially the initial decision of selecting the proper home to achieve a good resident-facility fit. Persons contemplating a move to AL should learn about assisted living in general; decide what aspects of AL are important to them; visit homes of different sizes and types; spend time in the homes being considered; find out about all aspects of the homes, including care, activities, meals, the physical environment, and especially facility philosophy about resident choice; express their views to family and friends; and in general seek an optimum person-environment fit. Residents should also be encouraged to ask for help when needed and allow others to support them. Who should be responsible for educating potential residents is not clear; we only believe their quality of life in assisted living would be vastly improved if they were much more involved in the choices that put them there and guide their everyday lives.

For Families

Families are a key element of the community of care. When the elder has dementia or is very physically debilitated, the family often must exert tremendous energy to see that providers do their jobs and to fill in the inevitable gaps in care, and often they must assume responsibility for all decisions. Our particular concern is when families mistakenly assume that the elder is too impaired to participate or is irrelevant to the process. The decision to move is perhaps the most crucial. Whatever the elder's mental or physical state, families should solicit her or his opinion about both whether and where to move. The family may have concluded that moving is imperative, but forcing the move without adequate consultation and preparation can create alienation not only between the elder and family members but also between the elder and her or his new home.

Whether the elder can be involved or not, families should be advised and helped to follow the same careful procedures for choosing an assisted living facility recommended for residents. Once the elder has become a resident, families should be understanding of the provider's role and responsibilities; they should share with the provider pertinent information about the resident's preferences and needs and work to form a partnership with the provider. Communication between family and provider is important, as are family expressions of appreciation to providers for their efforts. Actual help with the work of care, especially transportation, goes a long way to keep providers going. Families should also support the resident's self-care, both verbally and by providing the resources necessary for it, such as assistive devices, portable toilets, and the like. They should help to educate the resident about self-care as well as offer motivation. They should restrain their own instincts to "do for" the resident and try to assist only when needed, accepting the residents' possibly imperfect ways of doing for themselves.

For Providers

Our recommendations for providers are offered respectfully, because we recognize the magnitude and complexity of their job, and we do not lightly assume these suggestions could easily be incorporated. Nevertheless, we believe that many of them, if adopted, could actually reduce providers' workload or produce better outcomes for residents and families and thus create greater job satisfaction for the providers themselves.

First, we recommend that providers direct their marketing efforts primarily to potential residents rather than to families. This might increase residents' involvement in the decision making right from the start. We suggest they provide as much information about their home as possible to aid the assessment of resident-facility fit, that they encourage prospects to visit several other facilities, and that they encourage potential residents and families to spend time in their home. We suggest providers also try to learn as much as possible about potential residents to facilitate a good resident-facility fit and encourage families to involve the resident as much as possible in each phase of the moving process. Once the move is complete, providers should continue to learn about the resident in order to provide choices that are meaningful.

Based on our findings regarding Oak Manor residents, African American (and other) providers would be well advised to capitalize on the stated preferences of African American clients for a distinctively African American cultural milieu. At least those middle-class residents of Oak Manor were appreciative of what Eugene Ellis called "the common thread of culture," the shared experience and outlook he found with his fellow residents. Other than having a racially and economically similar clientele and decorating with African-theme motifs, it is not clear, however, what any particular owner could do to promote the African American lifestyle. Clearly, social class differences among the six homes produced markedly different cultural environments, despite the "common thread" of African Americanism.

We urge providers to do everything in their power to support residents' self-care. To do this, we suggest they assess residents' self-care abilities, using both a formal tool that can capture partial abilities and informal means, including interviews with residents and their families and direct observation. We suggest providers consider adopting a negotiated service agreement with residents and families, or at least an informal equivalent. Providers should teach residents the knowledge and skills required for self-care and provide resources to accomplish it, as well as to encourage and motivate. Providers should help only when needed and should assist, rather than do, when possible. We understand that it is usually easier for providers to perform tasks themselves than to wait for the resident to do them, but the rewards in resident confidence and improved abilities should compensate for those costs. We also encourage providers to allow residents to support one another when possible and to provide opportunities for physical activity and a supportive physical environment. Finally, it is crucial to train staff in the importance of self-care and how to support it.

Providers should understand the concept of kin-work and its value in supplementing and supporting their own caregiving efforts. Better outcomes can be achieved when providers and families work together. Providers should take care to specify their expectations of family responsibilities, both informally and with documents. Providers should learn about family members and their circumstances in order to understand the resident better. Family members should be included in the home's social activities; they should receive regular communication about life in the home through newsletters and calendars of activities; and they should be kept informed about the resident and her or his needs. Finally, providers must view their task as more than bed and body work. Their prime goal should be to assist residents in preserving their former identities and in finding new patterns, new friends, and new meaning in their new living arrangement. One key to achieving this goal should be the bridges to the larger community formed by the various day programs and community churches. Providers should seek to take full advantage of these programs for the sociability, mental stimulation, and physical activity they provide.

For Communities

The communities surrounding assisted living facilities are sometimes either ignorant of their existence or overtly hostile to their presence. These are destructive stances that can only weaken community structures and neighborhood bonds. Strong communities recognize the common stake of all their residents and accommodate diversity. Assisted living homes in the midst of residential neighborhoods, as all the small homes in this study are, can enrich, rather than deplete, their surroundings. We suggest that, rather than viewing Cora Greene's facility as a problem and an eyesore, the Ashby Grove neighborhood gentry seek to support it and incorporate it into the life of the community. Class differences certainly militate against that outcome, but we believe constructive engagement to be the preferable strategy to that of hostile takeover. A positive response by the community might actually enliven and solidify the neighborhood. Volunteers from community groups in Ashby Grove now help low-income elders maintain their properties, and such services would have similar value if extended to owners of low-income ALFs.

Larger, more affluent homes, like Oak Manor, attract a variety of community groups, such as schools, Girl Scouts, and college fraternities and sororities; such groups should be encouraged to reach out to the smaller homes, as well. Because of the marginal status of these homes, community groups also should be educated concerning their importance, as well as their crucial need for assistance. Evidence shows that community outreach can successfully increase support of this kind (Stone, 2000).

Local health care professionals and students enrolled in health care training programs also should be encouraged to volunteer their services in low-income AL settings. The mental health day program serving Greene's had help from nursing students and local eye care professionals, who provided weekly blood pressure checks, foot care, and eye exams. Oak Manor received services from a university geriatric hospital, and another upscale ALF participant in Study II used doctors enrolled in a residency training program at County Hospital to provide on-site care. Clearly, such programs would benefit residents of small low-income ALFs, as would similar services from dental schools.

Because some of the programs used by small ALFs, such as those providing low-cost dentures and assistive devices, are not well advertised, a directory of available services would be quite useful to small-home providers. This information could be distributed through local ombudsman programs and state regulatory agencies (for example, at mandatory training sessions). These agencies also should consider developing more supportive relationships with AL providers. Although some providers have had positive experiences with representatives of these programs, others, like Cora Greene, feel threatened. Ms. Greene no longer attends training sessions provided by the state regulatory agency specifically for small homes because she believes regulators show greater respect toward large-home providers. Her experience is consistent with findings from other studies of small ALFs (Morgan, Eckert, & Lyon, 1995; Perkins et al., 1998).

We are heartened at the variety of community programs available to the residents of these six homes and by providers' efforts to use them to the residents' benefit. However, we also learned of resistance by some county agency personnel to allowing assisted living residents to attend their senior centers. These seniors are in most ways just like their peers who arrive on the county van; they simply come from a congregate rather than a single-family residence, and some of them are driven by their paid caregivers. They certainly derive similar benefits from the senior center, as do the owners and staff of their homes, who receive much-needed respite and time for other duties. We strongly recommend that agencies not discriminate against residents of congregate care facilities in the provision of services.

For Policy Makers

The goal of all our recommendations for a new public policy toward assisted living homes in the African American community is the preservation and strengthening of small homes. We are supportive of the larger facilities, too, but we believe they already have the advantages of size, visibility, and adequate resources to survive and thrive. Their middle-class market is growing and will become more aware of their existence and more accepting of their service. Small homes, however, appear to be struggling to provide quality care to their market among the poor and working class; some small homes are closing, and others are in jeopardy. Several steps could be taken to reverse this trend.

First, small homes should be governed and evaluated by a different set of regulations than large, modern, purpose-built facilities. With each new standard of comfort or safety, small-home providers must spend more to retrofit their generally older structures, money they might be spending to provide activities for residents or raising salaries for their minimum-wage workers or even considering the addition of limited employment benefits for them. Dollars spent on fire doors and sprinkler systems in a three-bedroom house might better be spent improving the quality of care.

With each new record-keeping requirement, owners have struggled to find time to do the paperwork, generally stealing either from their direct care responsibilities or their own downtime, which they usually need desperately. Many providers describe their work as physically and emotionally demanding, even draining, while providing very little income and low return on investment. These are not conditions conducive to long-term commitment by owners or retention of employees. Advocates for the elderly are well intentioned when they push for better physical environments, stricter enforcement, and more accountability, but older persons of limited means are far better served by calibrating the standards to fit the available resources than by hiking expectations beyond the ability of that market to reach them.

Georgia is one of only six states (along with Arkansas, Kansas, Mississippi, Tennessee, and West Virginia) that do not provide a state supplemental payment to recipients of Supplemental Security Income who live in assisted living. Some states (for example, Hawaii) provide several hundred dollars a month, which then allows providers to charge higher rates, permitting improvements in the quantity and quality of care that can be provided. Although the SSP amount in some states is so small it has little practical effect on care, the idea is sound. The political concern must be that providers might simply raise their rates to capture the SSP payment amount and pocket the money, passing along little or nothing in the way of better care to residents. Our knowledge of small-home providers leads us to believe that a reasonable amount of SSP funds would find its way into improvements of care, and thus SSP payments would be an excellent investment of public funds for this population.

In this time of scarce resources at all levels of society, local communities and states must search for new and creative ways to support ALFs, particularly those serving low-income residents. Pennsylvania and New Jersey have used lottery revenues to expand community-based programs, and in Hamilton County, Ohio, the local Area Agency on Aging successfully advocated for a levy to fund these services (Stone, 2000). Other ways of providing financial relief for low-income providers might involve indirect methods. Low-income AL providers who are home owners could be considered for homestead exemptions, similar to those available to older residents in many states. Since this study ended, property taxes for Greene's have doubled, and earlier research has shown the financial damage to ALFs caused by neighborhood gentrification (Eckert & Morgan, 2001; Morgan, Eckert, & Lyon, 1995).

In Georgia only about 15% of Community Care Services Program funds is used to pay for assisted living services (Community Care Services Program, 2003). While no one can say what might be a proper mix of home care services provided to recipients living on their own and what Georgia calls alternative living services, we do believe that the amount allowed for each resident-day of assisted living care is low and should be increased.

Transportation was a huge problem for the small homes. Liability insurance was so costly that none of these providers could afford it. Therefore, some did not provide transportation for their residents at all, though some did, using their personal vehicles while "praying all the way, don't nothing happen." We would support a proposal to redefine "necessary" transportation for health reasons more broadly than only a trip to the doctor, so that transporting impaired, Medicaid clients living in assisted living for any therapeutic purpose would be covered. As Medicaid already pays for some nonmedical care, such as homemaker services, because it is necessary to keep the recipient living independently at home, it should be possible to treat transportation services for ALFs in the same way.

The final public policy concern we mention is one we have argued before (Ball & Whittington, 1995): the exploitation of low-skill, largely minority and female workers by the long-term care system. Those who work in AL share much the same difficult conditions and low wage compensation as those caregivers who work in nursing homes and home care services. This is especially true of the staff workers but also is true to some extent of the owners. Of course, the argument is made that such labor does not require much skill or training, and many otherwise unemployable people are available to take these jobs, so the pay is naturally low. We acknowledge these realities but make two rebuttal points. First, the approach is incredibly shortsighted. As we noted of home care work 10 years ago, "We should remember the ironic similarities between the home care workers we observed and their clients. By continuing to employ mainly semi-skilled workers, paying them little and providing few health or pension benefits, and by affording them little meaning and satisfaction in their work, we are quite literally creating the poor, disabled, older home care clients of the future. Our welfare system is feeding on itself. It is insuring that this chain-letter of dependency will be forwarded to the next generation" (Ball & Whittington, 1995, 244). Our business people understand intuitively the concept and benefits of investment; our policy makers, reflecting society's biases against the poor and uneducated and the taxpayers' current unwillingness to pay more taxes, apparently do not.

Our second point is that assisted living workers should be much better trained to provide a kind of care that is now uncommon—one beyond the physical care typical of most homes, focused on preserving the personality, the identity, and the will of the resident. Not strictly mental health care, it would nevertheless focus much more attention on the socioemotional state of residents and concern itself with the person's definition of quality of life. While some of the small-home owners saw this approach as part of their task, they were not always fully equipped to accomplish it. Some workers in the larger homes also shared this perspective but often did not have the time to enact it. Some had not yet adopted this expanded concept of the work.

A quality-of-life model of care is possible because it would not replace physical care but rather would be integrated with it and require little extra staff time or effort. It would require only training, commitment, support, and reinforcement—in other words, public investment. We should invest in a new approach to training long-term direct care workers, one that will redefine their work as professional and important and allow for a realignment of values. Physical care, comfort, and safety should be considered basic, a given, similar to lunch breaks, air conditioning, and security in our schools. Just as the main work of teaching is intellectual and developmental, a primary job of long-term care should be socioemotional. Socioemotional care would require advanced—but not extensive or expensive—training in how to care for an older person's identity, or soul. Most of us believe that quality of life is more important to us than quantity; we affirm that principle every time we sign an advance directive. We have hypothesized and are in the process of testing an idea that care workers value the same things as care recipients—independence and autonomy, self-care and control. What if we created care environments that permitted those values to be expressed and possessed by all participants, care giver and receiver alike? Would residents' morale improve if they were allowed to make choices about how they live? Would caregivers be more satisfied with their jobs if they were allowed more discretion and were reinforced in their beliefs in the importance of their work? Clearly, some of the small-home owners we studied already do. Would residents value the care more highly if they perceived it as coming from a committed professional? Would workers enjoy the work more if they could see that the result was deeply pleasing and beneficial to the persons being cared for? Is it possible to reconceptualize our care system to take souls into account?

References

Administration on Aging. 2002. *A profile of older Americans, 2002*. Washington, D.C.: Department of Health and Human Services.

Agich, G. 1993. *Autonomy and long-term care*. New York: Oxford University Press.

American Seniors Housing Association. 1999. *The state of seniors' housing*. Washington, D.C.: Coopers & Lybrand Associates.

Arbor, S., & M. Evandrou. 1997. Mapping the territory: Ageing, independence and the life course. In *Ageing, independence, and the life course*, ed. S. Arbor & M. Evandrou, 9–26. London: Jessica Kingsley Publishers.

Baldwin, N., J. Harris, R. Littlechild, & M. Pearson. 1993. *Residents' rights: A strategy in action for older people*. Aldershot, U.K.: Avebury.

Ball, M., M. Perkins, F. Whittington, B. Connell, C. Hollingsworth, S. King, et al. 2004a. Managing decline in assisted living: The key to aging in place. *Journal of Gerontology: Social Sciences* 59B:S202–12.

Ball, M., M. Perkins, F. Whittington, C. Hollingsworth, S. King, & B. Combs. 2004b. Independence in assisted living. *Journal of Aging Studies* 18:467–83.

Ball, M., & F. Whittington. 1995. *Surviving dependence: Voices of African American elders*. Amityville, N.Y.: Baywood Publishers.

Ball, M., F. Whittington, M. Perkins, V. Patterson, C. Hollingsworth, S. King, et al. 2000. Quality of life in assisted living facilities: Viewpoints of residents. *Journal of Applied Gerontology* 19:304–25.

Baltes, M. 1994. Aging well and institutional living: A paradox? In *Aging and quality of life: Charting new territories in behavioral science research*, ed. R. Abeles, H. Gift, & M. Ory, 185–201. New York: Springer Publishing.

Baltes, P., & M. Baltes. 1990. Psychological perspectives on successful aging: The model of selective optimization with compensation. In *Successful aging: Perspectives from the behavioral sciences*, ed. P. Baltes & M. Baltes, 1–34. Cambridge: Cambridge University Press.

Barken, B. 1995. The regenerative community: The Live Oak Living Center and the quest for autonomy, self-esteem, and connection in elder care. In *Enhancing autonomy in long-term care: Concepts and strategies*, ed. L. Gamroth, J. Semradek, & E. Tornquist, 169–92. New York: Springer Publishing.

Barnes, A. 1985. *The black middle class family: A study of black subsociety, neighborhood, and home in interaction*. Bristol, Ind.: Wyndam Hall Press.

Basu, D., & P. Werbner. 2001. Bootstrap capitalism and the culture industries: A critique of invidious comparisons in the study of ethnic entrepreneurship. *Ethnic and Racial Studies* 24:236–62.

Beck, C., & T. Vogelpohl. 1995. Cognitive impairment and autonomy. In *Enhancing autonomy in long-term care: Concepts and strategies*, ed. L. Gamroth, J. Semradek, & E. Tornquist, 44–57. New York: Springer Publishing.

Belgrave, L., & J. Bradsher. 1994. Health as a factor in institutionalization: Disparities between African Americans and whites. *Research on Aging* 16:115–41.

Belgrave, L., M. Wykle, & J. Choi. 1993. Health, double jeopardy, and culture: The use of institutionalization by African Americans. *Gerontologist* 33:379–85.

Bernard, S., S. Zimmerman, & K. Eckert. 2001. Aging in place. In *Assisted living: Needs, practices, and policies in residential care for the elderly,* ed. S. Zimmerman, P. Sloane, & K. Eckert, 224–41. Baltimore: Johns Hopkins University Press.

Binstock, R. 1999. Public policies and minority elders. In *Serving minority elders in the twenty-first century,* ed. M. Wykle & A. Ford, 5–24. New York: Springer Publishing.

Bitzan, J., & J. Kruzich. 1990. Interpersonal relationships of nursing home residents. *Gerontologist* 30:385–90.

Brody, E. 1981. "Women in the middle" and family help to older people. *Gerontologist* 21:471–80.

Brooks, S. 1996. Separate and unequal. *Contemporary Long-Term Care* 9:40–46.

Burton, L., B. Zdaniuk, R. Schulz, S. Jackson, & C. Hirsch. 2003. Transitions in spousal caregiving. *Gerontologist* 43:230–41.

Cagney, K., & E. Agree. 1999. Racial differences in skilled nursing care and home health use: The mediating effects of family structure and social class. *Journal of Gerontology: Social Sciences* 54B:S223–36.

Cantor, M. 1983. Strain among caregivers: A study of experiences in the United States. *Gerontologist* 23:597–604.

Capitman, J., & M. Sciegaj. 1995. A contextual approach for understanding individual autonomy in managed community long-term care. *Gerontologist* 35:533–40.

Carder, P. 2002. The social world of assisted living. *Journal of Aging Studies* 16:1–18.

Carder, P., J. Eckert, T. Piggee, A. Wright, K. de Medeiros, & S. Zimmerman. 2003. The real meaning of assessment in assisted living. Paper presented at the annual meeting of the Gerontological Society of America, San Diego, Calif., November 21–25, 2003.

Carder, P., & M. Hernandez. 2004. Consumer discourse in assisted living. *Journal of Gerontology: Social Sciences* 59B:S58–67.

Chapin, R., & D. Dobbs-Kepper. 2001. Aging in place in assisted living: Philosophy vs. policy. *Gerontologist* 41:43–50.

Chappell, N., & R. Reid. 2002. Burden and well-being among caregivers: Examining the distinction. *Gerontologist* 42:772–80.

Citro, J., & S. Hermanson. 1999. *Assisted living in the United States.* Washington, D.C.: American Association of Retired Persons, Public Policy Institute.

Clark, P. 1987. Individual autonomy, cooperative empowerment, and planning for long-term care decision making. *Journal of Aging Studies* 1:65–76.

———. 1988. Autonomy, personal empowerment, and quality of life in long-term care. *Journal of Applied Gerontology* 7:279–97.

Clarke, A. 1996. *Lest we forget: Atlanta's disappearing black neighborhoods.* Atlanta: Fulton County Commission.

Clausen, J. 1986. *The life course: A sociological perspective.* Englewood Cliffs, N.J.: Prentice-Hall.

Cohen, R. 2000. *The black colleges of Atlanta.* Charleston, S.C.: Arcadia Publishing.

Collopy, B. 1988. Autonomy in long-term care: Some crucial distinctions. *Gerontologist* 28:10–17.

———. 1990. Ethical dimensions of autonomy in long-term care. *Generations* 14 (Suppl.): 9–12.

————. 1995. Power, paternalism, and the ambiguities of autonomy. In *Enhancing autonomy in long-term care: Concepts and strategies,* ed. L. Gamroth, J. Semradek, & E. Tornquist, 3–14. New York: Springer Publishing.

Combs, B. L. 2002. The role of community day programs in the lives of low-income residents of assisted living facilities. Ph.D. diss., Georgia State University. *Dissertation Abstracts International* 63/06:2369.

Community Care Services Program. 2003. *Annual progress report.* Atlanta: Department of Human Resources, Division of Aging Services.

Cox, C., & A. Monk. 1996. Strain among caregivers: Comparing the experiences of African American and Hispanic caregivers of Alzheimer's relatives. *International Journal of Aging and Human Development* 43:93–105.

Cutchin, M., S. Owen, & P. Chang. 2003. Becoming "at home" in assisted living residences: Exploring place integration processes. *Journal of Gerontology: Social Sciences* 58B:S234–43.

Davidson, H., & B. O'Connor. 1990. Perceived control and acceptance of the decision to enter a nursing home as predictors of adjustment. *International Journal of Aging and Human Development* 31:307–18.

Dilworth-Anderson, P. 1992. Extended kin networks in black families. *Generations* 17:29–32.

Dilworth-Anderson, P., S. Williams, & T. Cooper. 1999. The contexts of experiencing emotional distress among family caregivers to elderly African Americans. *Family Relations* 48:391–97.

Doka, K. 2003. The spiritual gifts—and burdens—of family caregiving. *Generations* 27:45–48.

Dorsey, A. 2004. *To build our lives together.* Athens: University of Georgia Press.

Dowd, J. 1975. Aging as exchange: A preface to theory. *Journal of Gerontology* 30:584–94.

Eckert, K., D. Cox, & L. Morgan. 1999. The meaning of family-like care among operators of small board and care homes. *Journal of Aging Studies* 13:333–47.

Eckert, K., & L. Morgan. 2001. Quality in small residential care settings. In *Linking quality of long-term care and quality of life,* ed. L. Noekler & Z. Harel, 95–115. New York: Springer Publishing.

Eckert, K., S. Zimmerman, & L. Morgan. 2001. Connectedness in residential care: A qualitative perspective. In *Assisted living: Needs, practices, and policies in residential care for the elderly,* ed. S. Zimmerman, P. Sloane, & K. Eckert, 224–41. Baltimore: Johns Hopkins University Press.

Edin, K., & L. Lein. 1997. *Making ends meet: How single mothers survive welfare and low-wage work.* New York: Russell Sage Foundation.

Elder, G., Jr. 1985. Perspectives on the life course. In *Life course dynamics: Trajectories and transitions, 1968–1980,* ed. G. Elder Jr., 23–49. Ithaca, N.Y.: Cornell University Press.

Estes, C. L., J. Swan, & associates. 1993. *The long-term care crisis: Elders trapped in the no-care zone.* Newbury Park, Calif.: Sage Publications.

Evans, W. 1995. Effects of exercise on body composition and functional capacity of the elderly. In Workshop on sarcopenia: Muscle atrophy in old age, ed. J. Holloszy. Special issue, *Journal of Gerontology: Biological Sciences and Medical Sciences* 50A: 147–50.

Federal Interagency Forum on Aging-Related Statistics. 2000. *Older Americans 2000: Key indicators of well-being.* Washington, D.C.: Government Printing Office.

Fine, M., & L. Weis. 1998. *The unknown city: Lives of poor and working-class young adults.* Boston: Beacon Press.

Fonda, S., E. Clipp, & G. Maddox. 2002. Patterns in functioning among residents of an affordable assisted living housing facility. *Gerontologist* 42:178–87.

Forbes, S., & N. Hoffart. 1998. Elders' decision making regarding the use of long-term care services: A precarious balance. *Qualitative Health Research* 8:736–50.

Frank, J. 2002. *The paradox of aging in place in assisted living.* Westport, Conn.: Bergin & Garvey.

Gaugler, J., R. L. Kane, R. A. Kane, T. Clay, & R. Newcomer. 2003. Caregiving and institutionalization of cognitively impaired older people: Utilizing dynamic predictors of change. *Gerontologist* 43:219–29.

Gaugler, J., S. Leitsch, S. Zarit, & L. Pearlin. 2000. Caregiver involvement following institutionalization: Effects of replacement stress. *Research on Aging* 22:337–59.

Geertz, C. 1983. Thick description: Toward an interpretive theory of culture. In *Contemporary field research: A collection of readings,* ed. R. Emerson, 37–59. Prospect Heights, Ill.: Waveland Press.

Gibson, R., & J. Jackson. 1987. The health, physical functioning, and informal supports of the black elderly. *Milbank Quarterly* 65:421–54.

Gignac, M., C. Cott, & E. Bradley. 2000. Adaptation to chronic illness and disability and its relationship to perceptions of independence and dependence. *Journal of Gerontology: Psychological Sciences* 55B:362–72.

Goffman, E. 1959. *The presentation of self in everyday life.* New York: Anchor Books.

Gornick, M., P. Eggers, T. Reilly, R. Mentnech, L. Fitterman, L. Kucken, et al. 1996. Effects of race and income on mortality and use of services among Medicare beneficiaries. *New England Journal of Medicine* 11:791–99.

Grafstrom, M., & B. Winbald. 1995. Family burden in the care of demented and non-demented elderly: A longitudinal study. *Alzheimer's Disease and Associated Disorders* 9:78–86.

Groger, L. 1994. Limit of support and reaction to illness: An exploration of black elders' pathways to long-term care settings. *Journal of Cross-Cultural Gerontology* 9: 369–87.

———. 1995. Health trajectories and long-term care choices: What stories told by informants can tell us. In *The culture of long term care: Nursing home ethnography,* ed. N. Henderson & M. Vesperi, 55–70. Westport, Conn.: Bergin & Garvey.

Grossman, H., & A. Weiner. 1988. Quality of life: The institutional culture defined by administrative and resident values. *Journal of Applied Gerontology* 7:389–405.

Gurney, C., & R. Means. 1997. The meaning of home in later life. In *Ageing, independence, and the life course,* ed. S. Arbor & M. Evandrou, 119–31. London: Jessica Kingsley Publishers.

Hall, C. 1993. Long term care and the minority elderly. *Pride Institute Journal of Long Term Home Health Care* 12:3–8.

Harel, Z., & L. Noelker. 1995. Severe vulnerability and long-term care. In *Matching people with services in long-term care,* ed. Z. Harel & R. Dunkle, 5–24. New York: Springer Publishing.

Harmon, D. 1996. *Beneath the image of the civil rights movement and race relations: Atlanta, Georgia, 1946–1981.* New York: Garland Publishing.

Hasenfeld, Y. 1983. *Human service organizations*. Englewood Cliffs, N.J.: Prentice-Hall.

Hatch, L. 1991. Informal support patterns of older African-American and white women. *Research on Aging* 13:144–70.

———. 2000. *Beyond gender: Adaptation to aging in life course perspective*. Amityville, N.Y.: Baywood Publishers.

Hatchett, S., & J. Jackson. 1993. African American extended kin systems: An assessment. In *Family ethnicity: Strength in diversity*, ed. H. McAdoo, 90–108. Newbury Park, Calif.: Sage Publications.

Hawes, C., V. Mor, J. Wildfire, V. Iannacchione, L. Lux, R. Green, et al. 1995. *Analysis of the effect of regulation on the quality of care in board and care homes: Executive summary*. Research Triangle Park, N.C.: Research Triangle Institute and Brown University.

Hawes, C., & C. Phillips. 2000. *High service or high privacy assisted living facilities, their residents and staff: Results from a national survey*. Beachwood, Ohio: Myers Research Institute.

Hawes, C., C. Phillips, M. Rose, S. Holan, & M. Sherman. 2003. A national survey of assisted living facilities. *Gerontologist* 43:875–82.

Hawes, C., M. Rose, & C. Phillips. 1999. *A national study of assisted living for the frail elderly. Executive summary: Results of a national survey of facilities*. Beachwood, Ohio: Myers Research Institute.

Headon, A. 1992. Time costs and informal social support as determinants of differences between black and white families in the provision of long-term care. *Inquiry* 29: 440–50.

———. 1993. Economic disability and health determinants of the hazard of nursing home entry. *Journal of Human Resources* 28:297–317.

Hennessy, C. 1987. Risks and resources: Service allocation decisions in a consolidated model of long-term care. *Journal of Applied Gerontology* 6:139–55.

———. 1989. Autonomy and risk: The role of client wishes in community-based long-term care. *Gerontologist* 29:633–39.

Herd, P. 2001. Vertical axes on the long-term care continuum: A comparison of board and care and assisted living. *Journal of Aging and Social Policy* 13:37–56.

Hersch, G., J. Spencer, & T. Kapoor. 2003. Adaptation by elders to new living arrangements following hospitalization: A qualitative, retrospective analysis. *Journal of Applied Gerontology* 22:315–39.

Heumann, L., & D. Boldy. 1993. The basic benefits and limitations of an aging-in-place policy. In *Aging in place with dignity*, ed. L. Heumann & D. Boldy, 1–8. Westport, Conn.: Praeger Publishers.

Hickey, T. 1980. *Health and aging*. Monterey, Calif.: Brooks-Cole.

Hill, R. 1999. *The strengths of African American families: Twenty-five years later*. New York: University Press of America.

Hofland, B. 1990. Why a special focus on autonomy? *Generations* 14 (Suppl.): 5–8.

———. 1995. Resident autonomy in long-term care: Paradoxes and challenges. In *Enhancing autonomy in long-term care: Concepts and strategies*, ed. L. Gamroth, J. Semradek, & E. Tornquist, 15–33. New York: Springer Publishing.

Holstein, J., & J. Gubrium. 2000. *Constructing the life course*. Dix Hills, N.Y.: General Hall.

Holzapfel, S., C. Schoch, J. Dodman, & M. Grant. 1992. Responses of nursing home residents to intrainstitutional relocation. *Geriatric Nursing* 13:192–95.

Hopkins, P. 1989. Enforcement of the rights of residents of board and care homes. In *Preserving independence and supporting needs: The role of board and care homes,* ed. M. Moon, G. Gaverlavage, & S. Newman, 137–46. Washington, D.C.: American Association of Retired Persons.

House, B. 2000. Does economic culture and social capital matter? An analysis of African-American entrepreneurs in Cleveland, Ohio. *Western Journal of Black Studies* 24:183–92.

Howard, D., P. Sloane, S. Zimmerman, K. Eckert, J. Walsh, V. Buie, et al. 2002. Distribution of African Americans in residential care/assisted living and nursing homes: More evidence of racial disparity? *American Journal of Public Health* 92:1272–77.

Jackson, J. 1985. Aged black Americans: Double jeopardy re-examined. In *The state of black America, 1985,* ed. J. Williams, 143–75. New York: National Urban League.

Jackson, J., & C. Perry. 1989. Physical health conditions of middle-aged and aged blacks. In *Aging and health: Perspectives on gender, race, ethnicity, and class,* ed. K. Markides, 111–76. Newbury Park, Calif.: Sage Publications.

Jenkins, C. 2001. Resource effects on access to long-term care for frail older people. *Journal of Aging and Social Policy* 13:35–52.

Johnson, C., & B. Barer. 1997. *Life beyond 85 years: The aura of survivorship.* New York: Springer Publishing.

Kalymun, M. 1992. Board and care versus assisted living: Ascertaining the similarities and differences. *Adult Residential Care Journal* 6:35–45.

Kane, R. 1990. Everyday life in nursing homes: The way things are. In *Everyday ethics: Resolving dilemmas in nursing home life,* ed. R. Kane & A. Kaplan, 3–20. New York: Springer Publishing.

———. 1991. Personal autonomy for residents of long-term care: Concepts and issues of measurement. In *The concept and measurement of quality of life in the frail elderly,* ed. J. Birren, J. Lubben, J. Rowe, & D. Deutchman, 316–34. San Diego: Academic Press.

———. 1995. Autonomy and regulation in long-term care: An odd couple, an ambiguous relationship. In *Enhancing autonomy in long-term care: Concepts and strategies,* ed. L. Gamroth, J. Semradek, & E. Tornquist, 68–86. New York: Springer Publishing.

Kane, R., M. Baker, J. Salmon, & W. Veazie. 1998. *Consumer perspectives on private versus shared accommodations in assisted living settings.* Washington, D.C.: American Association of Retired Persons, Public Policy Institute.

Kane, R., and C. Levin. 1998. Who's safe? Who's sorry? The duty to protect the safety of clients in home and community-based care. *Generations* 22:75–81.

Kane, R., & K. Wilson. 2001. *Assisted living at the crossroads: Principles for the future.* Portland, Ore.: Jessie F. Richardson Foundation.

Kapp, M., & K. Wilson. 1995. Assisted living and negotiated risk. *Journal of Ethics, Law, and Aging* 1:5–13.

Kaufman, S. 1986. *The ageless self: Sources of meaning in late life.* Madison: University of Wisconsin Press.

Keith, J. 1977. *Old people, new lives: Community creation in a retirement residence.* Chicago: University of Chicago Press.

Kemper, P., & C. Murtaugh. 1991 Lifetime use of nursing home care. *New England Journal of Medicine* 324:595–600.

Lawton, M. 1980. *Environment and aging.* Monterey, Calif.: Brooks-Cole.

Lawton, M., & L. Nahemow. 1973. Ecology and the aging process. In *The psychology of adult development and aging,* ed. C. Eisdorfer & M. Lawton, 619–74. Washington, D.C.: American Psychological Association.

Lidz, C., K. Fischer, & R. Arnold. 1992. *The erosion of autonomy in long-term care.* New York: Oxford University Press.

Lincoln, Y., & E. Guba. 1985. *Naturalistic inquiry.* Newbury Park, Calif.: Sage Publications.

Logan, J., R. Alba, & B. Stulus. 2003. Enclaves and entrepreneurs: Assessing the payoff for immigrants and minorities. *International Migration Review* 37:344–88.

Lopez, S. R., & P. J. Guarnaccia. 2000. Cultural psychopathology: Uncovering the world of mental illness. *Annual Review of Psychology* 51:571–98.

Lustbader, W. 1991. *Counting on kindness: The dilemmas of dependency.* New York: Free Press.

Lyon, S. 1997. Impact of regulation and financing on small board-and-care homes in Maryland. *Journal of Aging and Social Policy* 9:37–50.

Mahoney, F., & D. Barthel. 1965. Functional evaluation: The Barthel index. *Maryland State Medical Journal* 14:61–65.

Manisses Communications Group. 1999. Georgia tightens belt as it restructures Medicaid services. *Mental Health Weekly* (August 2). www.findarticles.com/m0BSC/30_9/issue.jhtml (accessed December 10, 2003).

Manton, K., & X. Gu. 2001. Changes in the prevalence of chronic disability in the United States black and non-black population above age 65 from 1982–1999. *Proceedings of the National Academy of Science* 98:6354–59.

Markides, K. 1983. Minority aging. In *Aging in society: Selected reviews of recent research,* ed. M. Riley, B. Hess, & K. Bond, 115–37. Hillsdale, N.J.: Lawrence Erlbaum Associates.

———. 1989. Aging, gender, race, ethnicity, class and health. In *Aging and health: Perspectives on gender, race, ethnicity, and class,* ed. K. Markides, 9–21. Newbury Park, Calif.: Sage Publications.

Matthews, S. 1979. *The social world of old women: Management of self-identity.* Beverly Hills, Calif.: Sage Publications.

McHugh, K. E., & R. C. Mings. 1996. The circle of migration: Attachment to place in aging. *Annals of the Association of American Geographers* 86:530–50.

Mikhail, M. 1992. Psychological responses to relocation to a nursing home. *Journal of Gerontological Nursing* 18:35–39.

Milburn, N., & P. Bowman. 1991. Neighborhood life. In *Life in black America,* ed. J. Jackson, 31–45. Newbury Park, Calif.: Sage Publications.

Mitchell, J., & B. Kemp. 2000. Quality of life in assisted living homes: A multidimensional analysis. *Journal of Gerontology: Psychological Sciences* 55B:117–27.

Mitchell, J., & J. Register. 1984. An exploration of family interaction with the elderly by race, socioeconomic status and residence. *Gerontologist* 24:48–54.

Mockenhaupt, R. 1993. Self-care and older adults. *Generations* 17:5–6.

Mollica, R. 2002. *State assisted living practices and options: A guide for state policy makers.* Portland, Me.: National Academy for State Health Policy.

Mollica, R., & R. Jenkins. 2001. *State assisted living practices and options: A guide for state policy makers.* Portland, Me.: National Academy for State Health Policy.

Mollica, R., K. Wilson, B. Ryther, & H. Lamarche. 1995. *Guide to assisted living and state policy: A guide for states.* Portland, Me.: National Academy for State Health Policy.

Moos, R., & S. Lemke. 1994. *Group residences for older adults.* New York: Oxford University Press.

Morgan, L., K. Eckert, & S. Lyon. 1995. *Small board-and-care homes: Residential care in transition.* Baltimore: Johns Hopkins University Press.

Morrison, B. 1995. Research and policy agenda on predictors of institutional placement among minority elderly. *Journal of Gerontological Social Work* 24:17–28.

Mui, A. 1992. Caregiver strain among black and white daughter caregivers: A role theory perspective. *Gerontologist* 32:203–12.

Mui, A., & D. Burnette. 1994. Long-term care service use by frail elders: Is ethnicity a factor? *Gerontologist* 34:190–98.

Muller, J. 1995. Care of the dying by physicians-in-training: An example of participant observation research. *Research on Aging* 17:65–87.

Murtaugh, C., P. Kemper, B. Spillman, & B. Carlson. 1997. The amount, distribution, and timing of lifetime nursing home use. *Medical Care* 35:204–18.

Mutran, E. 1985. Intergenerational family support among blacks and whites: Responses of culture to socioeconomic differences. *Journal of Gerontology* 40:382–89.

Mutran, E., S. Sudha, P. Reed, M. Menon, & T. Desai. 2001. African American use of residential care in North Carolina. In *Assisted living: Needs, practices, and policies in residential care for the elderly,* ed. S. Zimmerman, P. Sloane, & K. Eckert, 92–114. Baltimore: Johns Hopkins University Press.

Namazi, K., & P. Chafetz. 2001. The concept, the terminology, and the occupants. In *Assisted living: Current issues in facility management and resident care,* ed. K. Namazi & P. Chafetz, 1–11. Westport, Conn.: Auburn House.

Namazi, K., J. Eckert, E. Kahana, & S. Lyon. 1989. Psychological well-being of elderly board and care home residents. *Gerontologist* 29:511–16.

National Center for Assisted Living. 2001. *Facts and trends: The assisted living source book.* Washington, D.C.: American Health Care Association.

Newens, A., D. Forster, & D. Kay. 1995. Dependency and community care in presenile Alzheimer's disease. *British Journal of Psychiatry* 167:777–82.

Newman, K. 1999. *No shame in my game: The working poor in the inner city.* New York: Knopf and the Russell Sage Foundation.

Noonan, A., & S. Tennstedt. 1997. Meaning in caregiving and its contribution to caregiver well-being. *Gerontologist* 37:785–94.

Office of the State Long-Term Care Ombudsman. 2004. Ombudsman: Long term care residents' advocate. In *2003 Annual report of the Georgia long-term care ombudsman program.* Atlanta: Georgia Department of Human Resources.

Ory, M., G. DeFriese, & A. Duncker. 1998. The nature, extent, and modifiability of self-care behaviors in later life. In *Self-care in later life: Research, program, and policy issues,* ed. M. Ory & G. DeFriese, xv–xxvi. New York: Springer Publishing.

Patterson, V., S. King, M. Ball, F. Whittington, & M. Perkins. 2003. Coping with change: Religious activities and beliefs of residents in assisted living facilities. *Journal of Religious Gerontology* 14:79–94.

Patton, M. 1990. *Qualitative evaluation and research methods.* Newbury Park, Calif.: Sage Publications.

Perkins, M., M. Ball, F. Whittington, & B. Combs. 2004. Managing the care needs of low-income board-and-care home residents: A process of negotiating risks. *Qualitative Health Research* 14:478–95.

Perkins, M., F. Whittington, M. Ball, & V. Patterson. 1998. The new world of assisted living: Can "mom and pop" facilities survive? Paper presented at the fifty-first annual meeting of the Gerontological Society of America, Philadelphia, November 20–24, 1998.

Perkins, M. M. 2002. Survival in a small African American–owned and –operated assisted living facility: A process of negotiating risks. Ph.D. diss., Georgia State University. *Dissertation Abstracts International* 63/06: 2369

Phillips, C., Y. Munoz, M. Sherman, M. Rose, W. Spector, & C. Hawes. 2003. Effects of facility characteristics on departures from assisted living: Results from a national study. *Gerontologist* 43:690–96.

Port, L., A. Gruber-Baldini, L. Burton, M. Baumgarten, J. Hebel, S. Zimmerman, et al. 2001. Resident contact with family and friends following nursing home admission. *Gerontologist* 41:589–96.

Pynoos, J. 1993. Strategies for home modification and repair. In *Aging in place,* ed. J. Callahan, 29–38. Amityville, N.Y.: Baywood Publishers.

Regnier, V., J. Hamilton, & S. Yatabe. 1995. *Assisted living for the aged and frail: Innovation in design and financing.* New York: Columbia University Press.

Regnier, V., & A. Scott. 2001. Creating a therapeutic environment: Lessons from northern European models. In *Assisted living: Needs, practices, and policies in residential care for the elderly,* ed. S. Zimmerman, P. Sloane, & J. Eckert, 53–77. Baltimore: Johns Hopkins University Press.

Reinardy, J., & R. Kane. 2003. Anatomy of choice: Deciding on assisted living or nursing home care in Oregon. *Journal of Applied Gerontology* 22:152–74.

Reschovsky, J., & H. Ruchlin. 1993. Quality of board and care homes serving low-income elderly: Structural and public policy correlates. *Journal of Applied Gerontology* 12: 225–45.

Rodin, J. 1986. Aging and health: Effects of the sense of control. *Science* 233:1271–76.

Rodman, H. 1971. *Lower-class families: The culture of poverty in Negro Trinidad.* New York: Oxford University Press.

Rosen, E., & K. Knafl. 2003. Older women's response to residential relocation: Description of transition styles. *Qualitative Health Research* 13:20–36.

Ross, M., A. Carswell, & W. Dalziel. 2002. Family caregiving in long-term care facilities: Visiting and task performance. *Geriatrics Today* 5:179–82.

Rowles, G. 1993. Evolving images of place in aging and "aging in place." *Generations* 17:65–70.

Rowles, G., & D. High. 1996. Individualizing care: Family involvement in nursing home decision making. *Journal of Gerontological Nursing 22*:20–25.

Rowles, G., & H. Ravdal. 2002. Aging, place, and meaning in the face of changing circumstances. In *Challenges of the third age: Meaning and purpose in later life,* ed. R. Weiss & S. Bass, 81–114. New York: Oxford University Press.

Rubinstein, R., J. Kilbride, & S. Nagy. 1992. *Elders living alone.* New York: Aldine de Gruyter.

Rutman, I., R. Baron, & S. Tatem. 1987. *Training board and care home providers: Regulatory requirements, state programs, training approaches, and curricula.* Rockville, Md.: Project Share.

Savishinsky, J. 1991. *The ends of time: Life and work in a nursing home.* New York: Bergin & Garvey.

Schiman, C., & A. Lordeman. 1989. *A study of the involvement of state long-term care ombudsmen programs in board and care issues.* Washington, D.C.: National Association of State Units on Aging and National Center for State Long-Term Care Ombudsman Resources.

Schoenberg, N., & R. Coward. 1997. Attitudes about entering a nursing home: Comparisons of older rural and urban African-American women. *Journal of Aging Studies* 11:27–47.

Settersten, R., Jr. 1999. *Lives in time and place: The problems and promises of developmental science.* Amityville, N.Y.: Baywood Publishers.

Shanas, E. 1979. Social myth as hypothesis: The case of family relations of old people. *Gerontologist* 19:3–9.

Shawler, C., G. Rowles, & D. High. 2001. Analysis of key decision-making incidents in the life of a nursing home resident. *Gerontologist* 41:612–22.

Shield, R. 1995. Ethics in the nursing home: Cases, choices, and issues. In *The culture of long term care,* ed. N. Henderson & M. Vesperi, 111–26. Westport, Conn.: Bergin & Garvey.

Small, N. 1993. Self-care in institutional settings. *Generations* 17:19–23.

Stack, C. 1974. *All our kin: Strategies for survival in a black community.* New York: Harper & Row.

Stack, C., & L. Burton. 1993. Kinscripts. *Journal of Comparative Family Studies* 24:157–70.

State Health Planning Agency. 1993. *Personal care homes in Georgia, 1993.* Atlanta: State Health Planning Agency.

Stearns, S., & L. Morgan. 2001. Economics and financing. In *Assisted living: Current issues in facility management and resident care,* ed. K. Namazi & P. Chafetz, 271–91.Westport, Conn.: Auburn House.

Stewart, A., & A. King. 1994. Conceptualizing and measuring quality of life in older populations. In *Aging and quality of life: Charting new territories in behavioral science research,* ed. R. Abeles, H. Gift, & M. Ory, 27–56. New York: Springer Publishing.

Stone, R. 2000. *Long-term care for the elderly with disabilities: Current policy, emerging trends, and implications for the twenty-first century.* New York: Milbank Memorial Fund.

Stone, R., G. Cafferata, & J. Sangl. 1987. Caregivers of the frail elderly: A national profile. *Gerontologist* 27:616–26.

Strauss, A. 1987. *Qualitative analysis for social scientists.* New York: Cambridge University Press.

Strauss, A., & J. Corbin. 1990. *The basics of qualitative research: Grounded theory procedures and techniques.* Newbury Park, Calif.: Sage Publications.

Taylor, L., F. Whittington, C. Hollingsworth, M. Ball, S. King, V. Patterson, et al. 2003. Assessing the effectiveness of a walking program on physical function of residents of an assisted living facility. *Journal of Community Health Nursing* 20:15–26.

Taylor, R. 1988. Aging and support relationships. In *The black American elderly,* ed. J. Jackson, 259–81. New York: Springer Publishing.

Taylor, R., & L. Chatters. 1986. Church-based informal support among aged blacks. *Gerontologist* 26:637–42.

Taylor, R., L. Chatters, & J. Jackson. 1997. Introduction to *Family life in black America,* ed. R. Taylor, J. Jackson, & L. Chatters, 1–13. Thousand Oaks, Calif.: Sage Publications.

Taylor, R., M. Thornton, & L. Chatters. 1992. Black America's perceptions of the socio-historical role of the church. *Journal of Black Studies* 18:123–38.

Thomas, W., & S. Thomas. 1928. *The child in America: Behavior problems and programs.* New York: Knopf.

Thornton, R., & P. Nardi. 1975. The dynamics of role acquisition. *American Journal of Sociology* 80:870–83.

Tornatore, J., & L. Grant. 2002. Burden among family caregivers of persons with Alzheimer's disease in nursing homes. *Gerontologist* 42:497–506.

U.S. Department of Health and Human Services. 2001. *Mental health: Culture, race, and ethnicity—a supplement to mental health: A report of the surgeon general.* Rockville, Md.: U.S. Department of Health and Human Services Administration, Center for Mental Health Services.

U.S. General Accounting Office. 1999. *Assisted living: Quality-of-care and consumer protection issues in four states.* Washington, D.C.: Government Printing Office.

Utz, R. 2003. Assisted living: The philosophical challenges of everyday practice. *Journal of Applied Gerontology* 22:379–404.

Valentine, B. 1978. *Hustling and other hard work: Life styles in the ghetto.* New York: Free Press.

Van Gennep, A. 1960. *The rites of passage.* Chicago: University of Chicago Press.

Wallace, S. 1990. Race versus class in the health care of African American elderly. *Social Problems* 37:517–34.

Wallace, S., L. Levy-Storms, R. Kington, & R. Anderson. 1998. The persistence of race and ethnicity in the use of long-term care. *Journal of Gerontology: Social Sciences* 53B:S104–12.

Walls, C., & S. Zarit. 1991. Informal support from black churches and the well-being of elderly blacks. *Gerontologist* 31:490–95.

Wentowski, G. 1981. Reciprocity and coping strategies of older people: Cultural dimensions of network building. *Gerontologist* 21:600–609.

Whittington, F., M. Ball, M. Perkins, B. Connell, J. Sanford, V. Patterson, et al. 1998. *Quality of life of veterans with disabilities living in assisted living facilities.* Report submitted to the VA Rehabilitation Research and Development Center on Aging. Atlanta: VA Medical Center.

Wieland, D., L. Rubenstein, & S. Hirsch. 1995. Quality of life in nursing homes: An emerging focus of research and practice. In *Quality care in geriatric settings,* ed. P. Katz, R. Kane, & M. Mezey, 149–94. New York: Springer Publishing.

Wolinsky, F., C. Callahan, F. Fitzgerald, & R. Johnson. 1993. Changes in functional status and the risks of subsequent nursing home placement and death. *Journal of Gerontology: Social Sciences* 48:S94–101.

Yates, M., S. Tennstedt, & B. Chang. 1999. Contributors to and mediators of psychological well-being for informal caregivers. *Journal of Gerontology: Psychological Sciences* 54B:P12–22.

Yee, D., J. Capitman, & M. Sciegaj. 1996. *National survey of assisted living programs and residents: Descriptive results.* Paper presented at the forty-ninth annual meeting of the Gerontological Society of America, Washington, D.C., November 17–21, 1996.

Young, H. 1998. Moving to congregate housing: The last chosen home. *Journal of Aging Studies* 12:149–65.

Zurcher. 1983. *Social Roles.* Beverly Hills, Calif.: Sage Publications.

Index